Providing Home Care

A Textbook for

Home Care Aides

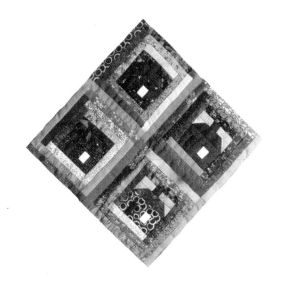

William Leahy, MD

WITH

Jetta Fuzy, RN, MS

Julie Grafe, RN, BSN

Hartman Publishing, Inc.

Table of

Contents

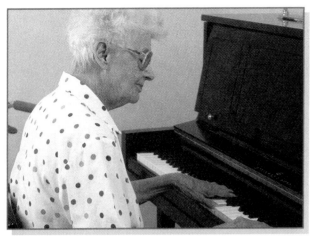

Table of

Procedures

Extensive listings of guidelines are included in our index.

Using This Book

Congratulations! The rewards of working in home health care begin right here—by learning important skills and knowledge to help your clients and yourself.

This book will help you master what you need to know to provide excellent, compassionate care to clients with very different needs. It will also teach you to take care of yourself and your career.

Understanding how the book is organized will help you make the most of this resource.

First, everything in this book, the student workbook, and even your instructor's teaching material is organized around LEARNING OBJECTIVES. A learning objective is a very specific piece of knowledge or a very specific skill. Every learning objective in this book is one that can be measured. Consider the following example: "List five important observations to make about changes in a client's skin." After you read the text following this learning objective, you should be able to DO just that—list five important observations to make about changes in a client's skin. After you have read that section of text, test yourself. Can you DO what the learning objective says? If you can, move on to the next assigned learning objective. If you cannot, just reread the section and try again.

Learning objectives help you organize what you need to learn and what you have learned. You won't need to guess what is important and what is not. If your instructor assigns a learning objective, you know it is important. If you can DO what the learning objective says, you know you have mastered the material.

For clarity, this book numbers the objectives within a chapter. So, if you miss a question on a test or cannot answer a workbook question, you can quickly find the section that will give you the help you need (See example on page viii).

Need help pronouncing a word? With each new word introduced in the text, both the pronunciation and the definition are included when the word is first used. We hope this is simpler than defining and pronouncing words in the back or the margins of the text. In-text definition also gives you examples of how the word is used.

Here are our rules for using the pronunciations:

Long vowels

A = AY	O = Oh or O
E = EE	U = oo or yoo
I = EYE	

Short vowels

a = a as in "above"	u = u as in "bud"
e = e as in "bet"	oo = oo as in "Sue"
i = i as in "sip"	yoo = as in "cute"
o = o as in "not"	oy = as in "oil"

Aides in home care have different titles depending on their state or their employer. This text uses the title *Home Care Aide*.

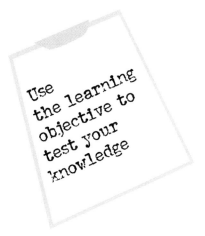

Use the learning objective to test your knowledge

to:

☑ 6. List five important observations to make about changes in a client's skin . . . .

☑ 7. List five guidelines for providing basic skin

Every chapter begins with learning objectives your instructor may assign. Every objective is "competency based," which means you can actually test yourself and know if you can do what the objective states.

❑ 6. List five important observations to make about changes in a client's skin

When the skin begins to break down, it becomes pale, white or a reddened color. The client may also complain of tingling or burning in the area. This white or reddened area does not go away, even when the client's position is changed. If pressure is allowed to continue, the area will further deteriorate, first breaking the skin surface, then eroding the next layer. The resulting wound is called a **pressure sore**, **bed sore**, or decubitus ulcer (dee-KYOO-bi-tus) (**Fig. 15-22**). Once a pressure sore forms, it can get bigger, deeper, and infected. Because pressure sores are difficult to heal, prevention is very important.

Report any of the following changes or abnormalities in the client's skin to your supervisor:

▶ pale, white or reddened areas, or blistered or bruised areas on the skin
▶ complaints of tingling, warmth, or burning of the skin
▶ dry or flaking skin
▶ itching or scratching
▶ rash or any skin discoloration
▶ swelling
▶ blisters
▶ fluid or blood draining from skin
▶ broken skin
▶ wounds or ulcers on the skin
▶ changes in an existing wound or ulcer (size, depth, drainage, color, odor)
▶ redness or broken skin between toes or around toenails

Within the chapter there will be a section teaching each learning objective. When you finish that reading, you should test yourself to see if you can "do" the objective.

In the space below, write five observations regarding changes in a client's skin that should be reported to a supervisor. (15-6)

_____

_____

_____

Workbook exercises and test questions have a reference to these objectives. The first number, 15, refers to the chapter of the book. The second number, 6, is the learning objective number. If you have trouble answering a question, you can return to the text covering that objective and reread the material.

Publisher's Acknowledgements

You cannot imagine how many people it takes to produce a great book. What follows is our best attempt to thank each person who helped make this project a reality.

All books need an author. Finding one who is passionate and knowledgeable is a publisher's most important work. William Leahy, MD became involved with home health aide education both out of an interest in the care his patients received and to give direction and meaning to the lives of young people in his community. After teaching the home health aide program at Bladensburg High School in suburban Maryland, he undertook the project of writing a better book. To his credit, he hired a registered nurse, working as a professional health journalist to help craft the project. His vision was to have learning and teaching material that could be used by the program he founded and subsequently, to use the royalties from the project to ensure the program's continuance.

Developing educational material for unlicensed health care workers demands the guidance of nurses who understand both educational theory and the practice of home health aide services. We found both in our Consulting Editors, Jetta Fuzy, RN, MS, and Julie Grafe, RN, BSN. Each drew from years of experience working in home care and education to develop a book that was current, appropriately leveled, and educationally sound.

We wanted a book tightly written around learning objectives, easily readable, and full of examples and concise explanations. Both of our Development Editors, Jennifer Plane Hartman and Michele Heskett, committed enormous time and talent toward the project. Celia McIntire, our staff Development Editor, John Davis, our designer, Susan Alvare, our Proofreader, and John Cole, who designed and composed the text, all deserve applause as well.

Reviewers offering suggestions for improvement ensure that books will work for the people who use them. During the three years of writing and reviewing this text, many nurses guided us. I hope they can now see the tremendous impact their comments had. A sincere thanks to each of them:

Betty J. Lipman, Former Primary Instructor, Home Health Aide Program, Dallas Chapter - American Red Cross; Barbara L. Haring,

Director, CNA/HHA Program, Central County Occupational Center, San Jose, CA; Inez Green, RN, C. Ross Educational Center, Milwaukee, WI; Marti Pizzini, Director of Nursing, Caregivers Plus, Inc., Laporte, IN; Mary Joan Greene, Education Coordinator, Central Alabama Home Health Services, Inc., Montgomery, AL; Maureen A. Williams, RN, C, MEd., Clinical Educator, Inova VNA Home Health, Inc., Arlington, VA; Linda Westerman, RN, MN, Staff Development Coordinator, Home Health of South Carolina, Inc., Rock Hill, SC; and Deloris Pederson, BSN, Health Occupations Instructor, Albuquerque TVI, Albuquerque, NM. Additional thanks go to Royal Prentice and Virginia Breeding of the Albuquerque Job Corps Center for coordinating student models for our photography.

See all the beautiful people in this book? Thanks to the following people for modeling for our wonderful photographer, Dick Ruddy, to shoot photographs that teach: Tom Hartman, Gail Hartman, Annie Chachere, Mary Plane, Robert Plane, Elliott Coghill Hartman, Warren Thomas Hartman, Nathan Couch, Aaron Couch, Melinda Cramer, Dennis Chavez, Nora Lucero, Rachel Floryance, Dimitri Floryance, Celia McIntire, John Davis, Dondi Hall, Erika Tapia, Jessica Acosta, Mirza Lee Perez, Leonard Shelca, Vicente Garcia, Kendera Heinrich, Brenda Tsosie, Diana Santiago, Yusteidy Rodriquez, Richard Medina, Denise Pacheco, Lenora Garcia, Adriennie DeMouchette, Antonia Bustos, Sarah Johnson, and last, but certainly not least, Tori Franklin.

A final word of thanks goes to Diane "Di" Goodman, without whom Hartman Publishing might not have found a wonderful author and a fantastic text.

Mark T. Hartman, *Publisher*
Hartman Publishing, Inc.

Notice to Readers

Though the guidelines and procedures contained in this text are based on consultations with health care professionals, they should not be considered absolute recommendations. The instructor and readers should follow employer, local, state, and federal guidelines concerning health care practices. These guidelines change, and it is the reader's responsibility to be aware of these changes and of the policies and procedures of her or his health care agency.

The publisher, author, editors, and reviewers cannot accept any responsibility for errors or omissions or for any consequences from application of the information in this book and make no warranty, expressed or implied, with respect to the contents of the book. The Publisher does not warrant or guarantee any of the products described herein or perform any analysis in connection with any of the product information contained herein.

Copyright Information

Thanks To

Our many reviewers, listed on page vii, for valuable suggestions on making this book the best it could be.

The Briggs Corporation for offering photographs of virtually every medical supply and piece of equipment in this book. Having one source for this material was enormously helpful and convenient. They can be reached at 1(800)247-2343.

Albuquerque Technical Vocational Institute for their assistance finding employed aides to model for our photography program and for consulting on content.

Albuquerque Job Corps Center and their nursing assistant program for assisting us with our photography program.

A+R Medical Supply in Albuquerque for the loan of medical equipment used in our photography.

Photography Credits

Medical equipment photography and record keeping forms on the following pages were provided courtesy of The Briggs Corporation: 12, 170, 179, 182, 187, 188, 191, 200 (fig14-28), 212, 214-215, 219, 261 (fig. 20-2), 272 (fig. 20-25), 290, and 314.

Photographs of pressure sores on page 88 and page 211 were provided and used with permission of the National Pressure Ulcer Advisory Panel

The wonderful, warm photography depicting clients and caregivers on the following pages is the work of Marilu Pittman, of CARING Magazine. Many of her photographs can be purchased through the National Association of Home Care: 2, 4, 13, 28, 84 (fig 8-4), 122, 134, 135, 139, 218, 257, and 285 (fig 20-33).

All photography of medical conditions included are used with permission of the copyright holder, Custom Medical Stock Photo, Inc. in Chicago, Illinois. Our thanks to them for the timely search of their tremendous collection of medical photography. Their photographs are used on the following pages: 3, 11, 76, 91 (9-9), 101, 103, 116 (fig 10-2), 213, 222, 224, 230, 234, 246, 261 (20-1), 262, and 277.

Photography on the following pages is copyrighted by Photodisc, Inc.: 83, 117, 119, 121, 123, 126 (fig 10-15), 130 (10-17), and 205.

All other photographs are the work of Dick Ruddy, Albuquerque, New Mexico.

Credits

Nursing Consultants: Jetta Fuzy, RN, MS and Julie Grafe, RN, BSN

Development Editors: Jennifer Plane Hartman and Michele Heskett

Copy Editor: Celia McIntire

Design and Composition: John Cole

Photography: Dick Ruddy

Illustration: Thaddeus Castillo, Mike Ramos, and John Davis

Medical Illustration: Electronic Illustrators Group

Medical Supply Photography: Courtesy of The Briggs Corporation

Printing and Binding: Courier

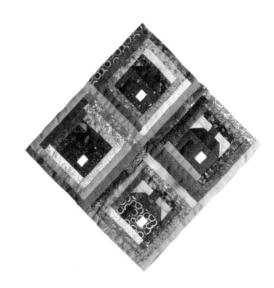

Quilts photographed for this text are the work of Barbara Bogan, used on the front cover, and Pat Keller, detail above.

SECTION I:
Understanding Home Care Aide Services

Chapter 1

Home Care Aide Services and the Health Care System

❑ 1. Describe the structure of the United States' health care system and describe ways it is changing

The health care system is something we often hear discussed. Perhaps you are training to become a home care aide because you know that health care is a growing field in the United States. When we talk about the health care system, we mean all the different kinds of providers, facilities, and payers involved in delivering medical care. **Providers** are people or organizations that provide health care, including doctors, nurses, clinics, and agencies. **Facilities** are places where care is delivered or administered, including hospitals, long-term care facilities or nursing homes, and treatment centers. **Payers** are people or organizations paying for health care services, including insurance companies, government programs like Medicare and Medicaid, and the individual patient or client. Together, all these people, places, and organizations make up our health care system.

When you need health care you probably go to a doctor's office, a clinic, or an emergency room. Where you decide to go for health care depends on who will be paying for your health care and how urgent your need for health care is. Most of the time, you will be seen and treated by a physician (MD), a registered nurse (RN), a nurse practitioner (NP), or a physicians' assistant (PA). If you need further care or treatment, it may be provided by a specialist (MD), a physical therapist (PT), speech therapist (ST), or any number of other kinds of health care workers. People who need continuing care may spend time in a hospital, rehabilitation center, or a nursing home. Some people who need continuing care will be cared for in their homes by a home care aide (HCA) or other home care professional (**Fig. 1-1**).

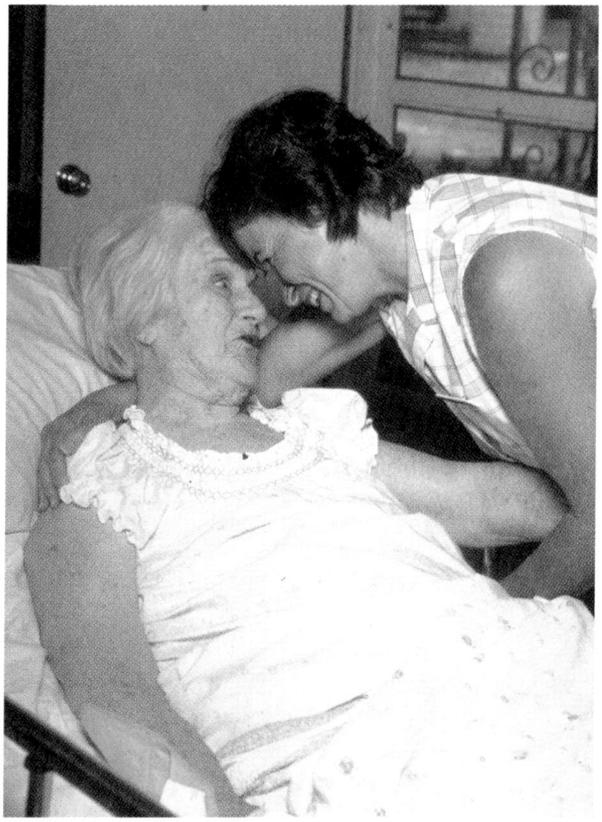

Who will pay for your care may determine where and what kind of care you receive. Increasingly, health care payers are controlling the amount and types of health care services people receive. **Traditional insurance companies** offer plans that pay for the health care of plan members, whether in the

Fig. 1-1. Home care aides provide continuing care in a person's home.

doctor's office, hospital or other facility, or at home. Most people covered by traditional insurance are part of a plan at their place of work. The costs of membership may be paid for by the employer, the employee, or shared by both. Traditional insurance plans usually provide excellent care for their members. However, the costs of providing this care have risen greatly and many employers and employees can no longer afford to pay for the most generous traditional insurance plans.

As a reaction to the increased costs of traditional insurance plans, many employers and employees now choose to belong to **health maintenance orga-**

nizations (HMOs). If you belong to an HMO, you must use a particular doctor or group of doctors except in case of emergency. The doctors working for HMOs are paid to provide care while keeping costs down. Thus they may see more patients, order fewer tests, or cut costs in other ways while still providing care.

Preferred provider organizations (PPOs) are another health care option many employers use to reduce costs. A PPO is a network of providers that contract to provide health services to a group of people. Employees are given incentives to use network providers, and employers are given reduced, fee-for-service rates for getting employees to participate in the network. A person in a PPO may still get health care outside the network of providers, but the employee must pay a higher portion of the cost.

If you become seriously ill, you may be admitted to a hospital for medical treatment. This decision is made by a doctor, and may have to be approved by your insurance company. The costs of hospital care have risen greatly, and to make up for it, health care payers are controlling who can be admitted to a hospital and for how long.

After release from the hospital, many people need continuing care. This is particularly true as people are released after shorter hospital stays. Continuing care may be provided in a skilled nursing facility, a long-term care facility, a rehabilitation hospital, or by a home health agency. The type of care depends on the medical condition and needs of the patient or client.

The major changes in our health care system are **rising costs of health care, increased use of expensive technology,** and **new ways to control costs of care.** As we develop new and better ways of caring for people, care becomes more expensive. Better health care helps people live longer, which leads to a larger elderly population that may need additional health care. New discoveries and expensive equipment have also driven health care costs higher (**Fig. 1-2**).

New ways to control expenses, such as HMOs and PPOs, are gradually replacing traditional insurance plans, affecting the amount and quality of health care provided. These cost control strategies are often called **managed care.** In the past the goal of health care was to make sick people well. Today it is to get sick people well in the most efficient (least expensive) way possible. The **growth of home health care** is in part a cost-controlling strategy, because it is generally less expensive to care for someone in the home than in a facility. Shorter hospital stays, another cost-controlling strategy, have also increased the need for home health care.

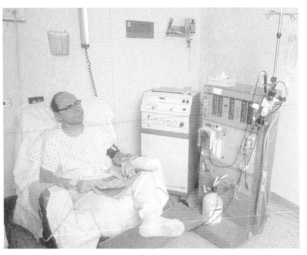

Fig. 1-2. Technology often makes it possible to offer better health care and extend people's lives, but sophisticated drugs and equipment are expensive.

❑ 2. Describe Medicare and Medicaid, and list when Medicare recipients may receive home care

Medicare was established in 1965 for people aged 65 or older. It now also covers people of any age with permanent kidney failure, and certain disabilities. Medicare currently covers approximately 38.1 million people, of whom almost 4 million are disabled and some 200,000 have kidney disease. Sixty percent (60%) of all home care is paid for by Medicare. Medicare has two parts: Hospital Insurance (Part A), and Medical Insurance (Part B). Part A helps pay for care in a hospital or skilled nursing facility or for care from a home health agency or hospice. Part B helps pay for physician services and various other medical services and equipment. Medicare will only pay for care it determines to be medically necessary. Medicaid, which pays for 15% of all home care, is a medical assistance program for low income people.

Medicare pays for intermittent, not continuous, home health services provided by a participating, or certified, home health agency. The participating agency must meet certain guidelines established by Medicare. To qualify for home health care, Medicare recipients must be homebound, or unable to leave home, and their doctors must determine that they need home health care. Medicare will pay the full cost of most covered home health care services; however, Medicare will not pay for round-the-clock home health care. Home health care frequently plays an important role when skilled care is needed on a part-time basis.

❑ 3. Explain the purpose of and need for home health care

Institutional health care delivered in hospitals and nursing homes is expensive. With increasing pressure to reduce costs, hospitals have begun to discharge patients earlier. Many of these people who are discharged have not fully recovered their strength and stamina; and many require skilled assistance or monitoring. Others need only short term assistance at home. Most insurance companies are willing to pay for a part of this care because it is less expensive than a prolonged hospital or nursing home stay.

The growing numbers of older people and chronically ill people are also creating a demand for home health care services. In a mobile society such as ours, family members who would normally be responsible for the care of aging or ill relatives frequently leave home to live and work in distant geographic areas. In addition, they often have other responsibilities or problems that interfere with their ability to provide care. For example, family members who work or who care for young children may be unable to look after aging relatives as they become frail and less functional. This has placed a great demand on nursing homes and long-term care facilities, some of which have had to create waiting lists. Even when these facilities are available, they may be too expensive for some families.

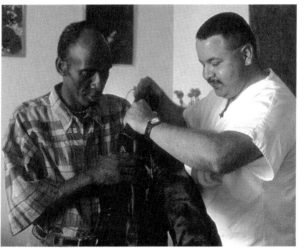

Fig. 1-3. Home care aides often provide care for people with chronic illnesses such as AIDS.

Most people who need some medical care prefer the familiar surroundings of home to an institution. They choose to live alone or receive care from a relative or friend. Home care aides can provide assistance to the chronically ill, the elderly, and family members who provide care and sometimes need relief from the physical and emotional stress of care giving. Many home care aides also work in assisted living facilities, which allow independent living in a homelike environment, with professional care available as needed.

As advances in medicine and technology extend the lives of people with chronic illnesses, the number of people needing health care will increase. Home services will be needed to provide continued care and assistance as chronic illnesses progress. For example, people with acquired immunodeficiency syndrome (AIDS), a chronic illness that is infecting more and more people throughout the world, will require in-home assistance (**Fig.** 1-3). They will also require disease-specific health care as their illnesses progress. Improvements in medications and better management of the disease have already demonstrated that the life expectancy of people with AIDS can be extended and their quality of life can be improved.

Perhaps the most important reason for health care in the home is that most people who are ill or **incapacitated** (disabled) feel more secure and comfortable when they are cared for at home. Health care in familiar surroundings improves mental outlook and physical well-being and has proven to be a major factor in the healing process.

❑ *4. List three key events in the history of homemaker-home care aide services*

The first home care aides were women who were hired to care for the homes and children of mothers who were sick or hospitalized in the early 1900s. During the Depression, in the 1930s, women were hired as "housekeeping aides," and paid by the government. When this government program was discontinued, some aides continued to work for local family and children's services, who provided services to families in need.

In 1959, a national conference on homemaker services was held. It was clear that there was a great need not only for homemaker or housekeeping services, but for personal, in-home care of sick people. Thus, the aide's role expanded to include personal care of the sick as well as care of the home and family.

In 1965, the Medicare program was created. Because many Medicare recipients need home care, home health services have been growing ever since. The

Fig. 1-4. Growth in the number of certified home health agencies, 1989 to 1997.

	Medicare Certified Home Health Agencies	Medicare Certified Hospice	Non-Medicare Certified Home Health Agencies
1989	5,676	597	4,824
1997	10,027	2,154	8,034

number of Medicare-participating home health agencies has grown from 6,000 in 1980 to over 10,000 in 1997 (**Fig.** 1-4). Medicare first began referring to homemakers as "home health aides."

In recent years, interest in home health care has increased in the United States for several reasons. Increased health care costs along with advances in capabilities have created a need for the affordable, continuing care that home care provides. The growing population of the elderly and people with chronic diseases, such as AIDS and Alzheimer's disease, has also created greater demand for home care.

Another reason home health care has grown so popular over the last fifteen years is the use of **diagnostic related groups** (**DRGs**) by Medicare and Medicaid. A DRG specifies the treatment cost Medicare or Medicaid will pay for various diagnoses (dye-ag-NOH-seez), or physician's determinations of an illness. Because a flat fee is assigned for each diagnosis, hospitals lose money if a person's stay is longer than what is allotted in the DRG. Hospitals generally make money if a person's treatment is completed more quickly than specified in the DRG. Home health care has grown to take care of the needs of people who are discharged from the hospital earlier than they would have been in the past. In the future, Medicare- and Medicaid-paid home health care may fall under a similar system.

Today, the process of training and monitoring home care aides is changing. In the last twenty years, the number of home care aides and the number of programs to train them has grown enormously. Many states are developing certification standards for programs that train aides. As the home health field continues to grow, the role of the home care aide will no doubt gain even greater recognition and respect (**Fig.** 1-5).

Fig. 1-5. Personal and home care aides, and home health aides are the two fastest growing occupations in the United States.

Occupation	Employment Change, 1994–2005		
	1994	2005	Percent
Personal and home care aides	179	391	119%
Home health aides	420	848	102%
Systems analysts	483	928	92%
Computer engineers	195	372	90%
Physical and corrective therapy assistants and aides	78	142	83%
Electronic pagination systems workers	18	33	83%
Occupational therapy assistants and aides	16	29	82%
Physical therapists	102	183	80%
Residential counselors	165	290	76%

The Health Care Finance Administration runs the Medicare and Medicaid programs at the federal level. In 1997, they proposed new rules for home health agencies that care for Medicare clients. These proposed rules include criminal background checks for newly hired aides, and they allow certified nursing assistants to work as home care aides.

❑ 5. Identify the basic methods of payment for home health services

Payment for home health care services is made to the home health agency when an agency has assigned or completed the services. Any of the following may be paying for the services (**Fig. 1-6**):

▶ Insurance company

▶ Health maintenance organization

▶ Medicare

▶ Medicaid

▶ The individual client or family

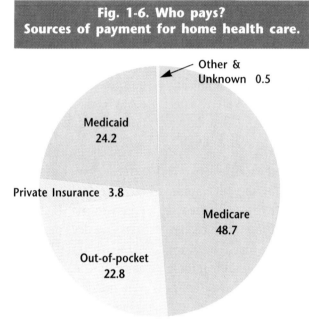

Fig. 1-6. Who pays? Sources of payment for home health care.

Other & Unknown 0.5

Medicaid 24.2

Private Insurance 3.8

Out-of-pocket 22.8

Medicare 48.7

Because Medicare pays for services after they have been given, and payment can be denied for a variety of reasons, it is very important for the home care aide to follow the care plan and document all work. Every home health agency has personnel who specialize in payment issues.

Major changes are taking place in the way agencies are paid for care their staff provides. For some clients, agencies will be paid following the delivery of services. For others, the agencies may be paid a fixed amount of money to care for a particular group of people. These clients may be part of an HMO or a government program that has contracted with the agency to provide care. Because all of an

agency's expenses, including wages for the home care aide, are being monitored very closely, how aides perform their jobs is carefully watched.

Most payers are moving toward systems that encourage agencies to improve the health and well-being of clients quickly and efficiently. The payment methods being eliminated are called "fee-for-service." Under fee-for-service plans, for example, an agency would be paid for all the necessary visits by a nurse, a home care aide, and a physical therapist to restore a client with recent hip replacement to full health and independence. The new payment methods might pay a fixed amount, based on averages across the country, for all the care this client will need. If the agency can achieve the goal for less cost than the payment, they make money. If the goal takes more visits than the average, they lose money.

❑ 6. Describe a typical home health agency

Many home care aides are employed by home health agencies. **Home health agencies** are businesses that have been organized to provide health care and personal services in the familiar surroundings of home. Health care services provided by home health agencies may include nursing care, specialized therapy, specific medical equipment, pharmacy and IV products, and personal care. Personal care services provided may include housekeeping, shopping, help with activities of daily living, and cooking.

Clients who are identified as needing home care are referred to a home health agency by their physicians. They can also be referred by a hospital discharge planner, a community social services agency, the state or local department of public health, the welfare office, a local agency on aging, or a senior center.

Clients and family members can also choose an agency that meets their needs. Often, an agency will have two divisions: one that is Medicare-certified, and one that serves clients not covered by Medicare (called "private pay"). Medicare clients must choose a Medicare-certified agency. Once an agency is chosen and the physician has made a referral, an agency staff member will perform an assessment of the client to determine how the care needs can best be met. The home environment will also be evaluated to determine whether it is suitable and safe for the client.

The number of services home health agencies provide depends on the size of the agency. Small agencies typically provide basic nursing care, personal care, and housekeeping services. Larger agencies may provide speech therapy, physical therapy, occupational therapy, and medical social work. Some of the more common services are listed below. A brief description of each service is provided in Chapter 2.

- physical therapy
- occupational therapy
- speech therapy
- medical-surgical nursing care, including management of clients with AIDS, diabetes (dye- ah-BEE-teez) management, instruction, care of tubes, and catheterization (kath-eh-ter- eye-ZAY-shun)
- intravenous (in-trah-VEE-nus) infusion therapy
- maternal, pediatric (pee-dee-A-trik), and newborn nursing care
- nutrition therapy/dietary counseling
- medical social work
- personal care, including bathing; taking vital signs; skin, nail and hair care; meal preparation; light housekeeping; ambulation; and range of motion exercises
- homemaker/companion
- medical equipment rental and service
- pharmacy (FAHR-mah-see) services
- hospice (HAH-spiss) services

All home health agencies have professional staff members who make decisions about what services

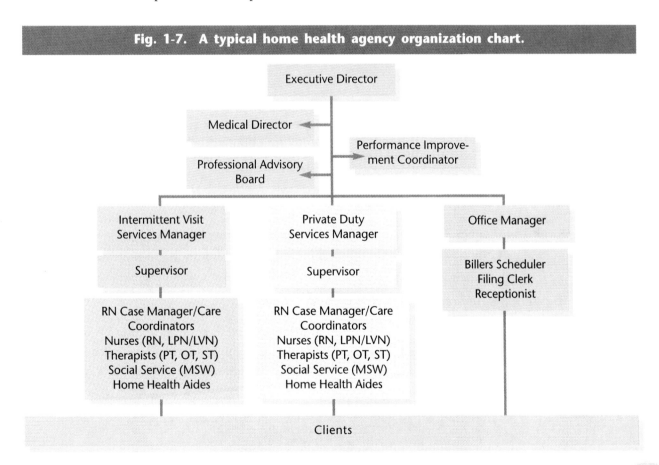

Fig. 1-7. A typical home health agency organization chart.

are needed. These professionals, who may be physicians, registered nurses, or other licensed professionals, will also reassess clients' needs for service, write care plans, and schedule services.

Once the agency's professional staff has determined the amount and types of care needed, assignments are given. A home care aide employed by the agency may be assigned to spend a certain number of hours each day or week with a client providing personal care and housekeeping services specified by the aide's supervisor. While the client care plan and the health care team assignments are developed by the supervisor or case manager, input from all members of the care team is needed. In home care, all HCAs are under supervision of the skilled professional: either a registered nurse, a physical therapist, or a speech therapist. **Figure 1-7**, on prior page, shows a typical home health agency organization chart, and more information about the care team and how the members work together is provided in Chapter 2.

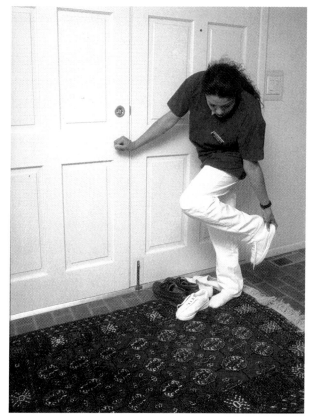

Fig. 1-8. As a home care aide, you are a guest in your clients' homes. You should respect each client's property and customs. For example, removing shoes is a custom in some homes.

❑ *7. Explain how working as an aide for a home health agency is different from working for a hospital, long-term care facility, or continuing care facility*

In some ways, working as a home care aide is similar to working as a nursing assistant, nurse's aide, or long-term care aide. Most of the basic medical procedures and many of the personal care procedures you perform will be the same. However, there are some aspects of working in the home that will be very different from working in a hospital or other care facility.

Housekeeping: You may have housekeeping responsibilities, including cooking, cleaning, laundry, and grocery shopping, for at least some of your clients.

Family contact: You may have a lot more contact with clients' families in the home than you would in a facility.

Independence: You will work independently as a home care aide. Although your supervisor will monitor your work, you will spend most of your hours working with clients without direct supervision. Thus you must be a responsible and independent worker to succeed as a home care aide.

Communication: Because you will be working independently, good written and verbal communication skills are important. You must keep yourself informed of changes in the client care plan, and you must keep others informed of changes you observe in the client and the client's environment.

Transportation: You will have to get yourself from one client's home to another. You will need to have a dependable automobile or know how to use public transportation. You may also face inclement weather conditions at times. Clients need your care—rain, snow, or sleet.

Safety: You must be aware of personal safety when you are traveling alone to visit clients. You may be visiting clients in high-crime areas. Be aware of your surroundings, walk confidently, and avoid dangerous situations, such as visits after dark.

Flexibility: Each client's home will be different, and you will need to adapt to the changes in environment. In a care facility, you know what supplies will be available and what kind of cleanliness and organization to expect at work. In home care, you may not know until you get there.

Working environment: Nursing homes are built to make care giving easier and safer. They have wide doors, large bathing facilities, and special equipment for transferring residents. If needed, other caregivers are close by and can help move a resident or answer questions you may have. In home care, the physical layout of rooms, stairs, lack of equipment, cramped bathrooms, rugs, clutter, even pets can complicate care giving.

Client's home: In a client's home, you are a guest and you need to be respectful of the client's property and customs (**Fig.** 1-8). The client is in control most of the time.

Clients' comfort: One of the best things about home care is that it allows clients to stay in the familiar and comfortable surroundings of their own homes. For most clients, this is a tremendous advantage that can help them recover or adapt to their condition more quickly.

Chapter 2

The Role of the Home Care Aide as a Member of the Care Team

Part 1
The Care Team

❑ 1. Identify the role of each health care team member

As a home care aide, you will work directly with clients and families in their homes. You will be part of a team of health professionals that includes physicians, nurses, social workers, therapists, and specialists. The team will work closely together to help clients recover from their illnesses or to do as much as they can for themselves when full recovery is not possible.

Because your clients will have different needs and problems, health care professionals with different kinds of education and experience will help care for them. Members of the health care team may include the following:

Home Care Aide (HCA): The home care aide performs delegated tasks, such as taking vital signs, and provides routine personal care, such as bathing clients or preparing meals. Because home care aides spend more time with clients than other members of the health care team, they act as the "eyes and ears" of the team. Observing and reporting changes in the client's condition or abilities to other team members is a **very important role of the HCA**.

Case Manager or Supervisor: Usually a **registered nurse**, a case manager or supervisor is assigned to each client by the home health agency. The case manager or supervisor, with input from other team members, formulates the basic care plan for the client and monitors any changes that are observed by the home care aide. The case manager also makes changes in the client care plan when necessary, after consulting with the physician and other team members.

Registered Nurse (RN): In a home health agency, a registered nurse coordinates, manages, and provides care. RNs also supervise and

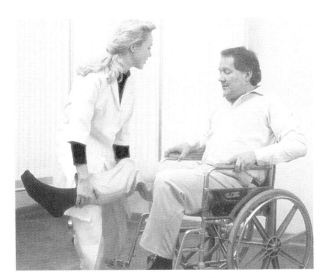

Fig. 2-1. A physical therapist is the member of the care team who is trained to administer therapy to promote healing, mobility, and pain relief.

train home care aides, and they develop the home care aid plan of care, or assignments. A registered nurse has graduated from a two- to four-year nursing program, has a certificate or college degree, and has passed a licensing examination administered by the state board of nursing. Registered nurses may have additional academic degrees or education in specialty areas.

Physician (MD): A physician's job is to diagnose disease or disability and prescribe treatment. MDs have graduated from four-year medical schools, which they attended after receiving a bachelor's degree. Many physicians also attend specialized training programs after medical school. A physician generally decides when patients need home health care and refers them to home health agencies.

Physical Therapist (PT): The physical therapist administers therapy in the form of heat, cold, massage, ultrasound, electricity, and exercise to muscles, bones, and joints in an effort to improve circulation of blood to the body part, promote healing, help the client regain or maintain mobility, and ease pain (**Fig. 2-1**).

Occupational Therapist. An occupational therapist helps clients understand and learn to compensate for disabilities. For clients in home care, an occupational therapist may assist in training clients for activities of daily living (ADLs), such as dressing, grooming, and bathing.

Speech Language Pathologist (pa-THAH-loh-jist). A speech language pathologist teaches exercises that will help the client improve or overcome speech impediments.

Registered Dietitian (RDT): A registered dietitian or nutritionist teaches clients and their families about special diets that will improve their health and help manage their illness.

Medical Social Worker (MSW): A medical social worker determines clients' needs and helps them get support services, such as counseling, meal services, and financial assistance. An MSW holds a master's or bachelor's degree in social work.

❑ 2. Define the client care plan and explain its purpose

The client care plan is individualized and developed to help achieve the goals of care for each client (**Fig. 2-2**). It designates tasks health care providers, including home care aides, must perform, states how often these tasks should be performed, and specifies how they should be carried out. For example, the HCA portion of the client care plan for a client who has had a stroke may list range of motion exercises to be performed daily; vital signs, such as temperature, pulse, and blood pressure to be taken at least once a day or more often if necessary; and diet and fluid requirements.

The purpose of the care plan is to give the health care provider a guide for helping the client attain and maintain the best level of health possible. Activities not listed on the care plan should not be performed without permission from the case manager or supervisor. The HCA care plan is part of this overall plan of care. It must be followed very carefully.

Throughout this text you will read how important it is to make observations and communicate them to your supervisor. Sometimes even simple observations are very important. The information you collect, such as vital signs, and the changes you observe in the client are all important in developing how that client's care plan needs to change.

Fig. 2-2. The client care plan is individualized for each client.

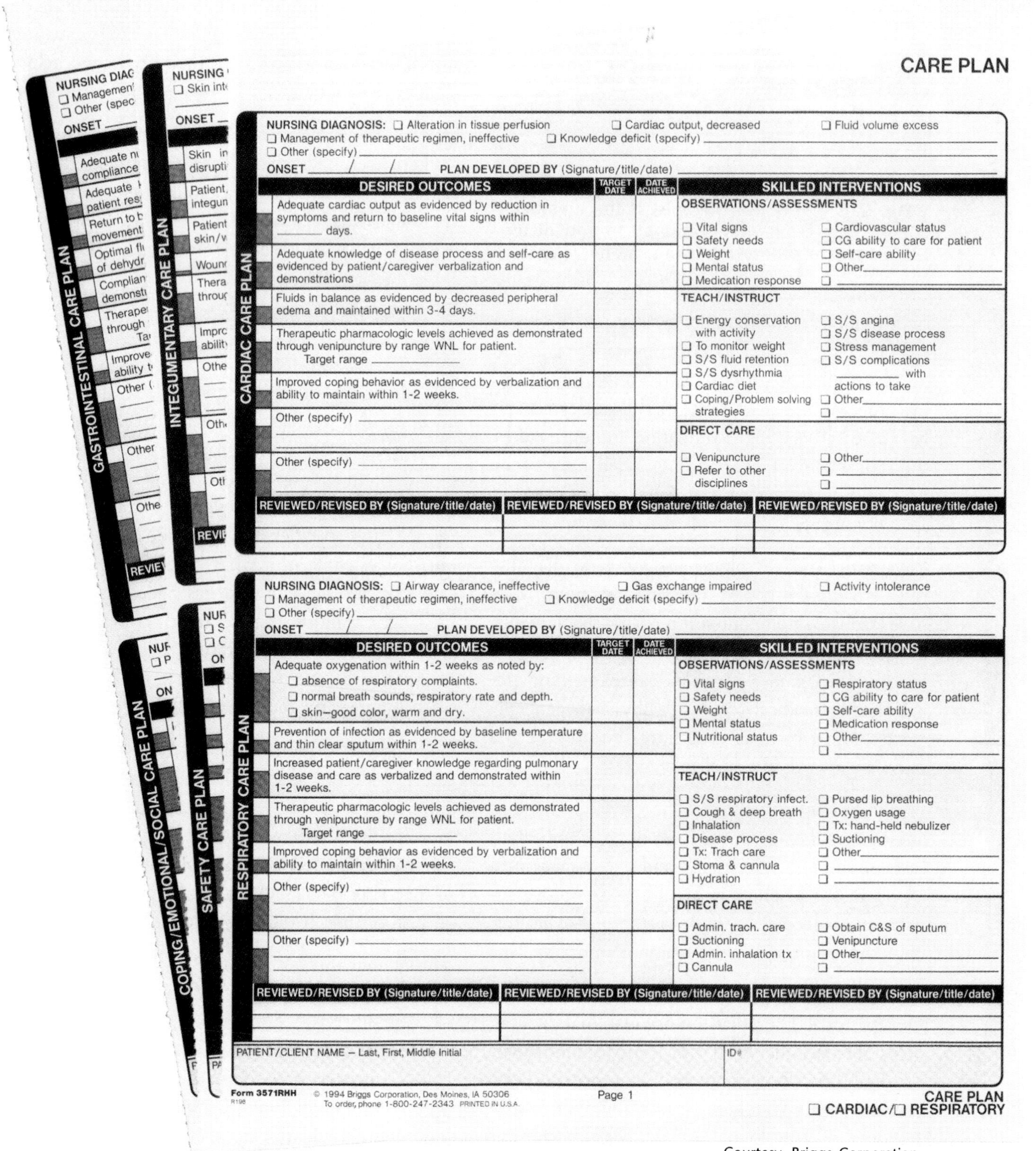

GASTROINTESTINAL CARE PLAN

INTEGUMENTARY CARE PLAN

COPING/EMOTIONAL/SOCIAL CARE PLAN

SAFETY CARE PLAN

CARE PLAN

CARDIAC CARE PLAN

NURSING DIAGNOSIS: ❑ Alteration in tissue perfusion ❑ Cardiac output, decreased ❑ Fluid volume excess
❑ Management of therapeutic regimen, ineffective ❑ Knowledge deficit (specify) ______
❑ Other (specify) ______
ONSET ___/___/___ PLAN DEVELOPED BY (Signature/title/date) ______

DESIRED OUTCOMES	TARGET DATE	DATE ACHIEVED
Adequate cardiac output as evidenced by reduction in symptoms and return to baseline vital signs within ______ days.		
Adequate knowledge of disease process and self-care as evidenced by patient/caregiver verbalization and demonstrations		
Fluids in balance as evidenced by decreased peripheral edema and maintained within 3-4 days.		
Therapeutic pharmacologic levels achieved as demonstrated through venipuncture by range WNL for patient. Target range ______		
Improved coping behavior as evidenced by verbalization and ability to maintain within 1-2 weeks.		
Other (specify) ______		
Other (specify) ______		

SKILLED INTERVENTIONS

OBSERVATIONS/ASSESSMENTS
❑ Vital signs ❑ Cardiovascular status
❑ Safety needs ❑ CG ability to care for patient
❑ Weight ❑ Self-care ability
❑ Mental status ❑ Other______
❑ Medication response ❑ ______

TEACH/INSTRUCT
❑ Energy conservation with activity ❑ S/S angina
❑ To monitor weight ❑ S/S disease process
❑ S/S fluid retention ❑ Stress management
❑ S/S dysrhythmia ❑ S/S complications
❑ Cardiac diet ______ with actions to take
❑ Coping/Problem solving strategies ❑ Other______ ❑ ______

DIRECT CARE
❑ Venipuncture ❑ Other______
❑ Refer to other disciplines ❑ ______ ❑ ______

REVIEWED/REVISED BY (Signature/title/date)	REVIEWED/REVISED BY (Signature/title/date)	REVIEWED/REVISED BY (Signature/title/date)

RESPIRATORY CARE PLAN

NURSING DIAGNOSIS: ❑ Airway clearance, ineffective ❑ Gas exchange impaired ❑ Activity intolerance
❑ Management of therapeutic regimen, ineffective ❑ Knowledge deficit (specify) ______
❑ Other (specify) ______
ONSET ___/___/___ PLAN DEVELOPED BY (Signature/title/date) ______

DESIRED OUTCOMES	TARGET DATE	DATE ACHIEVED
Adequate oxygenation within 1-2 weeks as noted by: ❑ absence of respiratory complaints. ❑ normal breath sounds, respiratory rate and depth. ❑ skin—good color, warm and dry.		
Prevention of infection as evidenced by baseline temperature and thin clear sputum within 1-2 weeks.		
Increased patient/caregiver knowledge regarding pulmonary disease and care as verbalized and demonstrated within 1-2 weeks.		
Therapeutic pharmacologic levels achieved as demonstrated through venipuncture by range WNL for patient. Target range ______		
Improved coping behavior as evidenced by verbalization and ability to maintain within 1-2 weeks.		
Other (specify) ______		
Other (specify) ______		

SKILLED INTERVENTIONS

OBSERVATIONS/ASSESSMENTS
❑ Vital signs ❑ Respiratory status
❑ Safety needs ❑ CG ability to care for patient
❑ Weight ❑ Self-care ability
❑ Mental status ❑ Medication response
❑ Nutritional status ❑ Other______ ❑ ______

TEACH/INSTRUCT
❑ S/S respiratory infect. ❑ Pursed lip breathing
❑ Cough & deep breath ❑ Oxygen usage
❑ Inhalation ❑ Tx: hand-held nebulizer
❑ Disease process ❑ Suctioning
❑ Tx: Trach care ❑ Other______
❑ Stoma & cannula ❑ ______
❑ Hydration ❑ ______

DIRECT CARE
❑ Admin. trach. care ❑ Obtain C&S of sputum
❑ Suctioning ❑ Venipuncture
❑ Admin. inhalation tx ❑ Other______
❑ Cannula ❑ ______

REVIEWED/REVISED BY (Signature/title/date)	REVIEWED/REVISED BY (Signature/title/date)	REVIEWED/REVISED BY (Signature/title/date)

PATIENT/CLIENT NAME – Last, First, Middle Initial | ID#

Form 3571RHH R198 © 1994 Briggs Corporation, Des Moines, IA 50306 To order, phone 1-800-247-2343 PRINTED IN U.S.A. Page 1

CARE PLAN ❑ CARDIAC/❑ RESPIRATORY

Courtesy, Briggs Corporation.

❑ 3. Describe how each team member contributes to the care plan

Care planning should involve input from the client and/or the family, as well as health care professionals who assess the client's physical, financial, social, and psychological needs. After the physician prescribes treatment, agency professionals, such as the supervisor, nurses, and other care team members, formulate the care plan (**Fig. 2-3**).

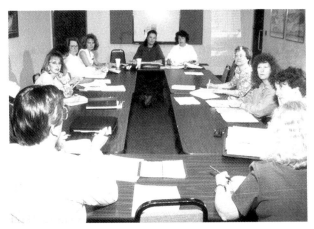

Fig. 2-3. The care team formulates the care plan.

In formulating the care plan, many factors are considered, including the client's health and physical condition; diagnosis and treatment; and whether additional services and resources, including transportation, equipment, or supplementary income, are needed. For example, a social worker may arrange transportation for the client to and from appointments with his or her physician.

The psychological (sye-ka-LOJ-ik-ul) and socioeconomic (soh-shee-oh-ee-ka-NOM-ik) status of the client and the client's family are other important factors. The agency will assess how the client and family members are reacting to the medical problems. Family members may be absent or unavailable for some clients. For example, a client may have only elderly and ailing relatives to help with care, or family members may have jobs to go to or children to care for. Some families may not have strong ties among members, or relatives may be unwilling to assist in care. For some families, problems like alcoholism and substance abuse can make it difficult

to provide care. Housing and financial resources may also be inadequate. The medical social worker may be sent to the home to assess the situation, make appropriate referrals to other community services, and assist with long-term care planning.

While the client care plan and assignments are developed by the supervisor, input from all members of the care team is needed. For instance, a 250-lb, elderly client may request a tub bath and the supervisor may assign it. The home care aide may find that the client has no adaptive equipment and is unsteady or unable to move to the tub. The assignment puts the home care aide and the client at risk of injury. The home care aide *must* communicate that the assignment needs to be changed to a sponge bath or shower, or that the client needs to obtain adaptive equipment. The supervisor is responsible for reassessing the assignment and making necessary changes to the care plan.

Multiple care plans may be necessary for clients whose care is provided by a variety of professionals. In such a situation, the supervisor or case manager will be responsible for coordinating the client's

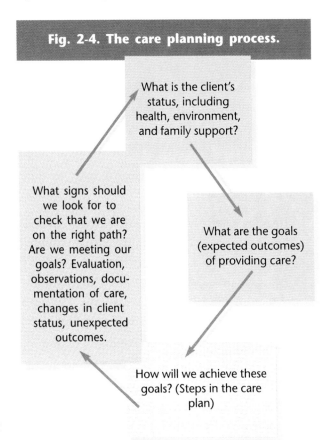

Fig. 2-4. The care planning process.

What is the client's status, including health, environment, and family support?

What are the goals (expected outcomes) of providing care?

How will we achieve these goals? (Steps in the care plan)

What signs should we look for to check that we are on the right path? Are we meeting our goals? Evaluation, observations, documentation of care, changes in client status, unexpected outcomes.

overall care. There will be one care plan or assignment for the home care aide to follow, and separate care plans for other providers, such as the physical therapist, to follow.

Care plans must be kept up-to-date as the client's condition changes. By reporting observations and problems to the supervisor, home care aides play an important role in monitoring clients' conditions so that the care team can revise care plans to meet the clients' changing needs (**Fig.** 2-4).

**Part 2
The Home Care Aide**

❏ *4. Describe the role of the home care aide and explain typical tasks home care aides perform*

The role of home care aides in the health care field is to improve or maintain the health and well-being of clients. Home care aides accomplish this directly by providing or assisting with personal care, assisting with ADLs (activities of daily living), and performing health care tasks delegated by other members of the team. Home care aides also fulfill the goals of home health care indirectly by promoting self-care, reinforcing the teachings of other health team members, and promoting behavior that improves health, such as diet and exercise.

Home care aides provide services directly to their clients in two ways:

1. Providing care or assisting with self-care, depending on the care plan. A care plan may include bathing, grooming, feeding, assisting with range of motion (ROM) exercises and ambulation, reminding the client about medications, and measuring **vital signs** (temperature, pulse rate, respiratory rate, and blood pressure).

2. Maintaining a safe, secure, and comfortable home life for clients and families. This may include light housekeeping, food shopping, meal preparation, and doing laundry.

Home care aides are also role models. They promote clients' independence by practicing good housekeeping, nutrition, and health care skills. For example, by encouraging clients to do tasks for themselves, home care aides help ensure that health will be maintained between visits.

In addition, home care aides teach by example. By performing procedures and providing assistance efficiently and cheerfully, they provide family members with a model for care giving.

❏ *5. Identify tasks outside the scope of practice for home care aides in your state*

Laws and regulations on what aides can and cannot do vary from state to state. Some procedures, however, are never performed by home care aides under any circumstances. These tasks are said to be "outside the scope of practice" of a home care aide.

Home care aides:

Never administer medications unless trained and assigned to do so. Only a few states allow nurses to delegate this task to home care aides, and it always requires specialized training. However, home care aides may assist the clients with self-administered medications in certain situations.

Never insert or remove tubes or objects (other than a thermometer) in a client's body. These procedures are called "invasive," and are performed only by licensed professionals.

Never accept or ignore an assignment or request to do something outside the scope of practice, the job description, or the assignment sheet. In this situation a home care aide should explain to the person making the request why they cannot comply, and report the request to a supervisor.

Never perform procedures that require sterile technique. For example, changing a sterile dressing on a deep, open wound requires sterile technique.

Never diagnose or prescribe treatments or medications.

Never tell the client or the family the diagnosis or the medical treatment plan. This is the responsibility of the physician or nurse.

Your instructor or employer may provide a list of other tasks outside your scope of practice as a home care aide. In some cases, you may be trained to do a particular task that your employer does not want home care aides to perform. Be sure to know which tasks these are and never perform them. Many of these specialized tasks require more training than you receive in basic home care aide training. It is important to learn how to decline a task for which you have not been trained, or which is outside your scope of practice.

❏ 6. List the federal regulations that apply to home care aides

There are three basic federal regulations that apply to home care aides:

1. **Home care aides working in a Medicare-participating agency must have 75 hours of training and/or pass a competency evaluation before they begin work-**

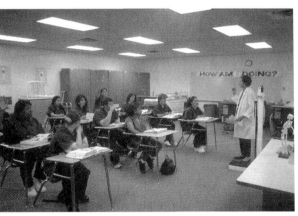

Fig. 2-5. Home care aides must complete 75 hours of training and/or pass a competency evaluation to work for a Medicare participating home health agency

ing. Training may be at a community college, high school, or home health agency (**Fig. 2-5**). State laws may require training in specific areas as well as certification through a standardized test. Proposed changes in these rules also include passing a criminal background check prior to employment, and demonstrating the ability to read, write, and give oral reports.

2. **Home care aides must have at least twelve hours of continuing education (in-service training) every year.** Home health agencies are required to offer continuing education courses for their employees, but it is **your** responsibility to successfully complete twelve hours of courses each year. An agency will not allow you to work if you have not met the twelve-hour in-service training requirement, and many states require more than twelve hours.

3. **Home care aides must comply with Occupational**

Safety and Health Administration (OSHA) rules about bloodborne pathogens, standard or universal precautions, and tuberculosis. OSHA is a federal government agency that sets rules and policies to protect workers from hazards on the job. Information on following these rules is covered in Chapter 5.

❏ 7. Describe the purpose of the chain of command

As a home care aide, you are carrying out instructions given to you by a nurse. The nurse is acting on the instructions of a physician or other member of the care team. This chain of command guarantees that your clients get appropriate health care and it protects you, your supervisor, and your employer from liability (lye-a-BIL-i-tee). Liability is a legal term that means someone can be held responsible for harming someone else. If something you do for a client hurts that person instead of helping him or her, but what you did was in the care plan and was done according to policy and procedure, then you are not liable, or responsible, for hurting the client. However, if you do something that is not in the care plan that hurts a client, you could be held responsible. That is why it is extremely important for you to follow the instructions in your care plan and for your agency to have a chain of command (**Fig. 2-6**).

As a home care aide you must have a full understanding of what you can and cannot do so that you do not harm a client or involve yourself or your employer in a lawsuit. Though some states **certify** that a home care aide is qualified to work, home care aides are not licensed health care providers. Everything you do in your job is delegated to you by a licensed health care professional. Because you are doing your job under the authority of another

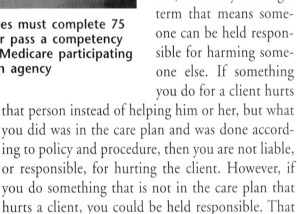

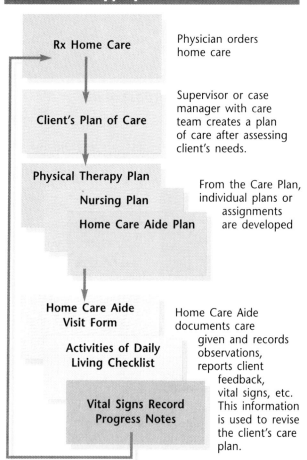

Rx Home Care — Physician orders home care

Client's Plan of Care — Supervisor or case manager with care team creates a plan of care after assessing client's needs.

Physical Therapy Plan

Nursing Plan

Home Care Aide Plan — From the Care Plan, individual plans or assignments are developed

Home Care Aide Visit Form

Activities of Daily Living Checklist

Vital Signs Record

Progress Notes — Home Care Aide documents care given and records observations, reports client feedback, vital signs, etc. This information is used to revise the client's care plan.

person's license, these professionals will show great interest in what you are doing and how you do it. They are not just being nosey. Every state grants the right to practice various jobs in health care through licensure, for instance granting a license to practice nursing, medicine, or physical therapy. When a licensed professional delegates a job to you, you are operating (doing your job) under their license. Their license to practice their profession is at risk every time you do your job.

Imagine you give an unlicensed driver permission to drive a car by letting them use your driver's license. However, if that driver is reckless or gets parking or speeding tickets, you pay the fines or possibly lose your license. Now imagine that the license is not to drive, but a license to make a living, for which you spent many years studying and practicing.

❑ 8. Identify examples of employers' policies and procedures and explain why they are important

When you work for a home health agency, you should either be given access to or told where to locate a list of **policies and procedures** that all staff members are expected to follow. A **policy** is a course of action that should be taken every time a certain situation occurs. For example, one very basic policy at most home health agencies is that the care plan must be followed. That means that every time you visit a client, what you do will be determined by the care plan. A procedure (proh-SEE-dyoor) is a particular method, or way, of doing something. For example, your agency will have a procedure for reporting information about your clients. The procedure tells you what form you fill out, when and how often to fill it out, and whom to give it to.

Common policies and procedures at home health agencies include the following:

Information given in a business relationship must remain confidential. Keeping information confidential means not telling anyone about it. This is not only an agency rule, but a law. The home health agency and all its employees must keep all information about clients and their families confidential. You should be careful where you keep your notes and assignment sheets. Keeping your paperwork in the open where someone could read it, or losing your notes or assignments, is a breach of confidentiality. Confidentiality also extends to the agency's personnel files and clinical records, which means your employer cannot give out information about you from your job application or other records.

The client's care plan must be followed. Home care aides should perform all tasks assigned to them in the care plan. They should not do any tasks that are not included in their job description or that have not been approved by the case manager or supervisor. If the client or family requests changes, they should be told to speak to the supervisor.

Report to the supervisor at regular arranged times and more frequently if necessary. For example, home care aides must report the following to their supervisors: important events or changes in clients and their families, an accident on the job, and anything that delays or prevents them from going to or completing an assignment.

Personal problems must not be discussed with the client or the client's family. Discussing your personal problems is unprofessional. You must act in a professional manner in order for clients to see you as someone whose job is to provide care, rather than as a friend or family member.

Be punctual and dependable. Employers expect this of all employees.

Deadlines for documentation and paperwork. Timely and accurate documentation is very important. This topic is discussed in detail in Chapter 4.

Delivery of client care. You should provide all client care in a pleasant, professional manner.

Do not give or receive gifts. Gift giving and receiving is prohibited by most agencies because it detracts from the professional relationship and quality of service (**Fig. 2-7**). Gift giving can cause other problems as well. For example, a client may forget giving an object as a gift and report it as stolen. Some clients who give gifts may believe they deserve special treatment.

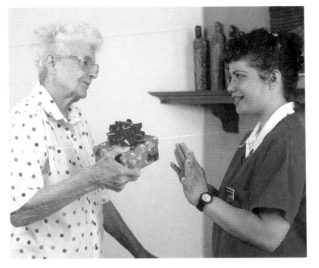

Fig. 2-7. Home care aides should not give or receive gifts, both because it is unprofessional and because it can lead to conflicts.

Your employer will have policies and procedures for every client care situation. These have been developed to give quality care and protect client safety. You must always follow your employer's policies and procedures.

For every task a home care aide performs, the agency's way to do it is spelled out, step by step, in the procedure. Though written procedures may seem long and sometimes complicated, each step is important.

This book includes general procedures for all the basic tasks you will do as a home care aide. The procedures are listed on page V. Always follow your employer's procedures when caring for clients.

Part 3
Professionalism

Professional means having to do with work or a job. The opposite of professional is personal, which refers to your life outside your job, for example, your family, friends, and home life. **Professionalism** is how you behave when you are on the job. It includes how you dress, the words you use, and the things you talk about. It also includes being on time, finishing your assignments, and reporting to your supervisor. For an HCA, professionalism means participating in care planning, being careful to make important observations, and reporting accurately. Following the policies and procedures of your agency is an important part of professionalism. Employees who behave in a professional way are respected by their clients, coworkers, and supervisors. Professionalism will help you keep your job and may help you earn promotions and raises.

❑ 9. List examples of a professional relationship with a client

Examples of a professional relationship with a client include:

▶ maintaining a positive attitude

▶ being cleanly and neatly dressed and groomed

- arriving on time, doing tasks efficiently, and leaving on time

- doing only the tasks assigned

- speaking politely and cheerfully to the client, even if you are not in a good mood

- never discussing your personal problems

- never giving or accepting gifts

- calling the client Mr., Mrs., Ms., or Miss, and his or her last name

- listening to the client

- always explaining the care you will provide before providing it

- always following care practices, such as handwashing, to protect yourself and the client

❑ 10. List examples of a professional relationship with an employer

A professional relationship with an employer includes:

- maintaining a positive attitude

- completing assignments efficiently

- consistently following policies and procedures

- documenting and reporting consistently and accurately

- communicating problems with clients or assignments

- reporting anything that keeps you from completing assignments

- asking questions when you do not know or understand something

- taking directions or criticism without getting upset

- being cleanly and neatly dressed and groomed

- always being on time

- participating in education programs offered

❑ 11. Demonstrate how to organize client care assignments efficiently

In order to finish all your assignments each day, you will have to work efficiently. To be efficient, you need to decide the order in which to do your tasks. For example, you are assigned to work with an elderly client from 2:00 to 4:00 pm on Monday. Your supervisor has told you that this client needs some housekeeping, dinner prepared, and personal care. When you arrive at the client's home, you see what tasks need to be done. It is a good idea to sit down and make a list of the tasks you will do and the order in which you will do them (Fig. 2-8).

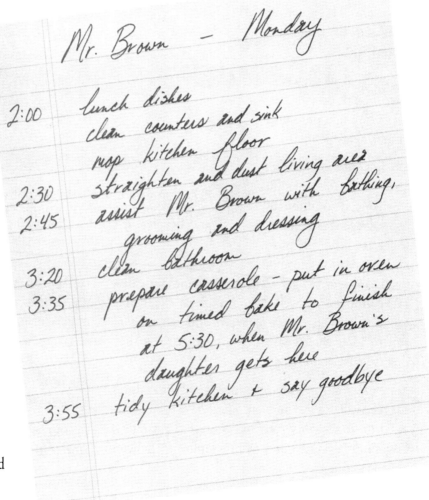

Fig. 2-8. Making a list of tasks to be done will help you organize to perform them efficiently.

Two hours is not a lot of time to do all those tasks, so you will have to work quickly and you will not have any extra time to turn on the television or sit down and have coffee. If you had not planned the tasks before you started, you might have spent too long cleaning the kitchen and never have gotten to make dinner. Making a list of tasks helps you be most efficient. It is also helpful to include the client in your planning. A client may not cooperate with your schedule if he or she has different priorities. It takes good communication, and sometimes negotiation, to arrange a schedule that works for you and the client.

If you run out of time with a client, you have to stay late to finish all your tasks. That makes you late to your next assignment. You are then left without enough time to do everything the next client needs, and you will upset that client's schedule. Completing assignments efficiently means you are not always running late. It lets you do your job calmly, which means you will probably do a better job.

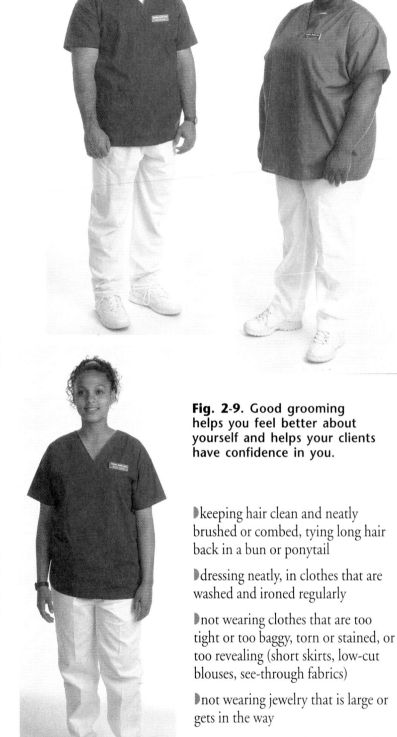

Fig. 2-9. Good grooming helps you feel better about yourself and helps your clients have confidence in you.

❏ 12. Demonstrate acceptable personal grooming habits

Good grooming makes you feel great, and it makes others feel good about you (**Fig. 2-9**). Grooming affects how confident clients feel about the care you give. Good employees have the following personal grooming habits:

▶ bathing or showering daily and using deodorant or anti-perspirant (use little or no perfume, as some clients may be intolerant of some odors)

▶ brushing teeth frequently and using mouthwash when necessary

▶ keeping hair clean and neatly brushed or combed, tying long hair back in a bun or ponytail

▶ dressing neatly, in clothes that are washed and ironed regularly

▶ not wearing clothes that are too tight or too baggy, torn or stained, or too revealing (short skirts, low-cut blouses, see-through fabrics)

▶ not wearing jewelry that is large or gets in the way

Your agency may have rules about your appearance. Be sure to know these rules and always follow them.

13. Identify personal qualities a home care aide must have

Home care aides must be:

Compassionate. Being compassionate (kum-PASH-on-et) means being caring, concerned, considerate, empathetic (em-pah-THEH-tik), and understanding. People who are compassionate understand other people's problems and care about them. Being empathetic means you can put yourself in another person's place to understand that person's problems and feelings.

Honest. A person who is honest tells the truth and can be trusted. Clients need to feel that they can trust the people who care for them. The care team will depend on your honesty in planning and implementing the care plan. Your employer counts on your truthful records of the care you provide, the hours you work, the time and mileage you spend traveling, and the observations you make.

Conscientious. People who are conscientious (kahn-shee-EN-shus) try to do their best in everything they do. They are always alert, observant, accurate, and responsible. Conscientious care of those who are ill involves making accurate observations, paying careful attention to the care plan, taking responsibility for actions, and reporting precisely to other members of the health care team (**Fig. 2-10**). For example, taking accurate measurements of *vital signs*, such as temperature, pulse, or respiration, is essential because other members of the health care team will make important treatment decisions based on the documented measurements. Without conscientious care, a client's health and well-being are in danger.

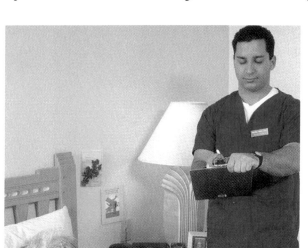

Fig. 2-10. Home care aides must be conscientious about documenting observations and procedures.

Dependable. Health care providers must be able to make and keep commitments. You must report to work on time each day that you are scheduled to work, skillfully perform the tasks that have been assigned, avoid too many absences, and keep your promises. Dependability is especially important in a home care setting, where the supervisor is not usually there to check on client care.

Respectful. Being respectful means seeing value in other people's individuality, including age, religion, culture, feelings, and beliefs. People who are respectful treat others politely and considerately. You should care about people's self-esteem and not do or say anything that will damage it. You must never let people down by gossiping about them, and you should respect the various cultures and practices of your clients.

Unprejudiced. As a home care aide you will work with many different people from different backgrounds. As a professional, you must give every one of your clients the same quality care regardless of age, sex, religion, race, or ethnic origin.

Non-judgmental. You may not like or agree with things that your clients or their families do or have done. However, your job is to care for each client according to the care plan, not to judge them, their words, their lifestyle, or their actions. Try to put aside your opinions and see each client as an individual who needs your care.

14. Identify responsibilities of an employer to the home care aide

Agencies are responsible for providing home care aides with the information they need about agency policies and procedures. Agencies are also responsible for making sure that home care aides are educated and able to perform all tasks assigned to them. Your employer should fulfill the following responsibilities to you:

Provide a written job description. The job description tells you what you are expected to do during your working hours (**Fig. 2-11**).

Provide competency testing and skills evaluation before you are sent to care for clients.

Provide initial training and continuing in-service training. Initial training should include an orientation to the policies and procedures of the agency. You should also be trained in the agency's documentation system. In-service training is not only a Federal requirement, but it keeps your skills fresh and helps you do an even better job. OSHA regulations require the employer to offer AIDS and Hepatitis B education as well.

Provide appropriate and adequate preparation for each assignment. The agency should give you the information you will need about each client and assignment. You should be told why the client needs service and what are the goals of care. If other health care professionals are involved, their jobs and responsibilities should also be explained to you.

Provide supervision. Supervisors will provide support and teach you how to do new tasks. They can help you find solutions to special problems and help you adjust to new situations. Supervisors will also routinely check with clients to assure the goals of the care plan are being met and that clients are satisfied with the care they are receiving.

Provide information about supervision. Your employer should tell you when and where you will meet with your supervisor and what you will discuss in these meetings. You should also be told how the supervisor can be reached for assistance, and when and why the supervisor will visit your clients' homes.

Provide adequate equipment and supplies for you to safely do your work. Your agency should always provide, for example, gloves you must sometimes wear to protect you and your client from infection.

Fig. 2-11. Your employer should provide you with a job description that defines your basic responsibilities on the job.

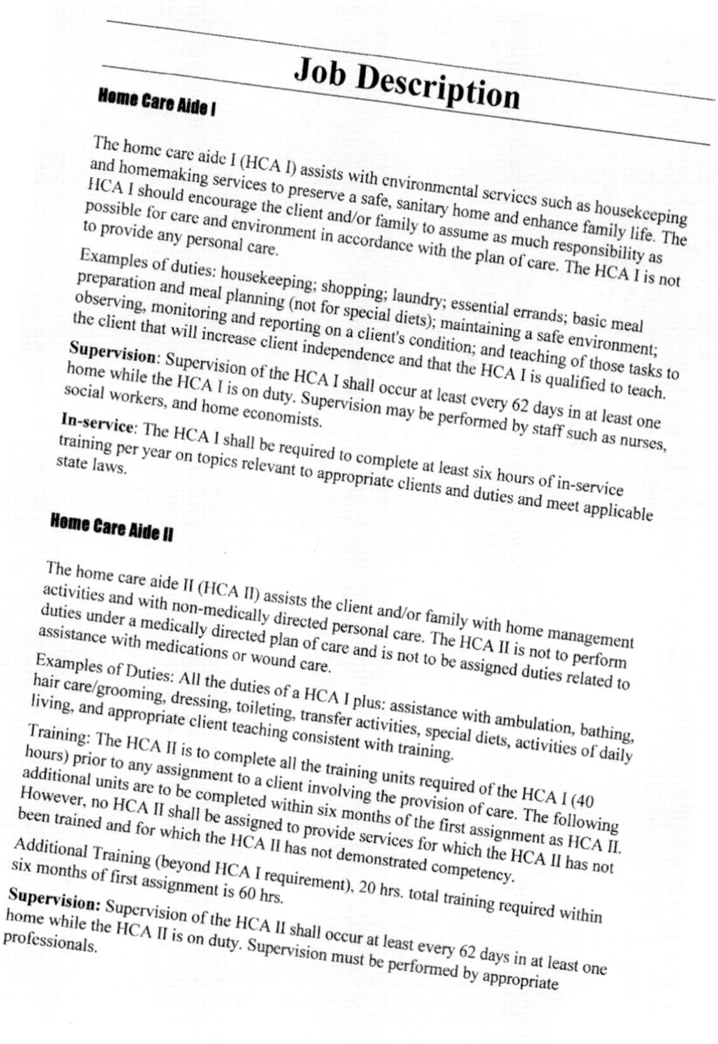

Job Description

Home Care Aide I

The home care aide I (HCA I) assists with environmental services such as housekeeping and homemaking services to preserve a safe, sanitary home and enhance family life. The HCA I should encourage the client and/or family to assume as much responsibility as possible for care and environment in accordance with the plan of care. The HCA I is not to provide any personal care.

Examples of duties: housekeeping; shopping; laundry; essential errands; basic meal preparation and meal planning (not for special diets); observing, monitoring and reporting on a client's condition; maintaining a safe environment; and teaching of those tasks to the client that will increase client independence and that the HCA I is qualified to teach.

Supervision: Supervision of the HCA I shall occur at least every 62 days in at least one home while the HCA I is on duty. Supervision may be performed by staff such as nurses, social workers, and home economists.

In-service: The HCA I shall be required to complete at least six hours of in-service training per year on topics relevant to appropriate clients and duties and meet applicable state laws.

Home Care Aide II

The home care aide II (HCA II) assists the client and/or family with home management activities and with non-medically directed personal care. The HCA II is not to perform duties under a medically directed plan of care and is not to be assigned duties related to assistance with medications or wound care.

Examples of Duties: All the duties of a HCA I plus: assistance with ambulation, bathing, hair care/grooming, dressing, toileting, transfer activities, special diets, activities of daily living, and appropriate client teaching consistent with training.

Training: The HCA II is to complete all the training units required of the HCA I (40 hours) prior to any assignment to a client involving the provision of care. The following additional units are to be completed within six months of the first assignment as HCA II. However, no HCA II shall be assigned to provide services for which the HCA II has not been trained and for which the HCA II has not demonstrated competency.

Additional Training (beyond HCA I requirement), 20 hrs. total training required within six months of first assignment is 60 hrs.

Supervision: Supervision of the HCA II shall occur at least every 62 days in at least one home while the HCA II is on duty. Supervision must be performed by appropriate professionals.

Chapter 3

Legal and Ethical Issues for Home Care Aides

❏ **1. List examples of legal and ethical behavior**

Our behavior is guided by **ethics** and **laws**. Ethics is the knowledge of right and wrong. An ethical person has a sense of duty and responsibility toward others, and always tries to do what is right.

If ethics tell us what we **should** do, laws tell us what we **must** do. Laws are usually based on ethics. Governments establish laws to help people live peacefully together and to ensure order and safety. When someone breaks the law, he or she may be punished by having to pay a fine or spend time in prison.

Ethics and laws are extremely important in health care. They protect people receiving care and guide people giving care. Home care aides and other health care providers should be guided by a code of ethics, and must know the laws that apply to their jobs.

Examples of legal and ethical behavior by home care aides include the following:

- being honest at all times— stealing, or lying about what care you provided or how long it took are examples of dishonesty
- protecting clients' privacy by never discussing their cases except with other members of the care team
- never accepting gifts or tips
- never becoming personally or sexually involved with clients or family members
- reporting abuse or suspected abuse of a client
- following the care plan/assignment
- never performing any task outside your scope of practice
- reporting all client observations and incidents to your supervisor
- documenting accurately and on time
- following OSHA rules about bloodborne pathogens, standard precautions, and tuberculosis

Clients and Providers Have a Right to Dignity and Respect

Home care clients and their formal caregivers have a right to not be discriminated against based on race, color, religion, national origin, age, sex, or handicap. Furthermore, clients and caregivers have a right to mutual respect and dignity, including respect for property. caregivers are prohibited from accepting personal gifts and borrowing from clients.

Clients have the right:
❖ to have relationships with home care providers that are based on honesty and ethical standards of conduct;
❖ to be informed of the procedure they can follow to lodge complaints with the home care provider about the care that is, or fails to be, furnished and about a lack of respect for property. (To lodge complaints with us call _____.
❖ to know about the disposition of such complaints:
❖ to voice their grievances without fear of discrimination or reprisal for having done so; and
❖ to be advised of the telephone number and hours of operation of the state's home care hot-line." which receives questions and complaints about local home care agencies, including complaints about implementation of advance directive requirements. The hours are _____ and the number is _____.

Decision making

Clients have the right:
❖ to be notified in advance about the care that is to be furnished, the types (disciplines) of the caregivers who will furnish the care, and the frequency of the visits that are proposed to be furnished;
❖ to be advised of any change in the plan of care before the change is made;
❖ to participate in the planning of the care and in planning changes in the care, and to be advised that they have the right to do so;
❖ to be informed in writing of rights under state law to make decisions concerning medical care, including the right to accept or refuse treatment and the right to formulate advance directives;
❖ to be notified of the expected outcomes of care and any obstacles or barriers to treatment*
❖ to be informed in writing of policies and procedures for implementing advance directives, including any limitations if the provider cannot implement an advance directive on the basis of conscience;
❖ to have health care providers comply with advance directives in accordance with state law requirements;
❖ to receive care without condition on, or discrimination based on, the execution of advance directives; and
❖ to refuse services without fear of reprisal or discrimina-tion

The home care provider or the client's physician may be forced to refer the client to another source of care if the client's refusal to comply with the plan of care threatens to compromise the provider's commitment to quality care.

Privacy

Clients have the right:
❖ to confidentiality of the medical record as well as information about their health, social, and financial circumstances and about what takes place in the home; and
❖ to expect the home care provider to release information only as required by law or authorized by the client and to be informed of procedures for disclosure.

Financial Information

Clients have the right:
❖ to be informed of the extent to which payment may be expected from Medicare, Medicaid, or any other payor known to the home care provider;
❖ to be informed of the charges that will not be covered by Medicare;
❖ to be informed of the charges for which the client may be liable;
❖ to receive this information, orally and in writing, before care is initiated and within 30 calendar days of the date the home care provider becomes aware of any changes; and
❖ to have access, upon request, to all bills for service the client has received regardless of whether the bills are paid out-of-pocket or by another party.

Quality of Care

Clients have the right:
❖ to receive care of the highest quality;
❖ in general, to be admitted by a home care provider only if it has the resources needed to provide the care safely and at the required level of intensity, as determined by a professional assessment; a provider with less than optimal resources may nevertheless admit the client if a more appropriate provider is not available, but only after fully informing the client of the provider's limitations and the lack of suitable alternative arrangements; and
❖ to be told what to do in the case of an emergency.

The home care provider shall assure that:

❖ all medically related home care is provided in accordance with physicians' orders and that a plan of care specifies the services and their frequency and duration; and

CONTINUES >

> CONTINUED FROM PREVIOUS PAGE

❖ all medically related personal care is provided by an appropriately trained home care aide who is supervised by a nurse or other qualified home care professional.

Client Responsibility

Clients have the responsibility:

❖ to notify the provider of changes in their condition (e.g., hospitalization, changes in the plan of care, symptoms to be reported);
❖ to follow the plan of care;
❖ to notify the provider if the visit schedule needs to be changed;
❖ to inform providers of the existence of any changes made to advance directives;
❖ to advise the provider of any problems or dissatisfaction with the services provided;

❖ to provide a safe environment for care to be provided; and
❖ to carry out mutually agreed responsibilities.

Additional Agency Information

To satisfy the Medicare certification requirements, the Health Care Financing Administration requires that agencies:

1. Give a copy of the Bill of Rights to each patient in the course of the admission process.
2. Explain the Bill of Rights to the patient and document that this has been done.
Agencies may have clients sign a copy of the patients Bill of Rights to acknowledge receipt. This patients Bill of Rights meets Federal Medicare requirements but may not meet state requirements. Agencies should develop an addendum if needed to meet additional state requirements.

Adapted from HCFA Proposed (1997) Conditions of Participation and National Association for Home Care Bill of Rights.

❑ 2. List examples of clients' rights and explain why they are important

The purpose of the Clients' Bill of Rights is to inform clients of their rights within the health care system and to provide an ethical code of conduct for health care workers. Home health agencies will give clients a listing of these rights and review each right with them.

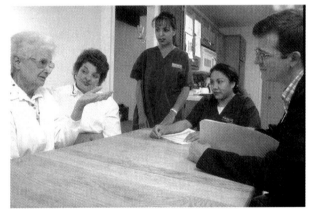

Fig. 3-1. Clients and their families should be involved in care planning

The first right listed in the Clients' Bill of Rights states that clients have the right to receive considerate, dignified, and respectful care. This also means that clients have the right not to be neglected or abused verbally, physically, or psychologically by their caretakers. **Neglect** is the failure of a caregiver to take proper care of a person. **Verbal abuse** is the use of words that do not show consideration and respect. **Physical abuse** refers to any treatment, intentional or unintentional, that causes harm to the client's body.

Psychological abuse is any behavior that causes the client to feel threatened and fearful. Many states require home health agencies to provide their clients with the abuse hotline numbers.

Home care aides must never abuse clients in any way. They must also try to protect their clients from others who abuse them. **If you ever see or suspect that a client is being abused by another caregiver or a family member, report this immediately to your supervisor.**

Two other basic clients' rights are the right to be fully informed of the goals of care and of the care itself, and the right to participate in care planning. Your employer should develop an agreement with each client about the goals of care before service is provided and should also make every effort possible to involve clients and their families in care planning (**Fig. 3-1**). Each of us knows how our bodies work best and what makes us comfortable or uncomfortable. People who feel in control of their bodies, lives, and health have greater self-esteem and are more likely to continue a treatment plan and to cooperate with caregivers. Clients also have a right to know what the agency expects to happen as a result of their care. These expected outcomes are sometimes called the goals of the care plan. Clients should be informed of obstacles or barriers to their care. For example, a client's consistent failure to eat enough healthy food can be an obstacle to getting well.

3. List examples of behavior supporting and promoting clients' rights

You can help protect your clients' rights in the following ways:

▶ Watch for and report to your supervisor any signs of abuse or neglect.

▶ Involve clients in your planning.

▶ Always explain a procedure before performing it.

▶ Never abuse a client physically, psychologically, or verbally.

▶ Respect a client's refusal of care, but report the refusal to your supervisor immediately.

▶ Tell your supervisor if a client has questions about the goals of care or the care plan.

▶ Never talk or gossip about a client.

▶ Never open a client's mail or look through his or her belongings (**Fig.** 3-2).

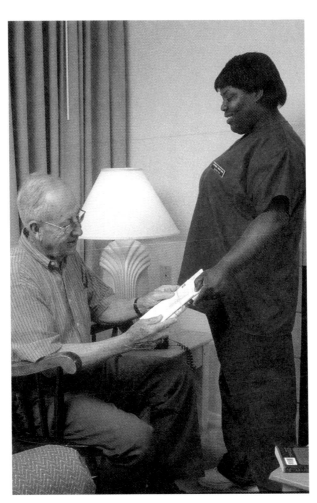

Fig. 3-2. Never look through a client's mail or belongings.

▶ Respect your clients' property.

▶ Report observations regarding a client's condition or care.

4. Explain the importance of maintaining confidentiality of client information

Confidentiality means keeping private things private. As a health care worker visiting clients' homes, you will probably learn a great deal of confidential information about your clients. You may learn about a client's state of health, finances, and personal and family relationships. You are both ethically and legally obligated to protect the confidentiality of this information, which means you should not tell anyone other than members of the health care team anything about your clients.

Maintaining confidentiality is a legal and ethical obligation. It is part of respecting your clients and their rights. Your clients have to trust you, and talking about them betrays this trust. **Invasion of privacy** is a legal term that means violating someone's right to privacy by exposing his or her private affairs, name, or photograph to the public without that person's consent. Discussing a client's care or personal affairs with anyone other than your supervisor or another member of the health care team could be considered an invasion of privacy, which violates civil law.

SECTION II
Building a Foundation: Before Client Care

Chapter 4

Communication

❑ **1. Define communication**

Communication is the process by which we exchange information with other people. It is a process of sending and receiving messages.

Learning Objectives

In this chapter you will learn to:

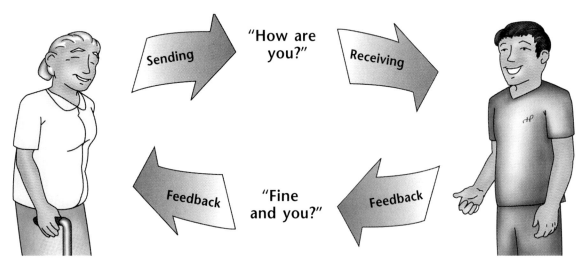

Fig. 4-1. The communication process consists of three basic steps: 1) sending a message; 2) receiving a message; and, 3) providing feedback.

People communicate by using signs and symbols, such as words, drawings, and pictures, and also by their behavior.

The simplest form of communication takes place between two people (**Fig. 4-1**). The person who communicates first is the "sender," sending a message. The person who receives the message is called the "receiver." Receiver and sender are constantly switching roles as they communicate.

In the third step, providing feedback, the person who receives the message repeats it or responds to it in some way. This lets the sender know that the message was received and understood. All three steps must be taken before the communication process is complete and the information has been exchanged. During a conversation, this three-step process is usually repeated over and over.

Effective communication is a critical part of your job as a home care aide. Home care aides must communicate with supervisors, members of the health care team, clients, and family members. A client's health and the family's trust may depend on how well you communicate your observations and concerns to your supervisor and to other caregivers. You will also need to be able to communicate clearly, respectfully, and diplomatically with clients and family members in stressful or confusing situations. Some family members may need your guidance in communicating clearly with each other or with the health care team.

❑ 2. Identify and use verbal and nonverbal communication

People can communicate, or exchange information, in many different ways. Communication is either verbal or nonverbal. Verbal communication involves the use of words or sounds, spoken or written. Nonverbal communication is the way we communicate without using words.

For example, nodding your head instead of saying yes is a kind of nonverbal communication. Shaking your head or shrugging your shoulders are other examples. Nonverbal communication also includes the *way* we say something using words. For example, you might say "I'll be right there, Mr. Dodd," and communicate that you are ready and willing to help. But if you say the same phrase in a different tone or emphasizing different words, you could communicate that you are frustrated and annoyed: "I'll *be* right *there*, Mr. Dodd!"

Body language is another form of nonverbal communication. Body movements, facial expressions, and posture can express different attitudes or emotions, including sadness, happiness, anger, and pain. Just as with speaking, you send messages with your body language, and other people receive them and interpret them. For example, slouching in a chair and sitting erect send two different messages (**Fig. 4-2**). Slouching sends the message that you are bored, tired, or hostile to the other person. Sitting up straight sends the message that you are interested and respect-

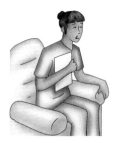 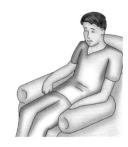

Fig. 4-2. Body language often speaks as plainly as words. Which of these people seems more interested in the conversation they are having?

ful. Take some time to look around and observe how people use body language to communicate.

Sometimes people send one message verbally and a very different message nonverbally. Nonverbal communication often tells us how someone is feeling, a message that may be quite different from what he or she is saying. For example, a client who tells you "I'm feeling fine today," but stays in bed and winces in pain, is sending two very different messages. This case shows how paying attention to nonverbal communication can help you give better care to your clients. You will need to communicate to your supervisor your observation that the client is staying in bed and appears to be wincing in pain despite what he or she says.

When communication is confusing or seems to involve conflicting messages, try to clarify it. Ask for an explanation of the message by saying something like "Mrs. Jones, you've just told me something that I don't understand. Would you explain it to me?" Or state what you have observed and ask if the observation is correct. For example, "Mrs. Jones, I see that you're smiling, but I hear by the sound of your voice that you may be depressed. Are you?" Taking the time to clarify communication can help you know your clients better and avoid misunderstandings.

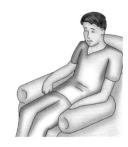

Fig. 4-3. How a person perceives your touch may depend on his or her cultural background.

It is also important to remember that nonverbal communication may depend on personality or cultural background. Some people are more animated when they speak, using lots of gestures and expression. Other people speak quietly or calmly, regardless of their moods. Depending on their cultural background, people may make motions with their hands when they talk, stand close to the person they are talking to, touch the other person, or make certain noises.

One cultural behavior that is sometimes a problem is that of accepted distance. People from some cultural groups stand further apart when talking than people from other groups. When one person shortens the distance, the other person may view it as a threat. Try to be sensitive to your clients' needs, and let them determine how close they want to be when talking to you.

You must also be aware of your own verbal and nonverbal messages. If you say "It's nice to see you today, Mrs. Rodriguez," but you don't smile or even look her in the eye, Mrs. Rodriguez will know that you aren't really all that happy to see her.

The use of touch and eye contact also varies with

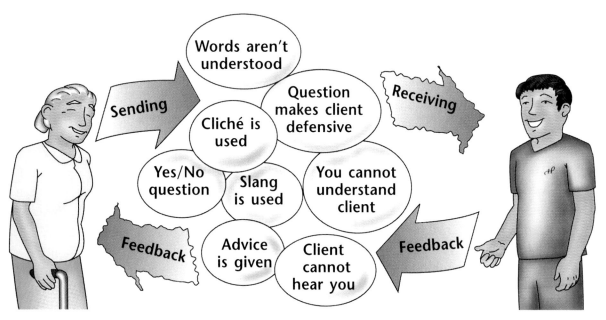

Fig. 4-4. Barriers to communication.

cultural background and with personality (**Fig. 4-3**). For some people, touching is welcome and expresses caring and warmth. For others, it seems intrusive, threatening, or even harassing. In the United States, we often talk about "looking someone straight in the eye" or speaking with each other "eye to eye." We regard eye contact as an indication of honesty. However, in some cultures, looking someone in the eye may seem bold or disrespectful.

Deciding what is nonverbal communication and what is individually or culturally determined behavior can be a challenge. However, it is an important part of understanding and communicating with people. It is especially important in a multicultural society (a society made up of many cultures), such as the United States. The key to using verbal and nonverbal communication effectively is to be aware of all the messages you are sending and receiving. As you practice listening and observing carefully, you will learn to understand your clients' needs and feelings.

❑ 3. Identify barriers to communication

Communication can be blocked or disrupted in many ways (**Fig. 4-4**). Following are some barriers and ways to avoid them:

Client does not hear you, does not hear correctly, or does not understand. Stand directly facing the client. Speak more slowly than you do with family and friends. Make sure each word is spoken clearly, especially if your client is hard of hearing or has a different native language. Speak in a low, pleasant voice. Do not whisper or mumble. If your client says he or she can't hear you, speak more loudly, but maintain a pleasant, professional tone of voice. If your client wears a hearing aide, check to ensure it is on and is working properly.

Client is difficult to understand. Be patient and take time to listen. Ask client to repeat or explain. Try to rephrase the message in your own words to make sure you have understood.

Message uses words receiver does not understand. Do not use medical terminology with your client or the family. Speak in simple, everyday words. Ask what a word means if you aren't sure.

Using slang confuses the message. Avoid using slang words and expressions that may not be understood or are unprofessional.

Using clichés makes your message meaningless. Clichés (klee-shays) are phrases that are used over and over again and don't really mean anything, for example "Everything will be fine," "It'll all work out," and "It's for the best." Instead of using a cliché, listen to what your client is really saying and respond with a meaningful message. For example, if a client is afraid of having a bath, say "I understand that it seems scary to you. What can I do to make you more comfortable?" instead of saying "Oh, it'll be over before you know it."

Asking "why" makes the client defensive. Avoid asking "why" when a client makes a statement. "Why" questions make people feel defensive. For example, a client may say she does not want to go for a walk today. If you ask "why not?" you may receive an angry response. Instead, ask, "Are you too tired to take a walk, or is there something else you want to do?" Your client may then be willing to discuss the issue.

Giving advice is inappropriate. Do not offer your personal opinion or give advice. Clients and family members should make important decisions on their own or with help from their doctors and nurses. Giving medical advice is not within the scope of your practice as a home care aide and could be dangerous. Giving advice about running the household when you have not been asked can seem pushy and intrusive.

Yes/no answers end a conversation. Unless you are seeking direct information, ask open-ended questions that need more than a yes or no answer. Yes and no answers bring any conversation to an end. For example, if you want to know what your client likes to eat, do not ask "Do you like vegetables?" Instead, try "Which vegetables do you like best?"

Nonverbal communication changes the message. Be aware of your body language and gestures when you are speaking. Be alert to nonverbal messages from your clients and clarify them. For example "Mr. Feldman, you say you're feeling fine but you seem to be in pain. Can I help?"

❑ *4. List ways to ensure that communication is accurate and complete*

In addition to avoiding the barriers to communication listed above, the following techniques will help ensure that you send and receive clear, complete messages.

Be a good listener. Allow the other person to express his or her ideas completely. When he or she is finished, restate the message in your own words to make sure you have understood.

Provide feedback as you listen. Active listening, a valuable part of communicating, involves focusing on the person who is sending the message and providing feedback. Feedback might be an acknowledgment, a question, or a repetition of the sender's message. By offering general but leading responses, such as "Oh?" or "Go on," or "Hmm," you are actively listening, providing feedback, and encouraging the sender to expand the message. For example, a client might tell you, "My son is having some problems at work." If you respond with "Oh really?" or "Tell me more," your client might disclose the fear that his or her illness has caused or contributed to the son's problems.

Bring up topics of concern. If you know of a topic that might be of concern to your client, raise the issue in a general, nonthreatening way. This allows the client to decide whether or not to discuss it. For example, if you have observed that your client is unusually quiet one day, you could say, "Mrs. Jones, you seem so quiet today." Or you may notice a certain emotion, and you would like to give the client an opportunity to discuss it; you might say, "Mrs. Jones, you seemed upset earlier. Would you like to talk about it?"

Let some pauses happen. Use silence for a few moments at a time to encourage the client to gather his or her thoughts and compose more messages.

Tune into other cultures. Learn the words and expressions of your client's culture. This shows that you respect the culture and are interested in what the client has to say, and it will help you understand your client's messages more fully. Be careful about using new words and terms yourself, however. Taken out of context, some words or expressions may have a different meaning than what you thought. The important thing is to understand words and expressions when others use them. Never be judgmental; accept people who are different.

Ask for more. When clients report symptoms, events, or feelings, have them repeat what they have said and ask them for more information.

❏ 5. Describe the difference between facts and opinions

A fact is something that is definitely true. For example, "Mr. Ford has lost four pounds this month." You can back up this fact with evidence: weighing Mr. Ford and comparing his current weight to his weight last month. An opinion is something someone believes to be true, but is not definitely true. "I think Mr. Ford looks thinner," is an opinion. So is "Mr. Ford has lost weight because he won't eat what I cook." These statements might be true, but you cannot back them up with evidence.

It is important to be able to separate facts from opinions. When a television commercial claims that a new cookie is 100% fat free, that is a fact. But when the actor on the commercial says the cookie tastes great, that is an opinion. You can be sure there is no fat in the cookie, but you really cannot be sure how it tastes unless you try it. Separating facts from opinions can help you make better decisions.

Separating facts from opinions will also make you a better communicator. When you give your opinion of a situation, you risk being wrong. If you say, "Mrs. Myers, drinking that coffee is going to keep you awake tonight," you may make your client mad. Also, you might be wrong: perhaps Mrs. Myers always drinks a cup of coffee and it does not affect her sleep, or maybe she does not sleep well because of a medication, not the coffee.

Using facts, you can communicate more effectively. "Mrs. Myers, many people find that the caffeine (kaf-EEN) in coffee keeps them awake at night. Would you like to try skipping your coffee today to see if you might sleep better?" Now Mrs. Myers has no reason to get mad at you, and you cannot be wrong, because it is a fact that caffeine keeps many people awake. Using facts instead of your opinion lets you communicate in a less threatening and more professional way.

When communicating with your supervisor and

Fact or Opinion?

For each statement, decide whether it is an example of a fact or an opinion:

Mrs. Connelly doesn't eat enough.

Mr. Moore looked terrible today.

Mr. Gaston had a fever of 100.7.

Ms. Martino needs to make some friends.

Ms. Martino hasn't had a visitor since last week.

The doctor says you have to walk once a day.

It's better to take your bath before you eat.

You'll get depressed if you stay in your pajamas all day.

It's not fair for you to give me a present.

My agency says I cannot accept a gift.

Your care plan calls for snacks between meals.

---

other members of the health care team, it is essential that you distinguish between facts and opinions. For example, "Mr. Morgan is acting like he had a stroke," is an opinion and could very well be wrong. Instead, report the facts: "Mr. Morgan has lost strength on his right side and his speech is slurred." When you need to report your opinion, introduce it with "I think..." Then it is clear that you are offering your opinion and not a fact you have observed.

❏ 6. Explain how to develop effective interpersonal relationships

Developing good relationships with your clients, their family members, and other members of the care team will allow you to provide excellent care.

While you should not try to become friends with your clients, you should try to develop a warm professional relationship with them based on trust. Good communication skills will help you get to know your clients and their needs. It will also help them learn to trust you.

In addition to the strategies we have already discussed, the following suggestions can help you communicate effectively and develop good relationships.

Avoid changing the subject when your client is discussing something, even if the subject makes you feel uncomfortable or helpless. For example, when a client says "I'm having so much pain today," do not try to avoid the topic by asking whether he feels like watching television. This makes the client feel that you are not interested in him or what he is talking about.

Do not ignore a client's request. Ignoring a request indicates laziness and a lack of concern, and it is considered negligent behavior. Honor the request if you can, otherwise, explain why the request cannot be fulfilled. Always report such requests to your supervisor.

Do not talk down to an elderly or disabled person or a child. Talk to your clients and their families as you would normally talk to any person, making adjustments if someone is hearing-impaired or visually impaired.

Sit near the person who has started a conversation. Sitting near a person shows that you find what he or she is saying important and worth listening to. Standing far away makes people feel that you do not have time to listen or that what they have to say is not important.

Lean forward in your chair when someone is speaking to you. Leaning forward lets the speaker know that you are receiving his or her message with interest. Pay attention to your nonverbal communication. If you fold your arms in front of you, you send the negative message that you are trying to distance yourself from the speaker.

Approach the person who is talking, even if you are in another room, and must move to do so. As with leaning forward in the chair, this tells the person you are interested in them and what they have to say.

Put yourself in other people's shoes, and try to understand what they are going through. This is called empathy (EM-pa-thee). Ask yourself how you would feel if you were confined to bed, or needed help to go to the bathroom. Don't tell clients you know how they feel, because you don't know exactly how they feel. But do say things like "I can imagine this must be scary and difficult for you."

Part 2
Communication Within the Agency

You will notice throughout this text the importance of communication among home health care staff. Because client care takes place outside a facility and members of the care team may not see each other very often, every aspect of communication is very important.

You must learn and follow your agency's guidelines for communication. You must know how to correctly and completely record the work you do and the observations you make. This part of Chapter 4 discusses some important aspects of communicating well.

Throughout the text, you will read more about your role in communicating change in a client to your supervisor. You will also read many helpful tips for communicating with various types of clients.

❏ 7. Demonstrate use of basic medical terminology and approved abbreviations

Throughout your training as a home care aide, you will learn medical terms that describe specific conditions. For example, the medical term for a runny nose is **nasal discharge**; a client whose skin is pale or blue is called cyanotic (sye-a-NOT-ik); a stroke is called a **CVA**, or cerebrovascular (ser-ee-bro-VAS-kyoo-lar) accident. When communicating with your clients and their families, you should use simple, non-medical terms. But when you communicate with your

a	without	hs	hours sleep
$\bar{a}$	before	hs	hours of sleep
abd	abdomen	I&O	intake and output
ac	before meals	NKA	no known allergies
AC	before meals	NPO	nothing by mouth
ad lib	as desired	O	oxygen
am	morning	OOB	out of bed
amb	ambulate	OP	right eye
AP	apical pulse	p	pulse
b.i.d.	twice daily	$\bar{p}$	after
B.M.	bowel movement	p.c.	after meals
BP	blood pressure	pc	after meals
$\bar{c}$	with	po	by mouth
C	Celsius degree	PRN	as necessary
c/o	complains of	q	every
CHF	congestive heart failure	qid	four times a day
CPR	cardiopulmonary resuscitation	qod	every other day
dc	discontinue	qs	quantity sufficient
dx or DX	diagnosis	R	respirations
F	Fahrenheit degree	ROM	range of motion
FBS	fasting blood sugar	$\bar{s}$	without
ft	foot	SOB	shortness of breath
FWB	full weight bearing	stat	at once
GI	gastrointestinal	tid	three times a day
H2O	water	VS	vital signs
hr.	hour	w/c	wheelchair

supervisor or other members of the health care team, using medical terminology will help you give more precise and complete information.

Abbreviations are another way to communicate more efficiently with other caregivers. Learn the standard medical abbreviations your agency uses and use them to report information briefly and accurately. You may also need to know these abbreviations to read your client assignments or care plans. Not all agencies allow the use of abbreviations or use standard abbreviations.

❏ 8. Explain how to give and receive an accurate oral report of a client's status

Home care aides providing care to Medicare clients must be able to read, write, and make brief and accurate oral and written presentations to clients, other caregivers, and staff. Oral or verbal reports of

a client's status are used in two ways. The first is to report something your supervisor needs to know about immediately. Signs and symptoms that should be reported will be discussed throughout this text. In addition, anything that endangers your client should be reported immediately, including any of the following occurrences or client conditions:

- falls
- chest pain
- severe headache
- difficulty breathing
- abnormal pulse, respiration, or blood pressure
- change in client's mental status
- sudden weakness or loss of mobility
- high fever
- loss of consciousness
- change in level of consciousness
- bleeding

- change in client's condition
- bruises, abrasions, or other signs of possible abuse
- problems with caregiver status

Another way oral reports are used is to discuss your experience with a client or family member and your observations of the client's condition and care. This type of informal oral report can be helpful in some situations. These reports should be facts, not opinions.

Even for oral reports, you should write notes for yourself before speaking to your supervisor. When reporting a fall or other immediate danger to your client, you should note the basic information so you don't forget to report any details. You will also have to make a written report later, so you'll need to be able to recall all the facts accurately. For a less formal discussion with your supervisor about a client's case, having written notes will help remind you of the points you want to make. Following an oral report, a home care aide should document when, why, about what, and to whom an oral report was given.

Sometimes your supervisor or another member of the health care team will give you a brief oral report on one of your clients. Listen carefully and take notes if you need to. Ask about any words or terms you don't understand. At the end of the conversation, restate what you have been told, to make sure you understand. Ask about any restrictions or limitations. An oral report from another home care aide who knows the client can be very helpful when you are new on a case.

Be careful of misinterpretations and misunderstandings when giving or receiving oral reports. If an oral report seems to require a change in your assignment sheet, request that the change be made.

❑ *9. Demonstrate ability to report and document factual, pertinent observations in written or oral form using senses of sight, hearing, touch, and smell*

When making any report, it is important that you collect the right kind of information before documenting it. As previously discussed, facts, rather than opinions, are most useful to your supervisor and the care team. Two kinds of factual information are appropriate in your reporting. **Objective information** is based on what you see, hear, touch, or smell. **Subjective information** is something you cannot or did not observe, but that the client reported to you. An example of objective information is "The client has lost two pounds." A subjective report of the same client might be "He says he has no appetite." Your supervisor and care team need factual information in order to make decisions about care and treatment. Both objective and subjective reports are valuable. The essential thing is to distinguish between what you observe and what the client reports to you.

The information you report should also be **pertinent** (PER-ti-nent). Pertinent means significant or useful. For example "Mrs. Lee had rice for lunch," is factual information, but it may not be very pertinent, unless she is allergic to rice or carbohydrates are restricted in her care plan. However, "Mrs. Lee refused to eat lunch," is both objective and pertinent information.

Some of the observations you report could be signs and symptoms of diseases or conditions. Throughout this text you will learn signs and symptoms for various conditions. You are **not** expected to make diagnoses based on signs and symptoms you observe. Your observations, however, can help other members of the care team stay alert to possible problems. Most of all, learn to notice and report any changes in your clients.

In order to report accurately, you must observe your clients, their families, and their homes accurately. To observe accurately, use as many senses as possible to gather information (**Fig. 4-5**). Some examples follow.

Sight: Are there changes in client's appearance, including rashes, redness, paleness, swelling, discharge, weakness, sunken eyes, posture or gait (walking) changes? Does the home appear disorganized or dirty? Have things been knocked over? Are there new stains or spills? Is food needed? Do safety hazards exist?

Hearing: Listen to what the client tells you about

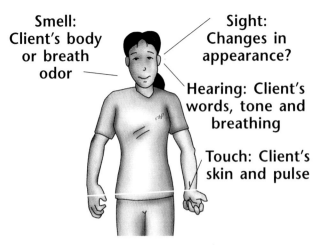

Smell: Client's body or breath odor

Sight: Changes in appearance?

Hearing: Client's words, tone and breathing

Touch: Client's skin and pulse

Fig. 4-5. Reporting what you observe means using more than one sense.

his or her condition, family, or needs. Is the client speaking clearly and making sense? Does the client show emotions such as anger, frustration, sadness? Is breathing normal, or does client wheeze, gasp, or cough? Listen to family members' observations about the client's needs or condition. Listen for noises in the home that suggest maintenance is needed (for example, leaking faucets or banging pipes). Is the atmosphere calm and quiet enough for your client to rest as needed? Does the volume of the radio or TV suggest your client may have a hearing impairment?

Touch: Does your client's skin feel hot or cool, moist or dry? Is pulse rate normal? Use your sense of touch to test the bath water and the home's heating or cooling.

Smell: Do you notice odor from the client's body? Odors could suggest inadequate bathing, infections, or incontinence (in-KON-ti-nens). Breath odor could suggest use of alcohol or tobacco, or indigestion. Odors in the home may suggest housecleaning or repairs are needed. Food odors could indicate spoilage.

Using all your senses will allow you to make the most complete report of a client's situation.

❏ 10. Explain the importance of maintaining current documentation

Maintaining current documentation means keeping a record of everything you do with your clients and everything you observe during a client visit. It is essential that you and your agency maintain current documentation for the following reasons:

1. It is the only way to guarantee clear and complete communication between all the members of the care team.

2. Documentation is a legal record of every part of a client's treatment. Medical charts can be used in court as legal evidence.

3. Documentation protects you and your employer from liability by proving what you did on every visit with your client.

Because you may see many clients in the course of a day, you cannot try to remember everything that each client ate, did, or said. Documentation gives you an up-to-date record of each of your clients' care. You must learn to document accurately, always taking the time to observe and record carefully. Always follow your agency's policies and procedures for documentation. The key to good documentation is doing it at the time the services are rendered. Because documentation is so important, you should never put it off until later.

❏ 11. Explain the legal implications of documentation

A medical chart is a legal document. What is written in the chart is considered in court to be what actually happened. If you worked in a client's home for four hours but never documented your visit, you could not necessarily prove that you actually visited the client. In general, if something does not appear in a client's chart, it did not legally happen. Failing to document your visits and activities with clients could cause very serious legal problems for you and/or your employer. It could also cause harm to your client. Remember, if you didn't document it, you didn't do it.

Medical charts are confidential. As discussed in Chapter 3, it is wrong and illegal to discuss information about your clients. It is important that you are aware of the legal implications of documentation and that you record all your activities completely.

❑ 12. Describe the correct way to complete visit records and incident reports

Your employer will have specific guidelines for you to follow in completing written reports of your work. Always follow your employer's guidelines. The information presented here is intended to be a general guide for completing the two types of reports that most employers require: visit records or notes, and incident reports.

Visit records, progress notes, or clinical notes, are the notes you make each time you visit a client. The purpose of these notes is to serve as a record of your visit and the care you provided. Visit records are also the place for you to document your observations of the client's condition, change, or progress (improvement). When writing visit records, observe the following rules:

1. Write your notes immediately after the visit, so everything is fresh in your mind. If you put off writing your notes, even for a few hours, you may forget important details.

2. Think through what you want to say before you begin writing. This will help you present your thoughts as briefly and as clearly as possible.

3. Write the facts, not your opinions about the client. For example, "Client has lost 2 lb. Did not finish lunch. Husband reports 'she has not been eating well,'" reports facts about the client's condition. It is more useful than "Client is thin and won't eat." When reporting something a family member told you, put the words in quotation marks (" "). Document the tasks that you performed, assisted with, or observed the client performing.

4. Write as neatly as you can. Use black ink.

5. If you make a mistake, draw one line through it and write the correct word or words. Above the crossed out mistake, write "error" and put your initials and the date (**Fig. 4-6**). Never erase something you have written, and never use white out.

6. Sign your full name, write your title (Home Care Aide, Aide, or HCA) and write the date after each day's visit notes.

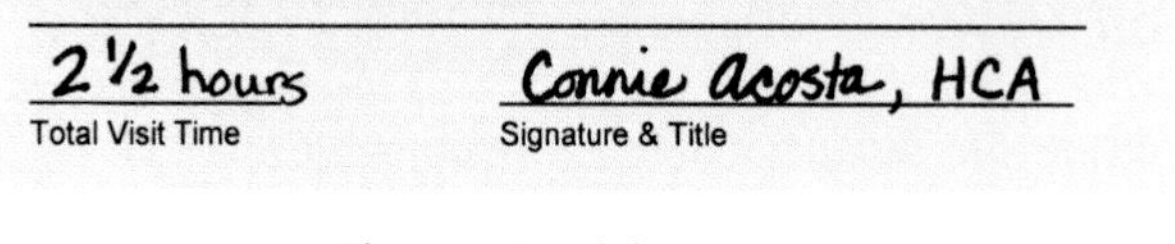

0930 Changed bed linens, picked up bedroom
0945 VS ~~BP 180/70 RA~~ error CA BP 150/70 RA

2 ½ hours   *Connie Acosta, HCA*
Total Visit Time   Signature & Title

Fig. 4-6. Visit Notes

7. Document as specified in the care plan.

Many home health agencies have aides use a "check-off" sheet, often called an ADL (activities of daily living) sheet or a visit form, for documenting care given (**Fig. 4-7**). Some companies train home care aides to submit visit records on a computer system, or have them "phone" in the note via the client's touch tone phone.

Incident reports must be completed when an accident or other significant event occurs during a visit. Report the incident as soon as possible, and definitely before leaving the client's home. Always check with your supervisor before completing the report. Every home health agency has its own policies and procedures for what kind of report should be completed in what situations and by whom.

In general, you should file a report when any of the following incidents occur:

▶ your client falls, drops something, or breaks something

▶ you break or damage something

▶ your client or a family member makes a request that is out of your scope of practice

▶ your client or a family member makes sexual advances or remarks

▶ anything happens that makes you feel uncomfortable, threatened, or unsafe

▶ you get injured on the job

▶ you are exposed to blood or body fluids

The purpose of an incident report is to document events that happen in the home and to protect yourself. If a client drops and breaks a favorite vase and then forgets what happened, you might be wrongly blamed for the incident. The report provides a written record of anything that happens and shows what your part in it was. Most agencies use incident reports in place of writing up the accident as a narrative on the visit form. You may be asked to document that you completed an incident report.

Fig. 4-7. Some agencies use check-off sheets to document care.

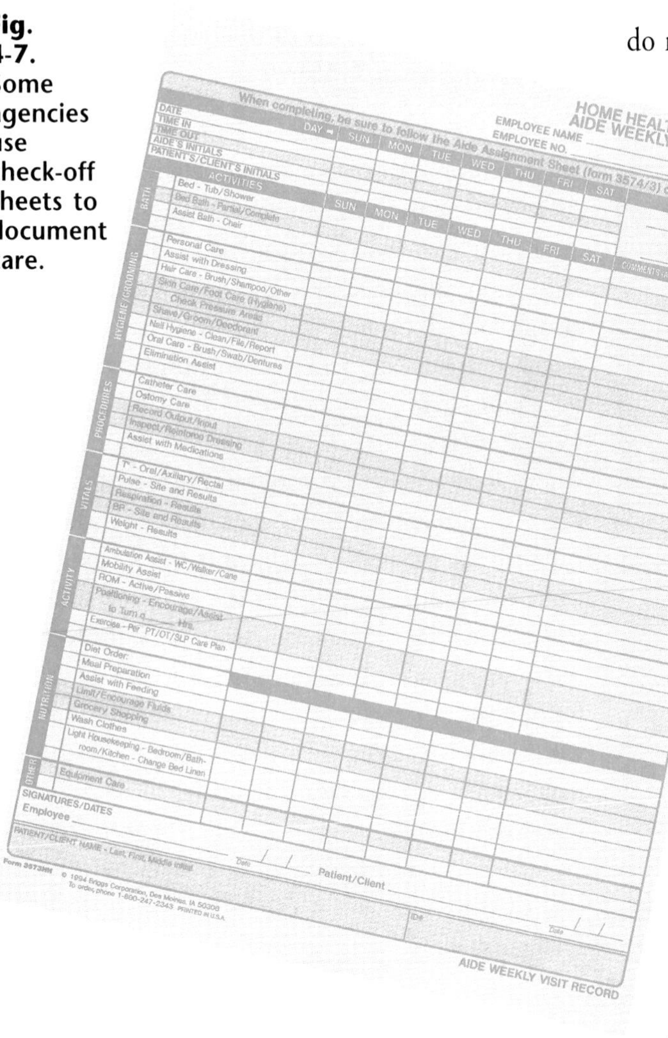

Part 3
Communication with Clients and Families

❏ 13. Demonstrate ability to use verbal and written information to assist with the client's care plan

As a home care aide, you will spend much more time with each of your clients than will most other members of the care team. Because of this, you will observe your clients closely and may notice things about them the nurses or doctor cannot know. Although you are not qualified to diagnose or recommend treatment, you will have a lot of valuable information about your clients that will help in care planning.

When you attend care planning meetings, sometimes called case management or case conferences, do not be afraid to speak up and share your observations of your clients. If you are not sure what is important to mention, try to find time to talk to your supervisor before the meeting and ask what you should report.

Writing accurate records of your visits makes important contributions to care planning. A thorough written record allows everyone to benefit from your observations and helps you remember details about each client.

❏ 14. Demonstrate effective communication on the telephone

You will use the telephone to communicate with your supervisor from clients' homes. Always ask permission before using a client's phone. You may also need to answer the phone for your clients, and know how to take messages for clients or family members.

When making a call, follow these steps:

1. Always identify yourself before asking to speak to someone. Never ask "Who is this?" when someone answers your call.

2. After you have identified yourself, ask for the person you need to speak with.

3. If the person you are calling is available, identify yourself again and state why you are calling. Planning your call before you pick up the phone will help you be as efficient as possible.

4. If the person is not available, ask if you can leave a message. Always leave a message, even if it is only to say you called. The message shows that you were trying to reach someone.

5. Leave a brief and clear message. Do not give more information than necessary. A basic message includes your name, the phone number you are calling from, how long you will be at that number, and a brief reason you are calling.

6. Thank the person who takes the message for you. Always be polite over the telephone, as you would in person.

—This is Ella Ferguson. I am calling from Mrs. Lee's house. She has a question about her medication and I need to know what to tell her.

—Her question is this: She forgot to take her pill this morning when she had breakfast. She wants to know if she should take two now with lunch.

—She should take one now and one with a snack around 3:00 pm? Okay, I'll tell her. I'll write in my visit notes that you told me to tell her to take one now, and one again with a snack at 3:00. I'll still be here then so I can help her remember.

—Thank you for your help, Ms. Crier. Goodbye.

If you could not reach Ms. Crier, your side of the conversation might go like this:

—Hello, this is Ella Ferguson calling. Is Ms. Crier there please?

—Could you take a message for me please?

—My name is Ella Ferguson, I'm an aide, and I am at Mrs. Lee's house. The number is 873-9042. I will be here until 4:30 this afternoon. I'm calling because Mrs. Lee has a question about her medication and I need to know how to answer it.

—Thank you very much. Goodbye.

When answering calls for clients, be sensitive to their privacy. Do not ask for more information than the client needs to return the call: a name and phone number is enough. Do not give out any information about your client. Simply say "Mr. Schmitt is not available right now. May I take a message?" Write down the name and phone number of the caller, and tell your client about the call.

❑ 15. Describe cultural diversity and religious differences

In the United States, people come from many different cultural backgrounds and religious traditions. As a home care aide you will have clients of different backgrounds and traditions than your own. It is important to respect and value each person as an individual. Sometimes it is easier to accept different practices or beliefs if you understand a little about them.

There are so many different cultures represented in the United States that they cannot all be listed here. A culture is a system of behaviors that people learn from the group of people they grow up and live with. One might talk about American culture being different from Japanese culture. But within American culture there are thousands of different groups with their own cultures: Japanese-Americans, African-Americans, and Native Americans, to name just a few. Even people from a particular region, state, or city can be said to have a different culture: the culture of the south is not the same as the culture of New York City.

Cultural background can determine how friendly people are to strangers, how they feel about having you in their houses, or how close they want you to stand to them when talking. Be sensitive to the cultural backgrounds of your clients. You cannot expect to be treated the same way by all your clients, and you may have to adjust your behavior around some of your clients. Regardless of cultural background, however, you must treat all clients with respect and professionalism and expect them to treat you respectfully as well.

Religious differences also influence the way people behave. Religion can be very important in people's lives, particularly when they are ill or dying. You must respect the religious beliefs and practices of your clients, even if they are different from your own. Never try to question your clients' religions or talk about your own beliefs. Understanding a little bit about the most common religious groups in America may be useful to you.

Christianity: Christians believe Jesus Christ was the son of God and that he died so their sins would be forgiven. Christians may be Catholic or Protestant, and there are many subgroups or denominations (such as Baptists, Episcopalians, Evangelicals, Lutherans, Methodists, or Presbyterians). Christians may go to church on Saturdays or Sundays; read the Bible, including the Old and New Testaments; take communion as a symbol of Christ's sacrifice; and be baptized as a symbol of their faith. Some Christians may try to share their beliefs and convert others to their faith. Religious leaders may be called priests, ministers, pastors, or deacons.

Judaism: Divided into Reform, Conservative and Orthodox movements, Jews believe that God gave them laws through Moses and in the Bible, and that these laws should order their lives. Jewish services are held on Friday evenings and sometimes Saturdays, in synagogues or temples. Some Jewish men wear a yarmulke (YAR-mul-ke), or small skullcap, as a sign of their faith. Some Jews observe special dietary restrictions. Jewish people may not do certain things, such as work or drive, on the Sabbath, which lasts from Friday sundown to Saturday sundown. Religious leaders are called rabbis (RAB-eyes).

Islam (IS-lahm): Muslims, or followers of Mohammed, believe that Allah (God) wants men to follow the teachings of the prophet Mohammed in the Koran (koh-RAN). Many Muslims pray five times a day facing Mecca, the holy city for their religion. Muslims worship at mosques (mosks) and generally do not drink alcohol. There are other dietary restrictions as well.

Other major world religions include **Hinduism** (HIN-doo-ism), practiced in India and elsewhere. **Confucianism** (kon-FYOO-shan-ism) is practiced in China and Japan, and **Buddhism** (BOO- dism) started in Asia but has followers in other parts of the world. All these religions are practiced in the United States, though they are not as common as the three discussed above.

❏ 16. List examples of cultural and religious differences that aides encounter

In addition to showing a general respect for different cultural and religious traditions, you should be aware of certain practices that might affect your work with clients. As mentioned above, many religious beliefs include **dietary restrictions**, or rules about what and when followers can eat. Many Jewish people eat kosher foods, do not eat pork, and do not eat meat products at the same meal with dairy products. Many Muslims do not eat pork or drink alcohol. Some Catholics do not eat meat on Fridays. Some people are vegetarians and do not eat any meat for religious or moral reasons. When planning and preparing meals for your clients, be aware of any dietary restrictions and honor them.

Some people's religious beliefs or cultural background may make them less comfortable being touched by others. Be sensitive to your clients' feelings. Of course you must touch clients in order to do your job, but recognize that some clients may feel more comfortable when physical contact is kept to a minimum.

❏ 17. List ways of coping with combative behavior

Clients may sometimes display combative (kom-BA-tiv), meaning violent or hostile, behavior. Such behavior may include hitting, pushing, kicking, or verbal attacks. Such behavior may be the result of disease affecting the brain. It may also be an expression of frustration with the circumstances, or it may just be part of someone's personality. In general, combative behavior is not a reaction to you, and you should not take it personally.

Always report combative behavior to your supervisor and document it. Even if you do not find the behavior upsetting, it is important for the rest of the health care team to be aware of it. Some ways of coping with combative behavior include the following.

1. Block physical blows or step out of the way, but *never* hit back. No matter how much a client hurts you,

or how angry or afraid you are, you must never hit, hurt, or threaten a client.

2. Leave the client alone if you can safely do so. Sometimes getting out of the room for a moment or two will calm everyone down. Call for help if you need to physically restrain someone. If you are afraid, leave the home and call your supervisor immediately.

3. Do not respond to verbal attacks. If you must respond, say something like, "I understand that you're angry and frustrated. How can we make things better?"

4. Consider what provoked the client. Did you do or say something that upset him or her? Sometimes something as simple as a change in caregiver or routine can be very upsetting to a client. Do not blame yourself, but try to learn from the situation and avoid it in the future.

❏ 18. List ways of coping with inappropriate behavior

Inappropriate behavior from a client includes trying to establish a personal, rather than a professional relationship. Examples include asking personal questions or revealing personal information, requesting visits or meetings on personal time, asking for or doing favors, giving tips or gifts, and loaning or borrowing money. It is also inappropriate for a client to ask a home care aide to perform tasks that would not be in the care plan, like scrubbing floors or cleaning the garage. Inappropriate behavior also includes making sexual advances and comments. Sexual advances include anything that makes you feel uncomfortable.

When clients or family members behave inappropriately, you should report the behavior to your supervisor, even if you think the behavior was harmless. Reporting is the only way to protect yourself, and it does not violate the client's privacy. Other ways to handle inappropriate behavior include the following:

1. If you think a light approach will work, say something like "I'm sorry, I'm not allowed to do that."

2. Address the behavior directly, saying something like "That makes me very uncomfortable." If the client persists, tell him or her that you will have to leave if the behavior continues.

3. Respond to personal questions by saying "I really can't talk about my personal life on the job." If the client is sharing thoughts or feelings that make you uncomfortable, say "That's not something I can help you with. If you'd like to speak with a social worker I can let the nurse/doctor know."

4. Firmly refuse gifts, tips, and favors, saying, "I really can't accept that. It's against the agency's rules."

5. Report inappropriate behavior to your supervisor if it continuously interferes with your client care and/or job satisfaction.

Working in people's homes, you may see family dynamics, including fighting, yelling, or verbal abuse. Report this kind of behavior to your supervisor.

Chapter 5

Infection Control and Standard Precautions

Asepsis (ay-SEP-sis) means sterility, or no infection is present. It refers to the clean and sanitary conditions you want to create in your clients' homes. In this chapter you will learn about the importance of preventing infection and how to protect yourself, your clients, and their families from disease.

Learning Objectives

In this chapter you will learn to:

There are many ways **pathogens** (PATH-oh-gens), the **microorganisms** (my-kro-OR-gan-izms) or germs that cause disease, can be transmitted to human beings. Microorganisms can be transferred from one person to another by touching, sneezing, coughing, or the exchange of body fluids (blood, semen, feces, urine, and others). Some microorganisms can also be transferred through contaminated food, water, or objects.

Transmission of most **infectious** (in-FEKT-shus) or contagious diseases can be prevented by always taking a few simple precautions. Washing your hands is an important and easy way to greatly reduce the spread of infection. All caregivers should wash their hands frequently. In this chapter and the chapter on housekeeping (Chapter 21), you will learn a great deal about infection control and medical asepsis. Practicing what you learn

Procedure 1: Handwashing for infection control

1. Assemble equipment:
   - bar or liquid soap provided by your employer
   - paper towels
   - warm running water
   - waste container

2. Turn on faucet and adjust water temperature. Keep your clothes dry, because moisture breeds bacteria.

3. Wet hands and wrists, keeping your hands lower than your elbows so water runs off your fingertips, not up your arm.

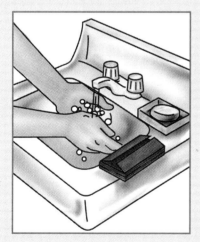

4. Use a generous amount of soap. Rub hands together and fingers between each other to create a lather. Rub the backs of your hands. Friction helps clean.

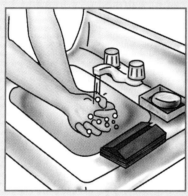

5. Continue to rub. Push soap under your fingernails and cuticles with a brush or by working them in the palm of your hand. Use soap above your wrist about two inches. Continue rubbing with friction for 15–30 seconds.

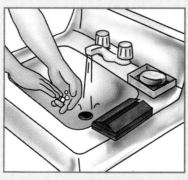

6. Being careful not to touch the sink, rinse thoroughly under running water. Rinse from just above the wrists down to fingertips. Do not run water over unwashed arm down to clean hands.

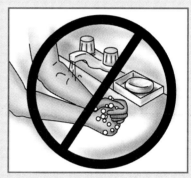

7. Using a clean paper towel, dry from tips of fingers up to clean wrists. Again, do not wipe towel on unwashed forearm and then wipe clean hands. Dispose of towel without touching waste container. If your hands ever touch the sink or waste container, start over.

8. Use a dry, clean paper towel to turn off the faucet, which is considered contaminated. Properly discard towel.

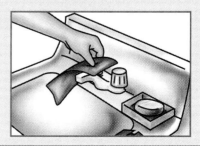

when caring for clients offers the best protection from infection—for everyone.

❏ 1. Identify when to wash hands

You should wash your hands:

▶ when arriving at a client's home

▶ before and after touching a client

▶ before and after meals or work in the kitchen

▶ after using the restroom

▶ after touching any item used by or for a client

▶ before you leave a client's home

▶ before entering the clean area of your supply bag

▶ every time you remove your gloves or any type of personal protection equipment (PPE), such as latex gloves

▶ after touching a surface that may be contaminated with any body fluid

❏ 2. Identify when to wear gloves

You must wear gloves when there is a chance you might come into contact with body fluids, open wounds, or **mucous** (MYOO-kus) membranes (the membranes that line body cavities such as the mouth or nose). Your agency will have specific policies and procedures on when to wear gloves. Learn and follow these procedures. If you are not sure whether to wear them, be cautious and wear them. Always wear gloves for the following tasks:

▶ anytime you might touch blood

▶ performing or assisting with mouth care or care of any mucous membrane

▶ performing or assisting with care of the **perineal** (payr-i-NEE-al) area (the area between the anus and the genitals)

▶ handling body fluids, such as vomitus, urine, feces, or saliva

▶ performing personal care on a client whose skin is broken by abrasions, cuts, rash, acne, pimples, or boils

▶ assisting with a client's personal care when you have open sores or cuts on your hands

▶ shaving a client

Procedure 2: Putting on gloves

1. Wash your hands following proper procedure.

2. If you are right handed, remove one glove from the box and slide it on your left hand (reverse, if left handed).

3. Pulling out another glove with your gloved hand, slide the other hand into the glove.

4. Interlace fingers to smooth out folds and create a comfortable fit.

5. Carefully look for tears, holes, or discolored spots, and replace the glove if necessary.

6. If wearing a gown, pull the cuff of the gloves over the sleeve of the gown.

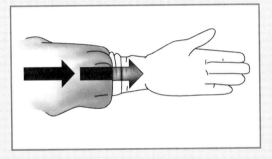

Remember you are wearing gloves to protect your skin from becoming contaminated. After a procedure your gloves are contaminated. If you open a door with the gloved hand, the door knob becomes contaminated. Later, when you open the door with an ungloved hand, you will be infected even though you wore gloves during the procedure. It is a common mistake, after carefully putting on PPE, to contaminate the room around you. Don't do it. Before touching surfaces, such as opening a door, remove one glove. Afterward, put on a new glove if necessary.

Procedure 3: Taking off gloves

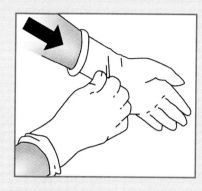

1. Touching only the outside of one glove, pull the first glove off by pulling down from the cuff.

2. As the glove comes off your hand it should be turned inside out.

3. With the fingertips of your gloved hand hold the glove you just removed. With your

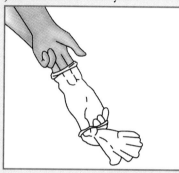

ungloved hand, reach two fingers *inside* the remaining glove, being careful not to touch any part of the outside.

4. Pull down, turning this glove inside out and over the first glove as you remove it.

5. You should be holding one glove from its clean inner side and the other glove should be inside it.

6. Drop both gloves into the proper container.

7. Wash your hands using proper procedure.

- disposing of soiled bed linens, gowns, dressings, and pads
- when feeding a client, gloves should be worn only if you have contact with the client's saliva, gums, and teeth

If you have cuts or sores on your hands, you must first cover these areas with bandages or gauze and then put on gloves. Disposable gloves are to be worn only once. They may *not* be washed or disinfected for reuse. Replace disposable gloves as soon as they are torn or overly contaminated. Wash hands before putting on fresh gloves. Some people are allergic to the latex used in certain gloves. If you notice a reaction, contact your supervisor immediately. Your employer will provide you with a kind of glove you can wear.

❑ 3. Identify when to use personal protective equipment (PPE)

Personal protective equipment (PPE), includes gowns, masks, and eye shields, as well as gloves. Your employer will provide you with PPE as necessary for your client assignments. The guidelines for wearing PPE are the same as for gloves. You should wear PPE if there is a chance you could come into contact with

body fluids, mucous membranes, or open wounds. Masks and eye shields are worn when splashing of body fluids or blood could occur. Masks should also be worn when caring for clients with respiratory illnesses. With some of your clients or for some types of care, this might mean you wear PPE all the time. Remember, if you are unsure of the risk, don't take any chances: wear PPE.

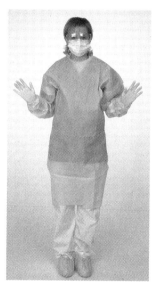

Fig. 5-9. Dress for the occasion!

❑ 4. Explain how to handle spills

Spills in the home, especially involving blood, body fluids, or glass, can pose a serious risk of infection. Clean spills using proper equipment and procedure.

Guidelines: Cleaning spills involving blood, body fluids, or glass

When blood or body fluids are spilled, put on gloves before starting to clean up the spill. In some cases, industrial strength gloves are best because they won't tear if you are also handling glass.

When glass has been broken, do not pick up any pieces, no matter how large, with your hands. Use a dustpan and broom or other tools.

If blood or body fluids are spilled on a hard surface such as a linoleum floor or countertop, clean immediately using a solution of one part house-

Procedure 4: Putting on a gown

1. Assemble the PPE you will wear.

2. Remove jewelry and wristwatch and place them on clean paper towel. If wearing long sleeves, push or roll them up.

3. Wash your hands using proper procedure.

4. Open gown. Slip your arms

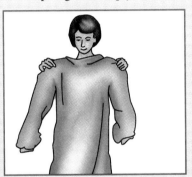

into the sleeves and pull the gown on.

5. Tie the neck ties into a bow so they can be easily untied later.

6. Reaching behind you, pull the gown until it completely covers your clothes and tie the back ties.

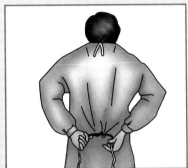

7. Remember, use gowns only once and then discard or remove for decontamination. If your gown ever becomes overly wet or soiled, remove it, check your clothing, and put on a new gown. The Occupational Safety and Health Administration (OSHA) requires non-permeable gowns, that is, gowns that liquids cannot penetrate, when working in a bloody situation.

8. Put on gloves *after* putting on gown.

Procedure 5: Putting on mask and eye shield

1. Assemble the PPE you will wear.

2. Remove jewelry and wristwatch and place them on clean paper towel. If wearing long sleeves, push or roll them up.

3. Wash your hands using proper procedure.

4. Pick up mask by the top strings or the elastic strap. Be careful not to touch the mask

where it touches your face. Never wear the same mask from one client to another.

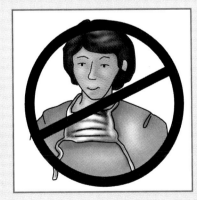

5. Adjust the mask over your nose and mouth. Tie top strings first, then bottom string. Masks must always be dry or they must be replaced. Never wear a mask hanging from only the bottom tie.

6. Put on eye shield.

7. Put on gloves *after* putting on mask and eye shield.

hold bleach to ten parts water. You can mix the solution in a bucket, and, with gloves on, wipe up the spill with rags or paper towels dipped in the solution. Or, mix the solution in a plastic spray bottle, and spray the spill before wiping. Be careful not to spill bleach or bleach solution on clothes, carpets, or bedding, as it can discolor and damage fabrics. Your employer may provide commercial sprays for cleaning spills.

▶ If blood or body fluids are spilled on fabrics such as carpets, bedding, or clothes, do not use bleach to clean the spill. Commercial disinfectants that do not contain bleach are available. If you have no disinfectant, wipe spills using soap and water and wearing gloves, then clean carpet with regular carpet cleaner. Use gloves to load soiled bedding or clothes into the washing machine and add bleach to the washer with the laundry detergent.

▶ Waste containing broken glass, blood, or body fluids should be properly bagged. Put the waste in one trash bag and close it properly. Then put the first bag inside a second, clean trash bag and close it. Waste containing blood or body fluids may need to be placed in a special biohazard waste bag and disposed of separately from household trash. Follow your agency's policy.

❏ *5. List three requirements for infection to spread*

To better understand how to prevent infection, it helps to understand how infections spread. The spread of infection requires three things:

1. A **source** of infecting microorganisms. The source can be a person (client or caregiver), a contaminated object or surface, plants, pets, or anything that can carry with it any germ.

2. A **susceptible** (sus-SEP-ti-bul) **host**. In this case a susceptible host means someone that could be harmed by the microorganism or germ. How likely it is that a microorganism will infect and harm someone depends on many things. A bacteria that contacts a paper cut on your finger can do much more harm than the same bacteria on an uncut finger. A healthy person who eats an undercooked egg may not ever get sick, but it could kill someone who has AIDS and has a poor immune system.

3. Finally, the infection needs a **means or mode of transmission**. This is the way the microorganism gets from the source to the susceptible host. Microorganisms can be transmitted in many ways:

▶ direct person-to-person contact

▶ indirect person-to-object-to person contact

▶ through the air

Infection control most often means preventing the transmission of infection. Washing your hands is the most effective way of preventing the spread or transmission of microorganisms. But there are many other methods you will learn in this chapter.

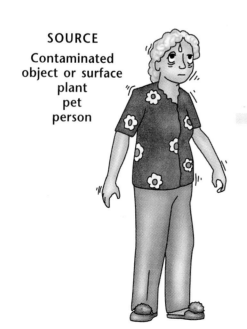

SOURCE
Contaminated object or surface
plant
pet
person

MEANS or MODE of TRANSMISSION
1. Direct person-to-person contact

2. Indirect object-to-person contact

3. Through the air

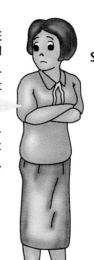

HOST
Susceptible person

❏ 6. Explain and follow standard precautions

Standard precautions, formerly called universal precautions, is a method of infection control defined by the Centers for Disease Control and Prevention, a government agency. Under state and federal laws, home care aides and other health care providers are required to follow certain precautions when caring for people. Standard precautions means treating all blood, body fluids, non-intact skin, and mucous membranes as if they were infected with an infectious disease. Following standard precautions is the only safe way of performing your job. You cannot tell by looking at your clients or their charts if they are infected with a contagious (infectious) disease, such as HIV, hepatitis, or influenza.

From 1987 to 1995, federal and state laws required all health care workers to follow certain precautions or safety measures when caring for people. These rules were called Universal Precautions because they applied to all people being cared for, even if they were not suspected of having a disease.

In 1995, the CDC issued new guidelines, called Standard Precautions. These precautions are very much like Universal Precautions. Standard Precautions means treating all blood, body fluids, non-intact skin (like abrasions, pimples, or open sores), and mucous membranes (openings of eyes, mouth, nose, rectum, or genitals) as if they were infected with an infectious disease.

Under Universal Precautions, some body fluids and mucous membranes were not included and some were. Standard Precautions is simpler to remember because it includes everything except sweat. It is also the best way to protect yourself from becoming infected with diseases, such as HIV/AIDS or hepatitis. Again, because you cannot tell if someone is infectious by looking at them or even by reading their charts, following Standard Precautions

is the only way to protect yourself.

Under standard precautions, "body fluids" include saliva, sputum (fluid coughed up), urine, feces, semen, vaginal secretions, and pus or other wound drainage.

Standard precautions include the measures listed below.

▸ **Wear gloves** if you are in a situation where you may come into contact with blood; any body fluids or secretions; broken skin (including abrasions, acne, cuts, sutures or stitches, and pinpricks); or mucous membranes (such as the linings of the mouth, nose, eyes, vagina, rectum, and penis). In the home, such situations may include mouth care; bathroom assistance; perineal care; assistance with a bedpan or urinal; ostomy care; cleaning up spills; cleansing basins, urinals, bedpans, and other containers that have held body fluids; and disposing of wastes.

▸ **Remove gloves immediately** when finished with procedure.

▸ **Wash your hands** before putting on gloves, and immediately wash your hands after removing your gloves.

▸ **Immediately wash all skin surfaces that have been contaminated** with blood and body fluids. Flush skin with running water for one minute.

▸ **Wear a disposable gown** if you may come into contact with blood or body fluids (for example, emptying a urinary drainage bag). If your client has a contagious illness, you should wear a gown even if it is not likely you will come into contact with blood or body fluids.

▸ **Wear a mask and protective glasses** if the possibility exists that you will come into contact with splashing blood or body fluids (for example, emptying a bed pan).

▸ **Wear gloves and use caution when handling razor blades, needles, and other sharp objects.** Discard these objects carefully in a puncture-resistant, biohazard container.

▸ **Avoid nicks and cuts** when shaving clients.

▸ **Carefully bag all contaminated supplies** and dispose of them according to your agency's policy.

- **Body fluids that are being saved for a specimen should be clearly labeled** with the client's name and a biohazard label, and kept in a container with a lid.

- **Never handle a client's needles or syringes.** Request that the client dispose of them in a hard, plastic biohazardous waste container.

- **Never attempt to put a cap on a needle or sharp.** Dispose of it in an approved container.

- **Contaminated wastes should be disposed of according to your agency's procedure and standard precautions.**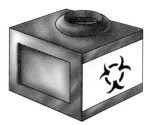

- **Waste containing blood or body fluids** is considered biohazardous waste and should be disposed of separately from household garbage. Your agency will have a policy on how to dispose of biohazardous waste.

❑ 7. Explain guidelines of care for clients with infectious diseases

When caring for clients with infectious bloodborne diseases, follow your employer's procedures. They will generally include the following guidelines.

- As with all client care, always follow standard precautions.

- Wash your hands frequently, especially after client care.

- Use gloves, gowns, masks, and eye shields when needed.

- Follow isolation procedures described in the assignment sheet for each client.

- Handle laundry, personal items, and waste carefully.

Remember that you can safely touch, hug, and spend time talking with clients who have bloodborne infectious diseases. They need the same thoughtful, personal attention you give all your clients. Follow standard precautions to protect yourself, but never isolate a client emotionally because he or she has an infectious disease.

Sometimes a client's plan of care will include **isola-**tion precautions. To isolate means to keep something separate, or by itself. When a client has or is suspected of having an infectious disease, special isolation precautions are required to keep the infection isolated, or separate from uninfected people, including you. These precautions will always be listed in the client's care plan and on your assignment sheet. It is for your safety and the safety of family members that these precautions must be followed.

There are several categories of isolation precautions. The type depends on the disease and how that disease is spread to other people. Isolation precautions are always *in addition* to standard precautions. Below is a list of isolation categories, the diseases they are intended to isolate, and some of the precautions that are appropriate.

Airborne precautions are taken to reduce the risk of spreading diseases such as tuberculosis, measles, and chicken pox. These diseases can be transmitted or spread through the air after being expelled by the client. The microorganisms are so small that they can attach to moisture in the air and remain floating for some time. For certain care procedures you may be required to wear a special mask to avoid being infected. A section on tuberculosis, with instructions for specific airborne precautions, is found later in this chapter (**Fig. 5-16**).

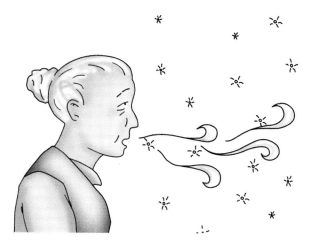

Fig. 5-16. Airborne diseases stay suspended in the air.

Droplet precautions are used when the disease-causing microorganism does not stay suspended in the air and usually travels short distances after being expelled. They can be generated by coughing, sneezing, talking, or suctioning. Droplet precautions can include wearing a face mask during care procedures and restricting visits from uninfected people. Cover your nose and mouth with a tissue when you sneeze or cough and ask clients, family, and others to do the same. If you sneeze on your hands, wash them

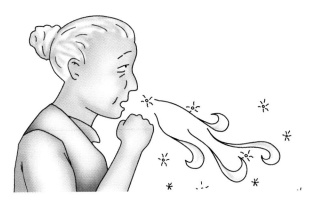

Fig. 5-17. Droplet precautions are followed when the disease causing microorganism does not stay suspended in the air.

promptly. Again, always follow your agency's procedures and the client's care plan (**Fig. 5-17**).

Contact precautions are taken when the client is at risk of transmitting or contracting a microorganism from touching an infected object or person. Exam-

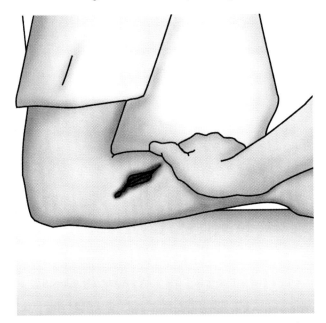

Fig. 5-18. Contact precautions are followed when the client is at risk of transmitting or contracting a microorganism from touching an infected object.

ples include bacteria that could infect an open skin wound or infection. Lice, scabies (a skin disease that causes itching), and conjunctivitis (pink eye) are other examples. Transmission can occur with skin to skin contact during transfers or bathing. Precautions include personal protective equipment and client isolation. Contact precautions require washing hands with antimicrobial soap, and not touching infected surfaces with ungloved hands or uninfected surfaces with contaminated gloves (**Fig. 5-18**).

Following are two important points to remember about all isolation precautions:

1. Always follow your agency's procedures and directions in the care plan.

2. It is the disease, not the person with the disease, that is being isolated. Communicate with your client, explaining why these special steps are being taken.

Guidelines for following isolation procedures with food trays, clothing, laundry, and other items

▶ Food should be served using disposable dishes and utensils that are discarded in specially marked bags and stored in covered garbage containers. When items cannot be discarded, they must be washed thoroughly in very hot water with detergent and bleach. Family members should use separate dishes and utensils.

▶ Wear disposable gloves when handling soiled laundry. Bag laundry in the client's room and carry it to the laundry area in the bag. Wash client's laundry separately. Use hot water and detergent.

▶ A solution of bleach and water (1:10) should be mixed in a clearly labeled, plastic spray bottle and stored in a safe place. The bleach solution can be used to clean up spills of blood or body fluids and to disinfect surfaces that may have been contaminated.

▶ A client in contact or airborne isolation should have a separate bathroom to use. If the client uses the same bathroom as other family members, it must be disinfected after the client uses it.

▶ Remember these isolation precautions are always used in addition to standard precautions described earlier.

FOCUS

Bloodborne and Airborne Pathogens

❑ 8. Explain how bloodborne diseases are transmitted

A bloodborne disease is transmitted by microorganisms carried in the blood. These microorganisms may also be present in body fluids, non-intact skin (such as open sores or acne), and mucous membranes.

Bloodborne diseases can be transmitted if infected blood enters your bloodstream, or if infected semen or vaginal secretions contact your mucous membranes. Mucous membranes include the linings of the vagina, penis, rectum, nose, and mouth. You can become infected with a bloodborne disease by having sexual contact with someone carrying that disease. It is not necessary to have sexual intercourse to transmit disease; other kinds of sexual activity can just as easily cause infection. Using a needle to inject drugs and sharing needles with others can also transmit bloodborne diseases. In addition, infected mothers may transmit bloodborne diseases to their babies in the womb or during birth.

In the health care setting, contact with infected blood or body fluids is the most common way to be infected with a bloodborne disease. Standard precautions, handwashing, isolation, and using PPE are all methods of preventing transmission of bloodborne diseases in the health care setting. Employers are required by law to help prevent health care workers from exposure to bloodborne pathogens. It is crucial that you understand and follow standard precautions and other procedures to protect yourself from bloodborne diseases.

❑ 9. Explain the basics about HIV and hepatitis infection

The major bloodborne diseases in the United States today are **HIV/AIDS** and hepatitis (hep-a-TYE-tis). HIV stands for human immunodeficiency (im-yoo-no-de-FISH-en-see) virus. When people are infected with HIV, the disease weakens their immune systems so that their bodies cannot effectively fight infections. After a number of years, a person with HIV usually develops acquired immune deficiency syndrome (AIDS). People with AIDS lose all ability to fight infection and can die from illnesses that a healthy body could handle.

Hepatitis refers to swelling (-itis) of the liver (hepa-) caused by infection. Liver function can be permanently damaged by hepatitis, which can lead to other chronic, life-long illnesses. Several different viruses can cause hepatitis; the most common are hepatitis A, B, and C. Hepatitis B and C are bloodborne diseases that can cause death. Many more people have hepatitis B (HBV) than HIV. The risk of acquiring hepatitis is greater than the risk of acquiring HIV. HBV poses a serious threat to health care workers. Your employer must offer you a free vaccine to protect you from hepatitis B. There is no vaccine for hepatitis C.

❑ 10. Identify high risk behaviors that allow the spread of HIV/AIDS and HBV

Behaviors that put people at high risk for HIV/AIDS or HBV infection include:

▶ Sharing used drug needles

▶ Having unprotected sex (not using latex condoms during sexual contact)

▶ Having sexual contact with many partners

▶ Engaging in any sexual activity that involves exchange of body fluids with a partner who has not been tested negative for HIV or who has had many sexual partners. Be aware that it may take 6 months to a year after coming into contact with the virus for an HIV test to show positive results.

Ways to protect against the spread of HIV/AIDS:

▶ **Never share needles** for injections of any type of drug.

- **Stay in a monogamous relationship** with a partner who has been tested negative for HIV. Monogamous means having only one sexual partner.

- **Practice abstinence.** Abstinence means not having sexual contact with anyone.

- **Practice safer sex** by using latex condoms during sexual contact.

- **Get tested** if you think you may have been infected with HIV. Infection may not show up for six months to a year, so get retested periodically if necessary. It is especially important that pregnant women get tested.

- **Follow standard precautions** at work to protect yourself.

❑ 11. Demonstrate knowledge of the legal aspects of AIDS, including testing

The right to confidentiality is especially important to people with HIV/AIDS, because others may pass judgement on people with this disease. A person with HIV/AIDS cannot be fired from a job because of the disease; however, a health care worker with HIV/AIDS may be reassigned to job duties with a lower risk of transmitting the disease.

HIV testing requires consent. That means no one can force you to be tested for HIV unless you agree. HIV test results are confidential and should not be shared with a person's family, friends, or employer without his or her consent. If you are HIV-positive, you might want to confide in your supervisor so your assignments can be adjusted to avoid putting you at high risk for exposure to other infections. Everyone has a right to privacy regarding their health status. Never discuss a client's status with anyone.

❑ 12. Identify community resources and services available to clients with HIV/AIDS

Depending on the community, many resources and services may be available for people with HIV/AIDS. These may include counseling, meal services, access to experimental drugs and any number of other services. Look in the phone book for resources available in your area, or speak to your supervisor if you feel a client with HIV/AIDS needs more help.

A social worker or another member of the care team may be able to coordinate services for clients with HIV/AIDS.

❑ 13. Explain three facts about tuberculosis and how it is transmitted

Tuberculosis (too-ber-kyoo-LOH-sis, or TB) is an airborne disease carried on mucus droplets suspended in the air. When a person infected with TB talks, coughs, breathes, or sings, he or she may release mucus droplets carrying the disease. TB usually infects the lungs, causing coughing, difficulty breathing, fever, and fatigue. If left untreated, TB may cause death.

There are two types of TB: 1) **TB infection**, also called **latent TB**, and 2) **TB disease**, also called **active TB**. Someone with TB infection carries the disease but does not show symptoms and cannot infect others. A person with active TB, or TB disease, shows symptoms of the disease and can spread TB to others. TB infection can progress to TB disease. The signs and symptoms of TB are shown in **Fig. 5-19.**

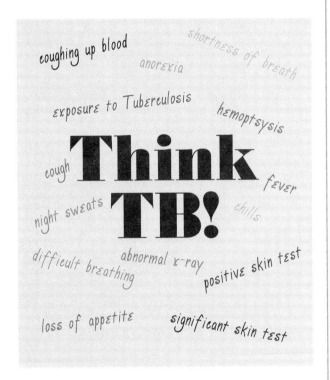

Fig. 5-19. Know the signs and symptoms of TB.

1. Wash hands.

2. Thread the top elastic strap through the top buckle. Repeat for the bottom elastic strap.

3. Place the bottom elastic strap around the head, just below the ears. Untwist the strap.

4. Pull the top strap over your head, resting it above your ears and at the top back of your head. Untwist the strap.

5. Adjust the strap tension by pulling the straps with both hands as shown.

6. Strap tension may be decreased without removing respirator from the head by pushing out on the back of the buckle.

7. Place your fingertips from both hands at the top of the metal nosepiece.

8. With both hands, mold the nose area to the shape of your nose by pushing inward while moving your fingertips down both sides of the nosepiece.

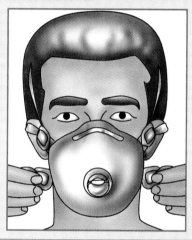

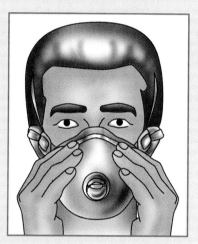

Pinching the nosepiece using one hand may result in improper fit and less effective respirator performance.

9. The seal of the respirator on the face should be fit-checked prior to wearing. To check the fit, cover the front of the respirator completely with both hands, being careful not to disturb the position of the respirator. Inhale sharply. A negative pressure should be felt inside the respirator. If any leakage is detected, readjust the position of the respirator and/or tension of the straps according to Steps 3, 4, and 5. Retest the seal. If you cannot achieve a proper fit, DO NOT enter the contaminated area. Contact your supervisor.

10. Wash your hands according to proper procedure.

TB is more likely to be spread in small, confined, or poorly ventilated places. TB disease is more likely to develop in people whose immune systems are weakened by illness, malnutrition, alcoholism or drug abuse. People with cancer and people with HIV/AIDS are especially susceptible to developing TB disease when exposed, because their immune system, which fights disease, is weakened.

❑ 14. List infection control guidelines for care of clients with known or suspected TB

1. Follow standard precautions and airborne precautions.

2. Wear a mask and gown during client care. A special mask, called a high efficiency particulate air (HEPA) respirator, may be needed. Some agencies use a less expensive N-95 mask. These masks filter out very small particles, such as the germs that cause TB. The procedure for putting on a HEPA respirator is outlined below.

3. Use special care when handling sputum or phlegm.

4. Ensure proper ventilation in the client's room. Open windows when possible.

5. Follow isolation procedures for airborne diseases if indicated in the care plan.

6. Help the client remember to take all medication prescribed. Failure to take all medication is a major factor in the spread of TB.

❑ 15. Explain the importance of reporting a possible exposure to an airborne or blood-borne disease

If you think you may have been exposed to TB, HIV/AIDS, or hepatitis at work, you must report this to your supervisor immediately. Fill out an **incident report** or a special **exposure report** form. Your employer will help you find out if you have been infected and take steps to prevent you from becoming sick. In order to protect your health and the health of your family members and other clients, you must report any potential exposures right away. Steps will also be taken to help prevent similar incidents from occurring again. Depending on the exposure, your agency may require tests and preventative measures to keep you healthy.

❑ 16. List three employer responsibilities and three employee responsibilities for infection control

Several state and federal government agencies have guidelines and laws concerning infection control. OSHA requires employers to provide for the safety of their employees through rules and suggested guidelines. The Centers for Disease Control issues guidelines for health care workers to follow on the job. Some states have additional requirements. Home health agencies consider these rules very carefully when writing their policies and procedures. It is very important that you learn these and follow them. They exist to protect you. Some of the infection control requirements for you and your employer are listed below.

Employer's responsibilities for infection control include the following:

1. Establish infection control procedures and an exposure control plan to protect workers.

2. Provide continuing in-service education on infection control, including bloodborne and airborne pathogens.

3. Have written procedures to follow should an exposure occur, including medical treatment and plans to prevent similar exposures.

4. Provide personal protective equipment for employees to use and train them when and how to properly use it.

5. Provide free hepatitis B vaccinations for all "at-risk employees." As a home care aide, you are considered at risk.

Employee's responsibilities for infection control include the following:

1. Follow standard or universal precautions.

2. Follow all agency policies and procedures.

3. Follow client care plans and assignments.

4. Use provided personal protective equipment as indicated or appropriate.

5. Take advantage of the hepatitis B vaccination.

6. Immediately report any exposure you have to infection.

7. Participate in annual education programs covering the control of infection.

Chapter 6

Safety and Body Mechanics

Part 1
Body Mechanics

❑ 1. Explain the principles of body mechanics

Health care providers use their bodies every day to help their clients. When you use your body in a way that causes stress and strain on muscles, you can cause permanent problems that not only cause pain, but also may prevent you from working. All people, including home care aides and their clients, benefit from learning to use good body mechanics to avoid injury.

Body mechanics is the way the parts of the body work together whenever you move.

When used properly, good body mechanics can save energy and prevent injury by enabling you to effectively push, pull, and lift objects or people who are not able to fully support or move their own bodies.

Understanding some basic principles will help you develop proper body mechanics.

Alignment: The concept of alignment is based on the word "line." When you stand up straight, a vertical line could be drawn right through the center of your body and your center of gravity (**Fig. 6-1**). When the line is straight, the body is in alignment. A body does not have to be standing up to be in alignment. When sitting or lying down, you should also try to have your body in alignment. This means that the two sides of the body are mirror images of each other, with body parts lined up naturally. You can maintain correct body alignment when lifting or carrying an object by keeping the object in front of you, pointing your feet and body in the direction you are moving, and avoiding twisting at the waist.

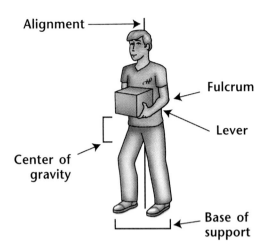

Alignment

Fulcrum

Lever

Center of gravity

Base of support

Fig. 6-1. Proper body alignment is important when standing and when sitting.

Base of support: The base of support is the foundation that supports an object. Something that has a wide base of support is more stable than something with a narrow base of support. For example, a tricycle is much harder to tip over than a bicycle or a unicycle. This is also true for the human body. The feet are the body's base of support. A person who is standing with legs apart has a greater base of support, and so is more stable, than someone standing with the feet close together.

Center of gravity: The center of gravity in your body is the point where the most weight is concentrated. This point will depend on the position the body is in. When you stand, your weight is centered in your pelvis.

A low center of gravity also gives a more stable base of support (**Fig 6-2**). Putting heavy books on the top of a narrow bookshelf will make the shelf top-heavy, and more likely to tip over. Putting heavy books on the bottom shelf and lighter books above lowers the center of gravity, making the bookshelf more stable. Bending your knees when lifting an object lowers your pelvis and, therefore, lowers your center of gravity. This gives you more stability and makes you less likely to fall or strain the working muscles.

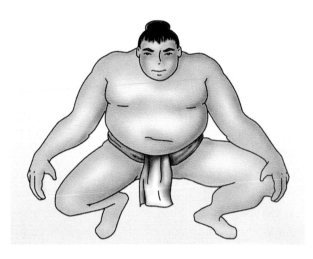

Fig. 6-2. This sumo wrestler knows that taking a wide stance and lowering his center of gravity make him much harder to knock over.

Fulcrum and lever: A **lever** moves an object by resting on a base of support, called a fulcrum. Think of a seesaw on the playground. The flat board you

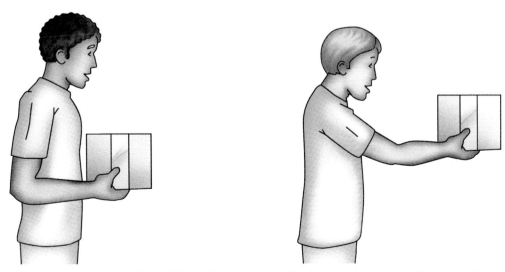

Fig. 6-3. Holding things close to you shortens the lever <u>and</u> moves the weight toward your center of gravity. In this illustration, whose arms will tire first?

sit on is the lever. The triangular base the board rests on is the fulcrum. When two children sit on opposite sides of the seesaw, they easily move each other up and down. They can do this because the fulcrum and lever of the seesaw are actually doing the work.

If you think of your body as a set of fulcrums and levers, you can find smart ways to lift without working as hard. Think of your arm as a lever with the elbow as the fulcrum. When you lift something, resting it against your forearm will shorten the lever and make it easier to lift than holding it in your hands (**Fig. 6-3**).

❑ 2. Apply principles of body mechanics to your daily activities

By applying the principles of body mechanics to your daily activities, you can avoid injury and use less energy to accomplish your duties. Some common examples of applying body mechanics include the following.

Lifting a heavy object from the floor. To lift a heavy object from the floor, spread your feet apart and bend your knees. Using the strong, large muscles in your thighs, upper arms, and shoulders, lift the object and pull it close to your body, to a point level with your pelvis. By doing this you are keeping the object close to your center of gravity and base of support. When you stand up, push with your strong hip and thigh muscles to raise your body and the object together.

Think about what would happen if you bent over from the waist. From this position, you would not only be lifting the object but also the entire upper half of your body, and all with the small muscles of the back (**Fig. 6-4**). This places great strain on those muscles and on the spinal column. Do not twist when you are moving an object. Always face the object or person you are moving. Pivot your feet instead of twisting at the waist.

Helping a client sit up, stand up, or walk. Whenever you need to support a client's weight, you can protect yourself by assuming a good stance. Your feet should be about 12 inches or hip width apart, one foot in front of the other, and knees bent. Your upper body should stay upright and in alignment. In this good stance, you have given yourself a wide base of support and a low center of gravity. If the client starts to fall, you will be in a good position to help support him or her. **Never** try to "catch" a falling client. In the event of a client falling, you should assist him or her to the floor or a level area.

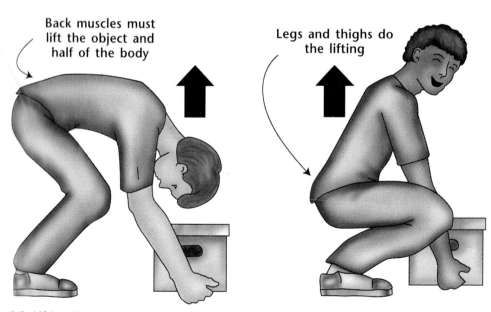

Back muscles must lift the object and half of the body

Legs and thighs do the lifting

Fig. 6-4. Lifting from a squat, with the back straight, allows the stronger muscles of the legs and thighs to do the lifting. In this illustration, which person is lifting correctly?

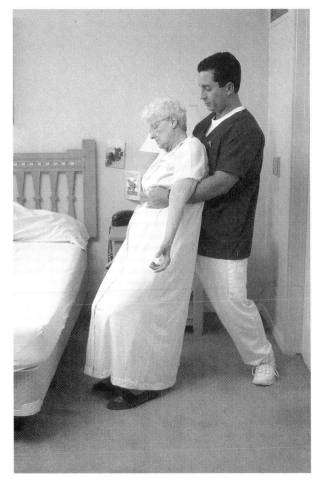

Fig. 6-5. Maintaining a wide base of support and low center of gravity will enable you to assist a falling client.

If you try to reverse a fall in progress, you will probably injure yourself and/or the client (**Fig. 6-5**).

Making a bed, or any job that requires bending. Anytime a task requires bending, you should use a good stance, bending your knees to lower yourself rather than bending from the waist. This allows you to use the big muscles in your legs and hips rather than straining the smaller muscles in your back. If you are making an adjustable bed, adjust the height to working level. If you are making a regular bed, you may need to put one knee on the bed, lean, or even kneel to support yourself at working level. Avoid bending at the waist.

Back strain or injury is one of the greatest risks a home care aide faces in every day work. Prevention is very important. Throughout this text you will learn correct procedures for assisting with client transfers, positioning, and ambulation. These procedures will include instructions for maintaining proper body mechanics. In addition, always keep the following tips in mind to avoid strain and injury:

- Start every physical task by thinking of ways to make it safer.

- Use a wide base of support (stand with your legs apart) when lifting. When standing for long periods, stand with feet apart and one foot slightly forward.

- Lower your center of gravity by bending your knees.

- Keep your back straight. **Do not** bend from the waist. Squat instead.

- Use both arms and hands when lifting, pulling, pushing, or carrying objects.

- Hold objects close to you when you are lifting or carrying them.

- Push, slide, or pull objects rather than lifting them.

- Avoid bending and reaching as much as possible. Move or position furniture so that you do not have to bend or reach.

- Avoid twisting at the waist. Instead, turn your whole body. Your feet should point toward what you are lifting.

- Teach your client and his or her family members how to use good body mechanics.

- Get help whenever possible for lifting or assisting clients.

- Let the client know what you will do so he or she can help if possible.

- Count to three and lift or move on three so everyone moves together.

- Report to your supervisor if your assignments include tasks you feel you cannot safely perform.

- Never attempt to lift an object or a client that you feel you cannot handle.

❑ 3. List ways to adapt the home to principles of good body mechanics

Following are several strategies that can help you apply good body mechanics in the home:

Have the right tools for a job. For example, if you cannot reach an object on a high shelf, use a step stool rather than climbing on a counter or straining to reach.

Have footrests and pillows available. You can make any position safer and more comfortable by using footrests and pillows to keep the body in alignment. For example, tasks that require standing for long periods can be more comfortable if you rest one foot on a footrest. This position flexes the muscles in the lower back and keeps the spine in alignment. When sitting, using a footrest allows comfortable positioning of the legs. Crossing the legs disrupts alignment and should be avoided. Using pillows can make any chair more comfortable. Use pillows behind the back or in the small of the back to keep back straight.

Keep tools, supplies, and clutter off the floor. Reduce the need for bending by keeping frequently used items on shelves or counters where they can be easily reached without lifting. Keeping things organized will also help you find what you need without straining.

Sit when you can. Whenever you can sit to do a job, do so. Chopping vegetables, folding clothes, and many other tasks can be done easily while sitting. For jobs like scouring the bathtub, kneel or use a low stool. Avoid bending at the waist.

Use gait or transfer belts when assisting clients with ambulation or transfers. In Chapter 12 you will learn correct procedures for safely assisting clients with ambulation and transfers.

> ## Part 2
> ## Safety in the Home

You must make sure the homes you work in are safe for your clients, their family members, and yourself. Working in a home that is unfamiliar or possibly neglected puts you at risk of injury if safety precautions are not taken. Do remember, however, that you are in the client's home. Unless an imme- diate danger exists, you should check with your supervisor and the client before making any significant changes in the environment.

A nurse or case manager will usually assess the safety of the homes you work in as part of the initial visit. However, you will spend more time in the home than any other member of the care team. You need to constantly be on the lookout for safety hazards and immediately report to your supervisor any hazards you observe.

❏ 4. Identify five common types of accidents in the home

Common types of accidents that occur in the home include the following:

Falls: Falls can be caused by an unsafe environment or by loss of abilities. Falls are particularly common among the elderly. Older people are often more seriously injured by falls because their bones are more fragile. Be especially alert to the risk of falls with your elderly clients.

Environmental factors that raise the risk of falls include clutter, throw rugs, exposed electrical cords, slippery floors, uneven floors or stairs, and poor lighting. Personal conditions that raise the risk of falls include loss of vision, gait or balance disturbances, weakness, paralysis or **paresis** (pa- REE-sis, or partial paralysis), and disorientation.

To guard against falls, clear all walkways of clutter, throw rugs, and cords (**Figs. 6-6 and 6-7**). Avoid waxing floors, and use non-skid mats or carpeting where appropriate. Immediately clean up spills on the floor. Mark uneven flooring or stairs with red tape to indicate a hazard, and improve lighting where necessary. The home care aide needs to be able to identify hazards and take action to remove them. In many cases, the home care aide will need to work with the client, the client's family, and/or other members of the care team to address the hazards.

Burns: Burns can be caused by stoves and electrical appliances, hot water, or heating devices. Small children, older adults, or people with loss of sensation due to paralysis are at greatest risk of burns.

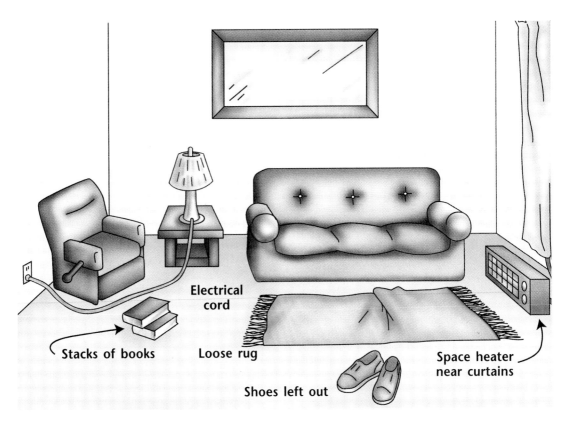

Fig. 6-6. Be aware of unsafe conditions in your clients' homes. This living room contains many tripping and fire hazards.

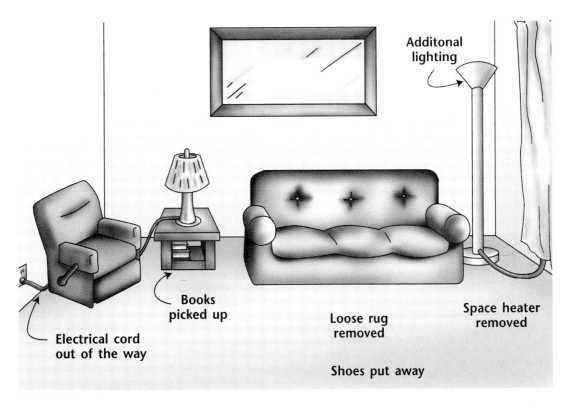

Fig. 6-7. By being observant, you can help prevent accidents. The hazards shown in the top picture have been removed in the above picture. Talk with your client about changes that need to be made to avoid hazards. If the client resists the changes, talk with your supervisor.

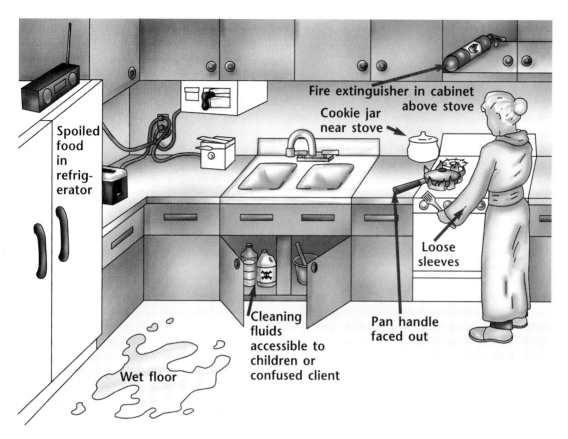

Fig. 6-8. Unsafe working conditions in the kitchen can lead to burns and other injuries.

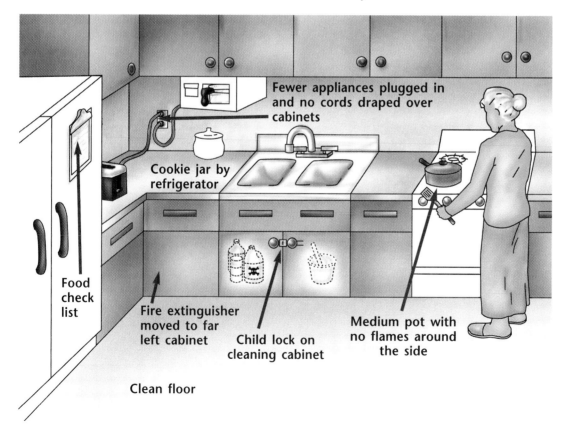

Fig. 6-9. Prevent burns, other injuries, and fires by following safe practices in the kitchen.

Section II: Building a Foundation: Before Client Care

To guard against burns, check that the stove and appliances are off when you leave. Roll up sleeves and avoid loose clothing when working at the stove (**Figs. 6-8 and 6-9**). Suggest that the hot water heater be set lower than normal (it should be set at 120-130° F) to avoid burns from scalding tap water. Always check water temperature with your finger or wrist before using. Keep space heaters away from clients' beds or chairs and draperies, and never allow space heaters to be used in the bathroom. Report frayed electrical cords or unsafe-looking appliances immediately.

Poisoning: Most homes contain many harmful substances that should not be ingested, including cleaning products, paints, medicines, toiletries, and glues. In homes with children, these products should all be locked up in special cabinets (**Figs. 6-10 and 6-11**). Confused clients, or those with limited vision, can confuse harmful items for non-hazardous items. Store them in separate places. All homes should have the number for the Poison Control Center posted by the telephone.

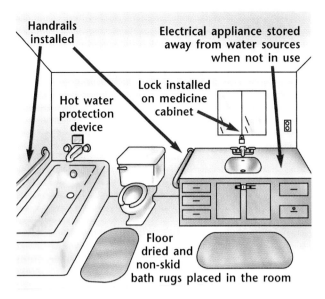

Fig. 6-11. In this bathroom, handrails, a hot water protection device, and medicine cabinet locks have been installed. Electrical appliances are put away when not in use. The floor is kept dry, and non-skid bath rugs have been brought in to reduce slipping hazards.

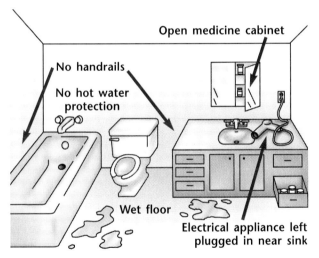

Fig. 6-10. The bathroom is full of safety hazards if it is not properly arranged and maintained.

Elderly people or clients who may have a diminished sense of taste or smell due to stroke or head injury are at risk of ingesting spoiled food. Check the refrigerator and cabinets frequently for foods that are moldy, rancid, sour or otherwise spoiled. Investigate any odors you notice. Clients with

dementia may hide food and let it spoil in closets, drawers or other places.

Cuts: Cuts typically occur in the kitchen or bathroom. Keep any sharp objects, including knives, peelers, graters, food processor blades, scissors, nail clippers, or razors out of reach of children. Lock sharp objects away if there is a client with confusion or dementia in the home. If you are preparing food, remember the rules: cut away from yourself, use a cutting board, and keep your fingers out of the way. Know proper first aid for cuts (see Controlling Bleeding, Chapter 7).

Choking: Choking can occur when eating, drinking or swallowing medication. Babies and young children who put objects in their mouths are at great risk of choking. People who are weak, ill, or unconscious may choke on their own saliva. A person's tongue can also become swollen and obstruct the airway.

To reduce the risk of choking, keep small objects out of the reach of babies and small children. Older children's toys that present a choking hazard must be kept away from a baby or toddler. Cut children's food into bite-sized pieces. Do the same for

Bathroom

▶ **Falls:** Use nonskid bathmats in tubs and showers. Request grab bars for the tub, shower, and toilet if the client is weak and unsteady.

▶ **Burns:** Check the temperature of bath water, shower water, and soaks with a bath thermometer or the inside of your wrist. Put away electrical appliances (such as hair dryers) when they are not in use. Do not allow electrical appliances to be used near a water source.

▶ **Drowning:** Do not leave young children unattended near any water, including bathtub, swimming pool, bucket or basin of water, puddle, pond, drainage ditch, toilet, or sink. Do not leave children who are ill and weak in a tub unattended. Do not leave clients who are dizzy, weak, or confused alone in the tub or shower.

▶ **Poisoning:** Suggest that all medications be stored in containers with childproof caps and in locked cabinets. Never tell children that medication is candy. Be sure all medicines are labeled and your client reads medicine labels with his or her eyeglasses if reading glasses are necessary. Store client's medications separately from medications taken by other members of the family. Discard old and unused medications.

▶ **Cuts:** Put away razors and any other sharp objects (such as nail scissors or clippers) when they are not in use.

Kitchen

▶ **Falls:** Be sure the high chair safety belt is fastened.

▶ **Burns:** Turn pot handles out of sight and toward the back of the stove. Stir food, especially if cooked in a microwave, to be certain it is uniformly warm and not too hot before serving. Cool hot liquids with an ice cube before serving, as appropriate.

▶ **Poisoning:** Keep emergency numbers, including the Poison Control Center, near the phone. Suggest that all household cleaning products and other chemicals be stored in locked cupboards or closets.

▶ **Cuts:** Keep cutlery put away. If you are using a knife and put it down for a moment, place it away from the edge of the counter or table (where it won't fall off or be in the reach of small children). Make sure the blade is pointed away from the counter or table edge. Keep other sharp kitchen tools in safe places, out of the reach of children.

▶ **Choking:** Do not give infants and toddlers popcorn, peanuts, hard candy, gum, or foods such as hot dogs or grapes. These items are easily aspirated (AS-pe-rayt-ed), or inhaled, causing choking. Cut all foods into small, bite-size pieces suitable for the age of the child. For elderly clients who have difficulty swallowing, serve softer foods and foods cut into small pieces. Encourage clients to take small bites of food, chew thoroughly, and eat slowly. Keep plastic storage bags out of reach. Discard plastic bags from drycleaners or other vendors.

Bedroom

▶ **Falls:** If available, keep a night-light or other soft lighting in the room to illuminate pathways. Do not leave children unattended on high surfaces, such as a crib, bed, or changing table or in a high chair or play pen. Do not turn your back when you are changing a child on a high surface. Be sure the crib side rails are raised before you leave the room.

▶ **Burns:** Do not allow clients to smoke in bed or when unattended. Especially do not allow smoking around oxygen tanks or equipment. When your client is unattended, place a call signal such as a bell nearby.

▶ **Poisoning:** Some window blinds have also been found to collect lead-contaminated dust, which can cause lead poisoning if ingested by children.

▶ **Cuts:** Be sure sharp objects, such as sewing scissors or letter openers, are put away- not left on a nightstand or in a chair, where they can cause injury.

▶ **Choking:** Report any cribs that have wide spaces between the slats. The infant's head could become wedged between them. Keep the crib away from drapes and blinds. Infants and toddlers can strangle on the cords. Do not prop up bottles for infants and toddlers. Keep pillows out of an infant's or toddler's crib to avoid suffocation. Examine all toys for loose or removable parts. Give children only age-appropriate toys.

Living area

▶ **Falls:** Request assistive devices for ambulation, such as walkers or canes, for clients who need support when walking. Talk to your supervisor about asking the family to have handrails installed where necessary. Keep the floors clear of sharp objects and loose rugs. Keep electrical cords and extension cords out of the way. Be sure shoes are sturdy and shoelaces are tied. Keep the floors free of clutter and spills. For small children, place safety gates, if available, at the tops and bottoms of stairs. Be certain the gates are secure and closed. Use hardware-mounted gates at the top of stairs rather than pressure gates.

▶ **Burns:** Suggest that electrical outlets be covered with baby-proof plugs. Keep lighters and matches out of reach and out of sight. Never smoke around children.

▶ **Poisoning:** Keep plants out of children's reach. Many common houseplants are poisonous.

▶ **Cuts:** Keep sharp objects out of children's reach. Do not allow children to run, jump, or play rough with any toy or object that could poke or stab.

▶ **Choking:** Do not permit young children to play with balloons or rubber bands. These objects are easily aspirated. Do not allow children to run and jump with food in their mouths.

Garage and outdoors

▶ Never leave children at home alone or alone in a vehicle.

▶ Make sure all children are fastened into an approved car seat as required by law. Child car seats should be placed in the back seat of the automobile. Children should never sit in the front seat of a car equipped with dual airbags.

▶ Supervise children at play.

▶ Keep walkways clear of toys and other obstructions, as well as snow and ice.

older people or those who have trouble using utensils. Position infants on their sides for sleeping after a feeding to reduce the risk of choking on spit up. Never put pillows, small toys, or other objects that could cause choking or suffocation in a baby's crib. Clients should eat in as upright a position as possible to avoid choking. Elderly clients with swallowing difficulties may have a special diet, such as thick liquids only (it is more common for people to choke on thin liquids). Know proper first aid for choking (see Chapter 7).

❑ 5. List five home fire safety guidelines and describe what to do in case of fire

1. **Recognize and report fire hazards.** Any of the following can be a fire hazard:

▶ wood stoves, kerosene, gas or electric heaters that appear old, damaged, or faulty

▶ unvented heaters used in small, enclosed areas or sleeping areas

▶ space heaters used near fabrics such as draperies, bedspreads, or towels, or used to dry clothing or towels

▶ flammable materials, such as gasoline, kerosene, or paint thinner, stored near stoves, heaters, furnaces, hot water heaters, or other appliances

▶ frayed or exposed electrical wires

▶ matches or lighters left within reach of children or incapacitated adults

▶ careless smoking, smoking in bed, cigarettes left burning, or confused clients smoking

2. Reduce hazards while you work. Follow these guidelines:

▶ Never work wearing loose or flowing clothing, especially around the stove. Roll up clients' sleeves and avoid loose clothing when client may be cooking or around the stove.

▶ Store potholders, dish towels, and other flammable kitchen items away from the stove.

▶ Never store cookies, candy, or other items that may attract children above or near the stove.

▶ Discourage careless smoking and smoking in bed. If clients must smoke, check to be sure that cigarettes are extinguished. Empty ashtrays frequently.

▶ Stay in or near the kitchen when anything is cooking or baking.

▶ Do not leave the dryer on when you leave the house. Lint can catch fire.

▶ Turn off space heaters when no one is home or everyone is asleep.

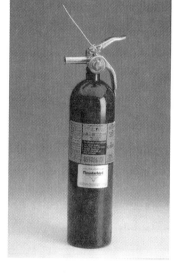

Fig. 6-12. Know where the extinguisher is stored and how to operate it.

3. Be sure there are working smoke alarms. Each floor of the home should have at least one smoke alarm. It is best to have one near bedrooms. Check monthly to see that alarms are working. Replace batteries when needed. It is helpful to choose an anniversary, birthday, or the day a time change occurs as the annual battery replacement date.

4. Have fire extinguishers on hand. Every home should have a fire extinguisher in the kitchen. Do not store the kitchen fire extinguisher near or above the stove, because you need to be able to get to it if the stove is on fire. It is a good idea to have another fire extinguisher somewhere else in the house, such as on the second floor. You should check that the homes you work in have fire extinguishers that have not expired. Know where the extinguisher is stored and how to operate it (**Fig. 6-12**).

5. In case of fire, RACE is a good rule to follow:

Remove clients from danger.

Activate 911.

Contain fire if possible.

Extinguish, or call fire department to extinguish.

In addition, follow these guidelines for helping clients and family members exit the building safely:

▶ Remain calm.

▶ Be sure all family members know how to exit in case of fire, and have a designated meeting place outside the home.

▶ If windows or doors have locking bars, keep keys in the lock or close by to allow escape in case of fire. Mark windows of children's rooms with stickers that indicate a child sleeps in the room.

▶ Remove anything blocking a window or door that could be used as a fire exit.

▶ If clothing catches fire, do not run. Drop to the ground and roll to extinguish flames.

▶ Do not try to put out a large fire. Get out of the house and call for emergency help. Fires can quickly get out of control.

❑ 6. Discuss the use of restraints for client safety

Certain kinds of physical restraints can be used to protect clients' safety. For example, bedrails keep clients from rolling out of bed. In the past some types of restraints have been abused by caregivers, leading to new restrictions and laws on the use of restraints. Check with your instructor or supervisor for laws and policies on the use of restraints.

Some restraints designed to safeguard clients can cause injury and even death if used improperly. In one case a restraint designed to hold a paralyzed woman in her wheelchair was improperly attached. When the woman slumped forward in her chair, the restraint tightened around her chest and prevented her from breathing. This woman died because of the incorrect use of a restraint intended to protect her safety.

Never use a restraint unless your supervisor has told you to do so, and you have been instructed in the proper use of the restraint. As with all care you give, follow the care plan.

Part 3
Personal Safety

❏ 7. Identify five ways to reduce the risk of automobile accidents

Since your work as a home care aide may require you to drive to and from clients' homes, you will need to protect your safety while driving. The following tips can help you do this:

Plan your route. Trying to read a map or directions while driving can be very dangerous. When you must drive to a new location, study the map or directions before you start your car. Plan the route you will take.

Minimize distractions. Simply paying attention to the road can help you avoid accidents. Keep your eyes on the road and your hands on the wheel. If music is distracting, don't listen in the car.

Use turn signals. Using your turn signals lets other drivers know what you are planning to do. Always use turn signals when preparing to turn or change lanes.

Use caution when backing up. Many accidents occur when drivers back up. When you must back up, look around you carefully, turning your head to both sides and looking behind your car. It is safest to turn your head and look behind you while backing up rather than relying on your rear view mirror.

Drive at a safe speed. Follow speed limits to be sure you are not driving too fast. Road conditions such as ice or heavy rain may mean you have to drive at a slower speed than indicated by the speed limit.

Always wear your seat belt: Although it may not help you avoid an accident, it will certainly help protect you if an accident occurs. Always buckle up, no matter how short the distance you must drive. Require your passengers to wear their seat belts as well.

❏ 8. Identify five guidelines for using your car on the job

Keep the following in mind when using your car on the job:

1. Park in safe, well-lit areas.

2. Lock doors, both when driving and when you leave your car.

3. Don't leave valuables in the car. If you must leave something in the car, put it out of sight, under a seat or in the trunk.

4. Have valid car insurance and carry the insurance card with you.

5. Keep your proof of registration or registration card with you, not in the car. If your car is stolen, you do not want the thief to have this important document.

6. Keep track of the miles you drive for work, and document them accurately. Lying about your mileage is the same as stealing from your employer.

7. Keep your car in good working order. Get your car serviced at the appropriate times, make sure you have good tires, and keep the gas tank full.

❏ 9. Identify guidelines for working in high crime areas

If an assignment takes you to an area where crime is a problem, use caution both while driving and when you leave your car. If you are using public transportation, be alert at all times. The following guidelines can help you avoid trouble:

▶ Park in well-lit areas, as close as possible to the home you are visiting.

▶ Try to leave valuables at home when you must work in a dangerous area.

- If possible, do not take your purse with you. If you must take it, hold your purse or bag tightly, close to your body.

- Lock your car and don't leave any valuables in it.

- Walk purposefully and confidently. Look as though you know where you are going (**Fig. 6-13**).

- Carry a whistle so you can make a loud noise to startle an attacker and get help.

- Carry your keys in your hand to unlock your car as soon as you arrive. If necessary, you can also use them as a weapon.

- Don't sit in your car, even with the doors locked. Drive away as soon as you reach your car.

- Try to avoid unsafe areas after dark.

- If you are concerned about your safety in a particular area, leave the area immediately and contact your supervisor.

- Do not approach a home where strangers are hanging around. Go to the nearest phone in a safe area, and call your supervisor.

- Call your client before you visit so they know approximately when to expect you.

- Never enter a vacant home.

- If necessary, ask your supervisor to arrange for an escort or another care provider to go with you.

- Be sure someone knows your schedule. Call the office at the end of your work day.

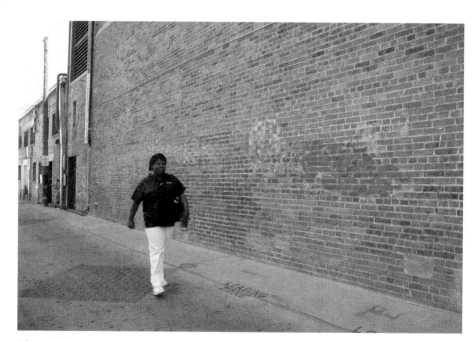

Fig. 6-13. Be cautious but look confident if you must enter a high-crime area.

Chapter 7

Emergency Care and Disaster Preparation

❑ **1. Demonstrate ability to recognize medical emergencies and respond appropriately**

Medical emergencies may be the result of accidents or sudden illnesses. In this chapter you will learn how to respond appropriately to medical emergencies. Heart attacks, stroke, diabetic emergencies, choking, automobile accidents, and gunshot wounds are all medical

Learning Objectives

In this chapter you will learn to:

emergencies. Falls, burns, and cuts can also be emergencies when they are severe.

When you come upon an emergency situation, it is important to remain calm, act quickly, and communicate clearly. Memorizing the following six steps will help you respond calmly and quickly in an emergency:

1. **Assess the situation.** Try to determine what has happened. Make sure you are not in danger. Notice the time.

2. **Assess the victim.** Ask the injured or ill person what has happened. If the person is unable to respond, he may be unconscious. If the person does respond, use his account along with your observations when you talk with emergency personnel. A person who has been injured or has suddenly become ill may not know or remember, or may be too embarrassed to say exactly what happened. Later in this chapter you will learn more about assessing a victim's condition.

3. **Get assistance.** Most emergencies will require that you or someone nearby call for emergency assistance immediately. Follow your agency's policies for who to call under what circumstances. Always have an emergency phone list near the telephone. Throughout this chapter, you will learn procedures for assisting in various emergencies. Each procedure includes instructions on when to call for help.

4. **Do no harm.** Make the injured or ill person as comfortable as possible. Moving a person who has had an accident can make an injury worse. Do not move the person unless he is in danger if he remains where he is (for instance, in case of a fire). Never perform lifesaving measures unless you are sure the person needs it. Never perform lifesaving measures unless you are trained to perform the procedure.

5. **Provide comfort and support.**
If the injured or ill person is conscious, he may feel panic about his condition. Listen to the person, and tell him what actions are being taken to help him. You must maintain a calm, confident manner to help reassure the injured or ill person that he is being taken care of.

6. **Report according to agency guidelines.** Once the emergency is over, you will have to file an incident/accident report with your agency. If you know in advance what information you will need to know to complete the report, you will be better able to remember important facts. Documenting emergencies accurately is very important to you and your agency.

❏ *2. Describe how to assess a person involved in a medical emergency*

The most serious medical emergencies involve one or more of the following:

▶ person is unconscious
▶ person is not breathing
▶ person has no pulse
▶ person is bleeding severely

To determine whether a person is conscious, tap the person and ask if she is all right. Speak loudly, and use the person's name if you know it. If the person does not respond, she is probably unconscious. Call for help right away, or send someone else to call for help. Later in this chapter you will learn more about reporting emergencies. After calling for help, return to the person and check for breathing, pulse, or severe bleeding, following these steps:

1. Check for breathing. Look for the chest to rise and fall, listen for sounds of breathing, and feel for the person's breath on your cheek.

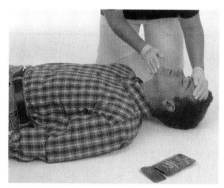

Fig. 7-1. Check the person's airway.

2. Check the person's airway. Tilt the head back slightly to open the airway (**Fig. 7-1**). Check for breathing again. If the person still is not breathing, give two rescue breaths (Procedure 1 discusses rescue breathing) before checking the pulse. If the person is breathing, she also has a pulse.

3. Check for pulse by feeling the carotid (ka-ROT-id) artery in the neck (**Fig. 7-2**). Determine if there is a pulse. If there is no pulse, make sure help is on its way. Initiate **cardiopulmonary resuscitation (CPR)** if you are trained and authorized to do so. CPR training is discussed later in this chapter.

4. If the person has a pulse but is still not breathing,

she may have inhaled or choked on something. If this has happened, the airway may be blocked, preventing breathing. Procedure 1 in this chapter describes how to clear an obstructed airway.

5. Check for severe bleeding. Look up and down the person's body. If you see blood spurting or running from any part of the body, or if you see a significant amount of blood on the person's clothes or on the ground, make sure help is on its way and then take steps to control bleeding. Procedure 3 in this chapter describes how to control bleeding.

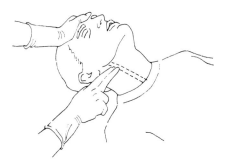

Fig. 7-2. Check pulse by feeling the carotid (ka-ROT-id) artery in the neck.

If a person *is* conscious and able to speak to you, she is breathing and has a pulse. Talk with the client about what happened, and check the person for injury. Symptoms to look for include severe bleeding, changes in consciousness, irregular breathing, unusual color or feel to the skin, odd bumps or depressions on the body, medical alert tags, and anything the clients says is painful. If one of these conditions exists, you may need professional medical help. Follow your agency's policies about whom to call in different situations.

❑ *3. Explain guidelines for reporting emergencies accurately and immediately*

If you need to call emergency medical services, call 911 or dial 0 for the operator to get emergency medical services. If you are alone, make the call yourself. If you are not alone, shout for help and have someone make the call for you and then return to you.

When calling emergency services, be prepared to give the following information:

▶ the phone number and address of emergency, including exact directions or landmarks if necessary

▶ the person's condition, including any medical background you know

▶ your name and position

▶ details of any first aid being given

The dispatcher you speak with may need other information or may want to give you other instruc-

tions. Do not hang up the phone until the dispatcher hangs up or tells you to hang up. If you are in a home, unlock the front door so emergency personnel can get in when they arrive.

If the person is breathing, has a normal pulse, is normally responsive, and is not bleeding severely, you may not need to call for emergency services. If a client has fallen, been burned, or cut himself but the damage seems to be minor, call your supervisor. Let the person answering the phone know that you are with a client and an accident has occurred. If your supervisor is not available, another member of the care team may be able to help you.

Later, you will need to document the emergency in your notes and complete an incident or an accident report. Try to remember as many details as possible, and remember to report the facts only. If a client had a heart attack, your notes should record the signs and symptoms *you* observed and the actions *you* took. Knowing the kind of information you will have to document will help you remember the important facts during the emergency (for instance, it is especially important to remember the time a client becomes unconscious).

❑ *4. Demonstrate knowledge of first aid procedures*

Your agency will probably arrange for you to be trained in **CPR** and **rescue breathing**. If your agency does not schedule you for training, ask about American Heart Association or Red Cross CPR training, or contact one of these agencies yourself. CPR is an important skill for home care aides to learn. If you are trained and you have a current card, perform CPR and rescue breathing when needed in an emergency. If you are not trained, do *not* attempt to perform CPR. Performing CPR incorrectly can further injure a person (for example, delivering chest compressions in the wrong place can result in a punctured lung).

Box 7-1. What to do if you suspect a heart attack

Signs of a heart attack include the following:

- skin, lips, or nailbeds that are pale or cyanotic (sye-a-NOT-ik), a bluish color
- shortness of breath or other difficulty breathing
- intense pain or pressure in the chest, shoulders, arms, jaws, or back
- sweating
- fast, slow, or irregular pulse
- denial that anything is wrong
- feeling that something is very wrong

You must take immediate action if a client experiences any of these symptoms. Follow these steps:

1. Place the client in a comfortable position. Encourage him to rest, and reassure him that you will not leave him alone.

2. Loosen clothing around the neck.

3. Call or have someone call emergency services, and call your supervisor.

4. Do not give the client liquids.

5. If the client takes heart medication, such as nitroglycerin, find the medication and offer it to the client. Never place medication in someone's mouth.

6. Monitor the client's breathing and pulse. If the client stops breathing or has no pulse, perform rescue breathing or CPR if you are trained to do so.

Procedure 1: Clearing an obstructed airway in a child or adult, performing the Heimlich (HIGHM-lick) maneuver, and rescue breathing

Clients who have difficulty chewing or swallowing, are confused, or have poor vision may be at risk of choking. An **obstructed airway** means the person cannot breathe normally because something is blocking the trachea (TRAY-kee-a), the tube through which air enters the lungs. When people are choking, they usually put their hands to their throats and

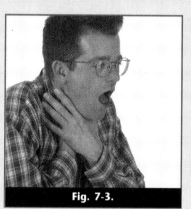

Fig. 7-3.

cough (**Fig. 7-3**). As long as the person can speak, breathe, or cough, do nothing. Encourage him to cough as forcefully as possible to get the object out. Stay with the person at all times, until he stops choking or can no longer speak, breathe, or cough.

If a person can no longer speak, breathe, or cough, you should call for help immediately. After calling for help return to the person. If he is still conscious, help push the object out by giving **abdominal thrusts:**

1. Ask the person if he is

choking. You must make sure he needs help before starting abdominal thrusts. If the person needs help, continue.

2. Stand behind the person and bring your arms under his arms.

3. Make a fist with one hand and place the flat, thumb side of the fist against the person's abdomen, above the navel but below the breastbone (**Fig. 7-4**).

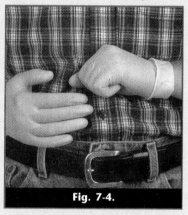

Fig. 7-4.

4. Grasp the fist with your other hand and pull both hands toward you and up, quickly and forcefully.

5. Repeat until the object is pushed out or the person

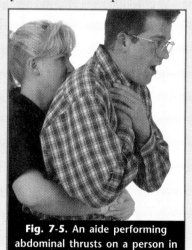

Fig. 7-5. An aide performing abdominal thrusts on a person in the upright position.

begins coughing forcefully again. Pause every five to ten thrusts to see if the victim can talk, breathe, or cough.

If the person becomes unconscious, help him or her to the floor gently, into a supine (SUE-pine) position, or lying on the back with the face up. Make sure help is on its way. A person who has become unconscious while choking probably has a completely blocked airway. He needs professional medical help immediately. While you wait for help to arrive, stay with the person and check for breathing as you learned to earlier in this chapter (see learning objective 2).

If the person is not breathing and you are trained to perform rescue breathing, begin to do so immediately. To protect yourself from infectious diseases, you should use a face shield or mask when performing rescue breathing. Face shields or masks are small enough to carry in your bag when you are working (**Fig. 7-6**). To perform rescue breathing, follow these guidelines:

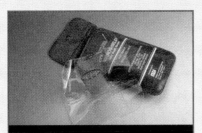

Fig. 7-6. Face shields or face masks protect you and the person you are helping from contacting body fluids.

6. Pinch the person's nose and form a seal with the face mask, shield, or your mouth over his mouth.

7. Breathe slowly into the face mask, shield, or the person's mouth for about 1 second, watching for the chest to rise (**Fig. 7-7**). If the chest rises, air is going in. Continue following these steps. If the chest does not rise, air is not getting in the person's lungs. Skip to step 11, below.

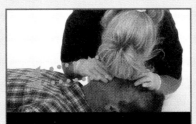

Fig. 7-7. Breath slowly into the face mask, shield, or the person's mouth for about 11/2 seconds, watching for the chest to rise. If the chest rises, air is going in.

8. Pause to let the air come back out, then give another breath.

9. Check for a pulse.

10. If a pulse is present but the person still is not breathing, give a slow breath about every 5 seconds, and check for pulse once a minute until the person starts breathing on his own or help arrives. If at any time no pulse is present, begin CPR if you are trained to do so, or wait for help to arrive.

If your breath won't go into the person's lungs, you need to check the person's airway and try to remove any obstructions. Retilt the person's head to open the airway, and check for breathing again. If the person is not

breathing, perform abdominal thrusts with the person in supine position:

11. Straddle the person's legs, facing his head, and place the heel of one hand on his abdomen just above the navel.

12. Interlace the fingers of both hands (**Fig. 7-8**).

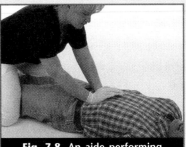

Fig. 7-8. An aide performing abdominal thrusts on a person in the supine position.

13. Press in and up with both hands, quickly and forcefully. Repeat up to five times. If the person vomits, roll him onto his side. Clear the vomit from his mouth, and resume abdominal thrusts.

14. Look in the mouth for any foreign objects. If you can see an object, reach in with your finger and sweep the object forward, out of the person's mouth (**Fig. 7-9**).

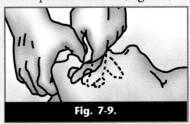

Fig. 7-9.

15. Check for breathing again.

16. If person is not breathing, repeat rescue breathing procedure above (return to step 6).

Continued on page 72

Continued from page 71

For a child who is choking, follow the same basic procedure as for an adult, with the following changes:

- If the child is small enough and there are no head or spine injuries, you can carry her to the phone and continue to give first aid while calling for help.

- The force of abdominal thrusts should be adjusted for the child's size.

- If you must give rescue breathing, give one breath every 3 seconds instead of every 5 seconds.

For an infant who is choking, you will need to give back blows and chest thrusts:

1. Lie the infant face down on your forearm, with his head lower than his chest. Support his head with your hand.

2. Using the heel of your hand, strike the infant between the shoulder blades five times. These are called **back blows** (**Fig.** 7-10).

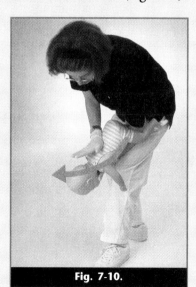

Fig. 7-10.

3. Put your other arm on top of the infant and switch arm positions, so that now the baby is chest up in your other arm (**Fig.** 7-11).

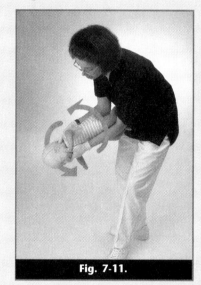

Fig. 7-11.

4. Place two or three fingers in the center of the breastbone and give five **chest thrusts**. Each chest thrust should push the chest down about 1 inch (**Fig.** 7-12).

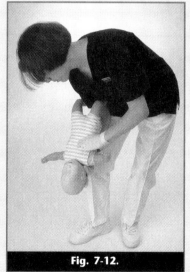

Fig. 7-12.

5. Repeat back blows and chest thrusts until the object is coughed up, the infant is breathing on his own, or he becomes unconscious.

6. If you must perform rescue breathing on an infant, seal his mouth and nose with your mouth, then follow the same procedure as for a child (1 breath every 3 seconds) (**Fig.** 7-13).

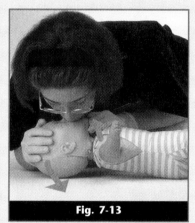

Fig. 7-13

Even if a person starts breathing on his own, he should receive medical attention if his airway has been obstructed. This is especially true for children and infants, because an object may still be lodged in the trachea.

Shock occurs when organs and tissues in the body do not receive an adequate blood supply. Bleeding, heart attack, severe infection, and conditions that cause the blood pressure to fall can lead to shock. Shock can become worse when the person is extremely frightened or in severe pain.

Shock is a dangerous, life-threatening situation. Signs of shock include pale or cyanotic skin, staring, increased pulse and respiration rates, decreased blood pressure, and extreme thirst. Always call for emergency help if you suspect a person is experiencing shock. To prevent or treat shock, do the following:

1. Have the person lie down in a supine position. If the person is bleeding from the mouth or vomiting, place her on her side (unless you suspect that the neck, back, or spinal cord is injured).

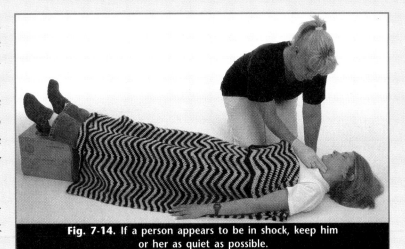

Fig. 7-14. If a person appears to be in shock, keep him or her as quiet as possible.

2. Control bleeding. Procedure 3, describes how to do this.

3. Check pulse and respirations if possible.

4. Keep the person as calm and comfortable as possible (**Fig. 7-14**).

5. Maintain normal body temperature. If the weather is cold, place a blanket around the person. If the weather is hot, provide shade.

6. Elevate the feet unless the client has a head or abdominal injury, breathing difficulties, or a fractured bone or back. Elevate the head and shoulders if a head wound or breathing difficulties are present. Never elevate a body part if a broken bone exists.

7. Do not give the person anything to eat or drink.

8. Call for emergency help. Victims of shock should always receive medical care as soon as possible.

Severe bleeding can cause death quickly and must be controlled. Call for help immediately, then follow these steps to control bleeding:

1. Put on gloves.

2. Hold a thick sterile pad, a clean pad, or a clean cloth such as a handkerchief, towel, or sanitary napkin against the wound (**Fig.** 7-15). Have the injured person use his bare hand until you can get a clean pad. Also have the client hold the pad if he is able until you can put on gloves.

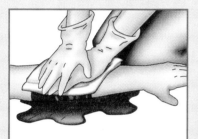

Fig. 7-15. Hold pad over wound and press down hard. Do not decrease pressure. If blood seeps through first pad, apply additional pads without removing the first.

3. Press down hard directly on the bleeding wound until help arrives. Do not decrease pressure. Put additional pads over the first pad if blood seeps through. Do not remove the first pad.

4. Raise the wound above the heart to slow down the bleeding. If the wound is on an arm, leg, hand, or foot, and there are no broken bones, prop up the limb on towels, blankets, coats, or other absorbent material.

5. If you cannot stop excessive bleeding, **pressure points** can be used as a last resort only. Press the artery against the bone just above the wound (**Fig.** 7-16). Do not use a pressure point for more than five minutes.

6. When bleeding is under control, secure the dressing to keep it in place, and check the person for symptoms of

shock (pale skin, increased pulse and respiration rates, decreased blood pressure, and extreme thirst; see Procedure 2). Stay with the person until medical help arrives.

7. Wash hands thoroughly when finished.

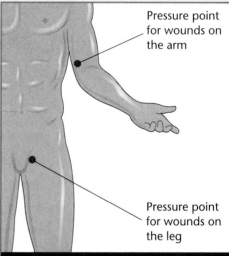

Pressure point for wounds on the arm

Pressure point for wounds on the leg

Fig. 7-16. Pressure points can be used as a last resort if you are unable to control bleeding with direct pressure on the wound.

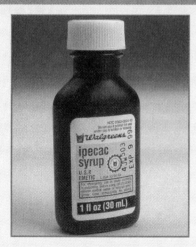

First aid kits in the home should contain syrup of ipecac (IH-pi-kak), activated charcoal, and Epsom salts for the treatment of accidental poisoning. Always have the poison control center phone number available and know if the client has syrup of ipecac in the house. Suspect poisoning when a client suddenly collapses, vomits, and has heavy, labored breathing. If you suspect poisoning, take the following steps:

1. Look for a container that will help you determine what the client has taken or eaten. Check the mouth for chemical burns and note the breath odor.

2. Call the local or state poison control center immediately. Follow instructions from poison control.

3. Notify your supervisor.

The severity of a burn depends on its depth, size, and location. There are three types of burns: superficial partial thickness burns, deep partial thickness burns, and full thickness burns (**Fig. 7-18**).

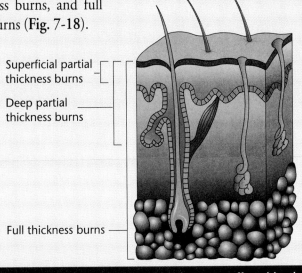

Superficial partial thickness burns

Deep partial thickness burns

Full thickness burns

Fig. 7-18. This cross-section of skin shows what layers are affected by the different types of burns.

Superficial partial thickness burns (first degree burns). Superficial partial thickness burns, like sunburns, involve just the epidermis (ep-i-DERM-is), or outer layer of skin. The skin becomes red, painful, and swollen, but no blisters occur.

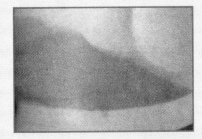

Deep partial thickness burns (second degree burns). Deep partial thickness burns extend from the epidermis to the next deeper layer of skin, the dermis (DERM-is). The skin is red, painful, swollen, and blisters occur.

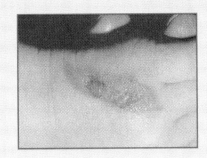

Full thickness burns (third degree burns). Full thickness burns involve all three layers of the skin and may extend to the bone. If the nerves are destroyed, no pain occurs. The skin is shiny and appears hard. It may be white in color.

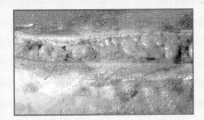

You should call for emergency help in any of the following situations:

- An infant or child, or an elderly, ill or weak person has been burned, unless burn is very minor.
- The burn occurs on the head, neck, hands, feet, face, or genitals, or burns cover more than one body part.
- Person who has been burned is having trouble breathing.
- The burn was caused by chemicals, electricity, or explosion.

To treat a minor burn:

1. Use cool, clean water (not ice) to decrease the skin temperature and prevent further injury. Ice will cause further skin damage. Dampen a clean cloth and place it over the burn.

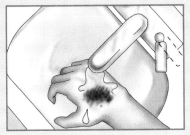

2. Once the pain has eased, you may cover the area with a dry, sterile gauze.

3. Never use any kind of ointment, salve, or grease on a burn.

Continued on 76

Continued from 75

For more serious burns:

1. Remove the person from the source of the burn. If clothing has caught fire, smother it with a blanket or towel to extinguish flames. Protect yourself from the source of the burn.

2. Check for breathing, pulse, and severe bleeding.

3. Call for emergency help.

4. Do not apply water. It may cause infection.

5. Remove as much of the person's clothing around the burned area as possible, but do not try to pull away clothing that sticks to the burn. Cover the burn with a thick, dry, sterile

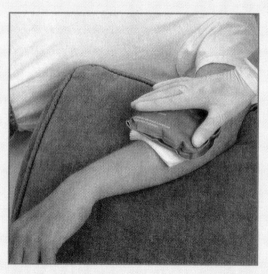

gauze if available, or a clean cloth. A dry, insulated cool pack may be used over the dressing. Again, never use any kind of ointment, salve, or grease on a burn.

6. Ask the person to lie down and elevate the affected part if this does not cause greater pain.

7. If the burn covers a larger area, wrap the person or the extremity in several thicknesses of a dry, clean sheet and apply an ice pack if possible. Take care not to rub the skin.

8. Wait for emergency medical help.

Procedure 6: Providing emergency treatment for seizures

Seizures or convulsions are involuntary, often violent, contractions of muscles. They can involve a small area or the entire body. Seizures are caused by an abnormality in the brain. They can occur in young children who have a high fever. Older children and adults who have a serious illness, fever, head injury, or epilepsy may also have convulsions.

The primary goal of a caregiver during a seizure is to make sure the client is safe. During a seizure, a person may shake severely, thrust arms and legs uncontrollably, clench his jaw, drool, and be unable to swallow. The following emergency measures should be taken if a client has a seizure:

1. Lower the person to the floor.

2. Have someone call for emergency medical help if needed. Do not leave the person during the seizure unless you must do so to get medical help.

3. Move furniture away to prevent injury.

4. Do not try to restrain the person.

5. Do not force anything between the person's teeth and do not place your hands in the person's mouth for any reason. You could be severely bitten.

6. Do not give liquids.

7. When the seizure is over, check breathing.

8. Call your supervisor. Report the length of the convulsion and your observations.

Fainting [syncope (SING-ke-pee)] occurs when the blood supply to the brain suddenly becomes insufficient, resulting in a sudden loss of consciousness. Fainting may be the result of hunger, fear, pain, fatigue, standing for a long time, poor ventilation, or overheating.

Signs and symptoms of fainting include dizziness, perspiration, pale skin, weak pulse, shallow respirations, and blackness in the visual field. If someone appears likely to faint, follow these steps:

1. Have the person lie down or sit down before fainting occurs.

2. If the person is in a sitting position, have him bend forward and place his head between his knees. If the person is in a supine position, elevate the legs.

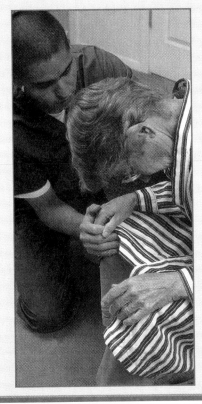

3. Loosen any tight clothing.

4. Have the person stay in position for at least five minutes after symptoms disappear.

5. Help the person get up slowly and continue to observe him for symptoms of fainting.

6. Call your supervisor and report the incident.

If a person does faint, lower him to the floor or other flat surface and position him on his back. Elevate his legs 8 to 12 inches, and loosen any tight clothing. Check to make sure the person is breathing. He should recover quickly, but keep him lying down for several minutes. Report the incident to your supervisor immediately. Fainting may be a sign of a more serious medical condition.

A nosebleed can occur spontaneously, when the air is dry, or when injury has occurred. The medical term for a nosebleed is epistaxis (ep-i-STAK-sis). If a client has a nosebleed, take the following steps:

1. Elevate the head of the bed or tell the client to remain in a sitting position. Offer tissues or a clean cloth to catch the blood. Do not touch blood or bloody clothes, tissues or cloths without gloves.

2. Put on gloves. Apply firm pressure over the bridge of the nose. Squeeze the bridge of the nose with your thumb and forefinger. Have the client do

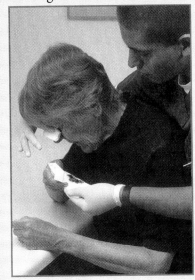

this until you are able to get gloves on.

3. Apply the pressure consistently until the bleeding stops.

4. Use a cool cloth or ice wrapped in a cloth on the back of the neck, the forehead, or the upper lip to slow the flow of blood. Never apply ice directly to skin.

5. Report the nosebleed to a supervisor.

Procedure 9:
Helping a client who has fallen

Falls can be minor or severe. All falls should be reported to your supervisor, and incident reports should be completed. In the case of a severe fall, call emergency medical services immediately. Take the following steps to help a client who has fallen:

1. Assess client's condition. Determine if client is unconscious, not breathing, has no pulse, or is bleeding severely. Get emergency medical help if any of these conditions exist.

2. Look for broken bones. Body parts lying in an unnatural position or bones protruding through the skin are indications.

3. If client seems unhurt, encourage her to stay down until you can check her condition thoroughly.

4. Ask client to move each body part separately to be sure there are no strains, sprains, or fractures.

5. If you find no evidence of injury, make the client as comfortable as possible.

6. Call your supervisor and report the fall immediately. Do not move the client until you have spoken with your supervisor.

Box 7-2.
Emergency Supplies

Keep enough supplies in your home to meet your needs for at least three days. Assemble a Disaster Supplies Kit with items you may need in an evacuation. Store these supplies in sturdy, easy-to-carry containers such as backpacks, duffel bags or covered trash containers.

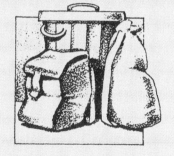

Include:

❑ A three-day supply of water (one gallon per person per day) and food that won't spill.

❑ One change of clothing and footwear per person, and one blanket or sleeping bag per person.

❑ A first aid kit that includes your family's prescription medications.

❑ Emergency tools, including a battery-powered radio, flashlight, and plenty of extra batteries.

❑ An extra set of car keys and a credit card, cash, or traveler's checks.

❑ Sanitation supplies.

❑ Special items for infant, elderly, or disabled family members.

❑ An extra pair of glasses.

❑ Keep important family documents in a waterproof container. Keep a smaller kit in the trunk of your car.

❏ 5. Identify emergency evacuation procedures

If a fire or other disaster occurs, you may need to get yourself, the client, and the client's family members out of the home immediately. Leaving in an emergency is called evacuation (ee-vac-yoo-AY-shun). Because you may not have a lot of time to think or plan in an emergency, you should know how best to evacuate each home you work in.

Plan for evacuation by doing the following:

▷ Locate all the doors and windows that could serve as exits in an emergency.

▷ In an apartment building, know where fire stairs are located. Elevators may be unsafe in an emergency.

▷ Know the location of disaster supplies if they are available in the home, including fire extinguishers, ladders for escape from upper floors, first aid kits or supplies, and utility shut off points.

▷ Discuss a plan for evacuation with your clients and their family members. Emphasize that everyone should keep calm in an emergency.

▷ Know who will be responsible for helping infants and children in emergencies.

▷ Agree on a place outside the home for everyone to meet after evacuation.

❏ 6. Demonstrate knowledge of disaster procedures

Disasters can include fire, flood, earthquake, hurricane, tornado, or severe weather. The disasters you may experience will depend on where you live and work. If you live in an area that is prone to disasters, call the local chapter of the Red Cross to learn more about how to prepare for and handle disasters. Know the policies of your agency concerning local disasters. There may be specific instructions for different geographical areas (for instance, designated shelters to go to).

The following guidelines apply in any disaster situation:

▷ Remain calm.

▷ Listen to radio or television bulletins to keep informed. A battery powered radio will allow you to stay informed if the power goes out.

▷ If a disaster is forecast (for example, a tornado or hurricane), be ready. Wear appropriate clothing and shoes. Have family members dressed and ready in case evacuation is necessary.

▷ Stay in contact with your supervisor or others if possible. Let someone know where you are, what conditions are, and where you will go if you must evacuate.

▷ Locate disaster supplies. Ideally, a disaster supplies kit should be assembled before disaster strikes. See **Box** 7-2 for a list of disaster supplies.

SECTION III
A Holistic Approach to Understanding Clients

Chapter 8

Basic Human Needs: Supporting Physical, Psychological, and Social Health

❑ *1. Identify basic human needs*

Although people differ in their genetic composition, physical appearance, cultural background, age, and social or financial status, all human beings have the same basic physical needs:

▶ food and water

▶ protection and shelter

▶ activity

▶ sleep and rest

▶ safety

▶ comfort, especially freedom from pain

As a home health aide, much of your role is to help your clients meet these basic physical needs. Activities of daily living (ADLs), such as eating, toileting, bathing, and grooming, are the ways we meet our most crucial physical needs. By assisting with ADLs or helping clients learn to perform them independently, you are helping clients meet their most basic needs.

In addition to physical needs, we also have **psychological** (sye-koh-LAJ-i-kal) needs, which involve social interaction, emotions, intellect, and spirituality. Psychological needs are not as easy to define as physical needs. However, research has shown that all human beings have the following psychological needs:

- love and affection
- acceptance by others
- security
- self-reliance and independence in daily living
- interaction with other people
- accomplishments and self-esteem

You should do what you can to help your clients meet these psychological needs as well as the physical ones. Satisfaction of psychological needs contributes to our physical, mental, and psychological growth and development. In fact, our health and well-being are determined by the degree to which our psychological needs are met. Frustration and stress, either physical, psychological, or both, commonly occur when basic needs are not met. This can lead to fear, anxiety, anger, aggression, withdrawal, apathy, and depression. Stress can also cause physical problems that may eventually lead to illness.

Abraham Maslow, a researcher of human behavior, categorized human needs into physical, psychological, and social needs. He arranged these needs into their order of importance, showing that our physical needs must be met before we can work on meeting our psychological or social needs. His theory is called Maslow's "Hierarchy of Needs." See **Box 8-1.**

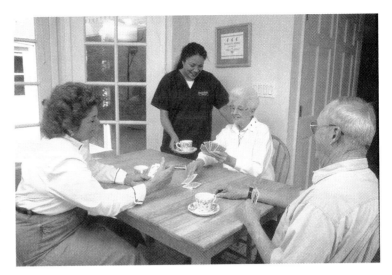

Fig. 8-1. Interaction with other people is a basic psychological need that does not disappear with age. Encourage your clients in any efforts to be with friends or relatives, or to make new friends. Remember how important social contact is to your clients, and accommodate visitors, even if doing so throws off your schedule.

❑ 2. Define holistic care

Holistic (hole-IS-tik) means considering a whole system, such as a whole person, rather than dividing the system up into parts and considering them independently. Holistic care involves caring for the whole person, the mind as well as the body, rather than treating the physical condition with no attention to psychological needs. A simple example of holistic care is taking time to talk with your clients while helping them bathe. You are meeting the physical need with the bath and meeting the psychological need for interaction with others at the same time.

Another way of practicing holistic care is considering psychological factors in illness as well as physical factors. For example, if Mr. Bollinger looks thin and fatigued, the cause might be depression rather than an infection. As a home care aide, you do not need to determine the cause of his condition, but by talking with him you might learn something that would help the rest of the care team. For example, you might learn that last year at this time his wife died, and he is still coping with that loss. You can and should share this information with the care team and document it.

Box 8-1.
Maslow's Hierarchy of Needs

Need for self-actualization: the need to learn, create, realize one's own potential.

Need for self-esteem: achievement, belief in one's own worth and value.

Need for love: feeling loved, accepted, belonging.

Safety and security needs: shelter, clothing, protection from harm, and stability.

Physical needs: oxygen, water, food, elimination, and rest.

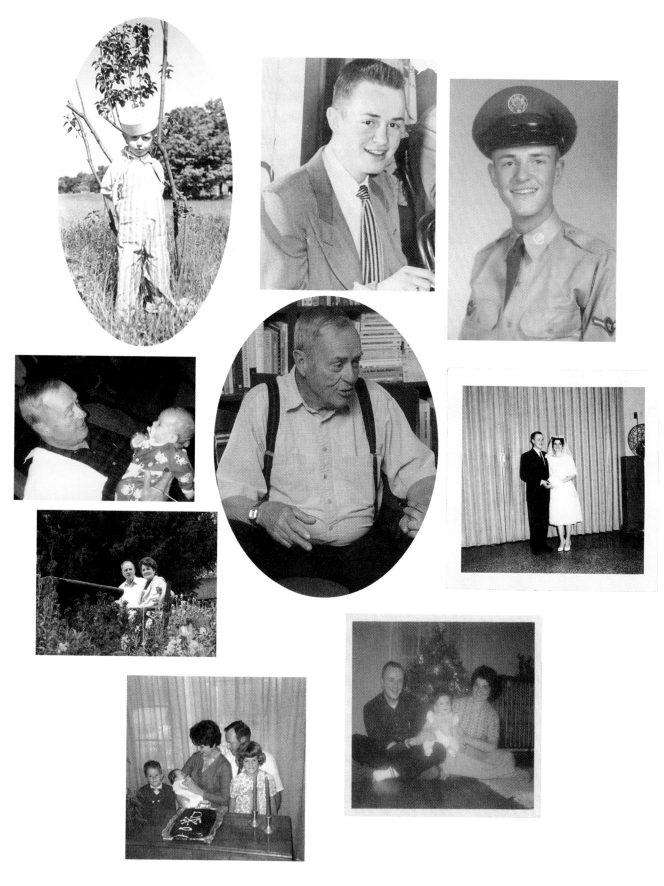

Fig. 8-2. Remember that clients are people, not just a list of illnesses or disabilities. They have many needs, just like you. Many have had rich lives with many wonderful experiences. Take time to experience and care for your clients as whole people.

❑ 3. Discuss family roles and their significance in health care

Families are the most important unit within our social system, and families play a huge role in many people's lives. Some examples of family types are listed below.

▶ Single parent families include one parent with a child or children.

▶ Nuclear families include two parents with a child or children.

▶ Blended families include widowed or divorced parents who have remarried, with children from previous marriages as well as from this marriage.

▶ Multigenerational families include parents, children, and grandparents.

▶ Extended families may include aunts, uncles, cousins, or even friends.

▶ Families may also be made up of unmarried couples of the same sex or opposite sexes, with or without children.

Today a family is defined more by a commitment to supporting each other than by the particular people involved. Your clients' families may not look

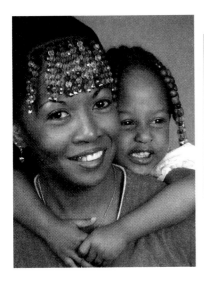
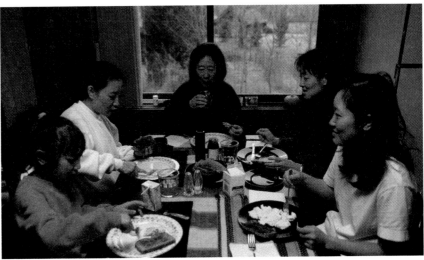
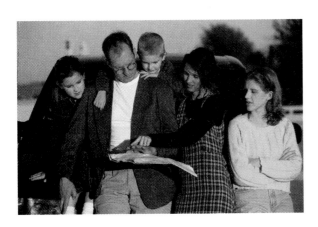
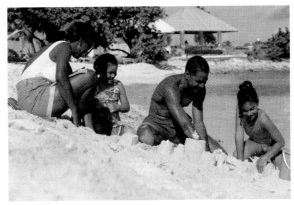
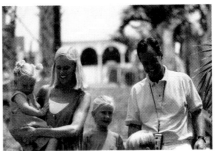

Fig. 8-3. Families come in many shapes and sizes.

like the kind of family you are used to. Clients with no living relatives may have friends or neighbors who function as a family. Whatever kinds of families your clients have, recognize the important role they can play in health care. There are many functions families or family members may serve, including any of the following:

▶ helping clients make care decisions

▶ communicating with the care team

▶ providing daily care when home care aide is not present

▶ giving support and encouragement

▶ connecting the client to the outside world

▶ giving assurance to dying clients that family memories and traditions will be valued and carried on

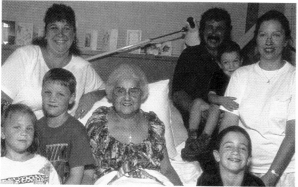

Fig. 8-4. Families play an important part in making sure the client is not isolated from the outside world.

❏ 4. Describe personal adjustments of the individual and family to illness and disability

Illness or disability require individuals and families to make adjustments. Making these adjustments may be more or less difficult depending on the family's emotional, spiritual, and financial resources. Some of the adjustments that illness or disability may require include the following.

▶ accepting the illness or disability and its long term consequences or results

▶ finding money needed to pay expenses of hospitalization or home care

▶ dealing with paperwork involved in insurance, Medicaid, or Medicare benefits

▶ taking care of tasks the client can no longer handle

▶ understanding medical information and making difficult care decisions

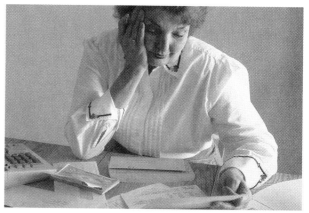

Fig. 8-5. Family members may have a hard time adjusting to the additional responsibilities when a loved one becomes ill or disabled.

▶ providing daily care when the aide can't be there

Be sensitive to the tremendous adjustments your clients and their families may be making. Help them by doing your job well, and refer them to your supervisor or another member of the health care team, such as a social worker, if you think more help is needed.

❏ 5. Identify community resources for individual and family health

The larger community — the local government or social service agencies, church or synagogue — can provide families with resources to help them through difficult times and help them resolve their problems. Such resources can include meal or transportation services, hospice care (HA-spis, or care for the dying), counseling, and support groups. Be familiar with resources available in your community. If clients or their families ask you for more help, refer them to these resources. If no one asks, but you think some help is needed, speak to your supervisor.

❏ 6. List three ways to respond to the emotional needs of your clients and their families

When clients or family members come to you with problems or needs, you may choose to respond in many ways. Your response will depend on how comfortable you feel with emotions in general, how well you know the client or family member, and what need or problem is brought up. Try to empathize (EM-pa-thyze), or understand how the person feels. The following are three good ways to respond in this situation:

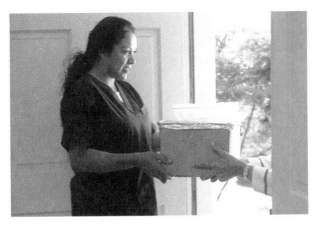

Fig. 8-6. Many communities offer "Meals on Wheels" or similar services to provide nutritious meals to people unable to cook for themselves. Being aware of the services available in your area can help improve your clients' situations.

Listen. Often just talking about a problem or concern can make it easier to handle. Sitting quietly and letting someone talk or cry may be the most help you can give in some situations.

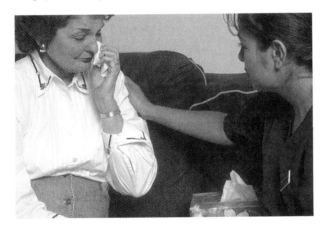

Fig. 8-7. Sometimes just listening to someone is the best way to provide emotional support.

Offer support and encouragement. Saying things like "You have really been under a lot of stress, haven't you?" or "I can imagine that really is scary," can provide a lot of comfort. Avoid using clichés (kli-SHAYS, or common phrases that really don't mean anything), like "I know how you feel," or "It'll all work out." You probably don't know exactly how the person feels, and things may not all work out. It is more comforting to the client if you acknowledge how hard the situation is rather than simply dismiss her feelings with a cliché.

Refer the problem to a social worker or your supervisor. When you feel that you cannot provide what the person needs, or when someone is asking you for help outside your scope of practice, get someone else on the care team to handle the situation. Say something like, "Mrs. Pfeiffer, I'm really not qualified to help you make a decision about your husband's care, but I can have my supervisor call you to talk it over."

❑ 7. Identify ways to help clients meet their spiritual needs

Helping clients meet their spiritual needs can help them cope with illness or disability and have a positive impact on their health and well being. While there are some things you can do to encourage clients to address these needs, spirituality is a sensitive area, and you must be careful not to offend your clients by making judgements or imposing your beliefs.

Following are some ways you can help clients meet their spiritual needs:

▶ Learn a little bit about your client's religion or beliefs.

▶ Accommodate practices such as dietary restrictions, and never make judgements about them.

▶ Get to know the priest, rabbi, or minister who visits or calls your client.

▶ If a client asks you, help find spiritual resources available in the area. The yellow pages usually list churches, synagogues, and other houses of worship.

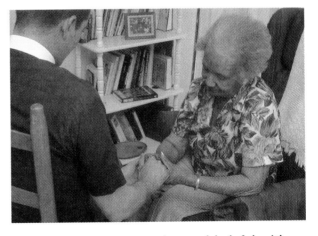

Fig. 8-8. Be encouraging and helpful with regard to your clients' spiritual needs. Do not impose your beliefs on clients or judge them for theirs. Do be open to your clients' beliefs and welcoming when they receive visits from a priest, rabbi, minister, or other spiritual leader.

Chapter 9

The Human Body in Health and Disease

You will learn to:

☑ 1. Describe the basic structure and function of each body system.

☑ 2. List the common disorders of each body system.

☑ 3. List signs and symptoms of common diseases and conditions of each body system.

☑ 4. Describe changes in each body system that must be reported to a supervisor immediately.

At some point in our lives, we are all affected by illness or injury. For most of us, the effects are acute (a-KYOOT), or intense and short-lived. For others, chronic (KRON-ik), or long-term problems occur that require special care. Many people who develop chronic illnesses or who suffer debilitating (dee-BIL-i-tay-ting) injuries (injuries that weaken or disable a person) are cared for at home by skilled caregivers, including home care aides. Because their bodies are unable to work as they should, these clients need assistance in meeting their basic needs.

Many of the illnesses or injuries you will see as a home care aide begin by affecting an organ in the body. An **organ** performs a specific function, for example, the heart pumps blood throughout the body. A group of organs works together as a **system** that performs a job for the body. All of the body's systems work together to make the body function. Because all the body's systems depend on each other for proper functioning, injury or disease in one part of a system affects other parts of that system, and eventually, other systems. Over time, a malfunctioning organ causes stress on other organs and systems, and a negative chain reaction occurs. This chain reaction can lead to failure of all the body's systems, and death (**Fig. 9-1**).

Each system in the body has a condition under which it works best. Homeostasis (hoh-mee-oh- STAY-sis) is the name for the condition in which all of the body's systems are working their best. In order for a body to be in homeostasis, its metabolism (me-TAB-oh-lism), or physical and chemical processes, must be operating at a steady level. When disease or injury occur, the body's metabolism is disturbed and homeostasis is lost. Changes in metabolic (me-tah-BOL-ic) processes are called **signs and symptoms**. For instance, changes in body temperature could indicate that the body is fighting an infection. Changes in pulse indicate that the body is trying to increase blood circulation to meet a new demand. Noticing and reporting changes in your clients is a very important part of your job, because the changes you notice could be signs of significant problems.

Each system in the body has its own unique structure and function. The body's systems can be broken down in different ways. In

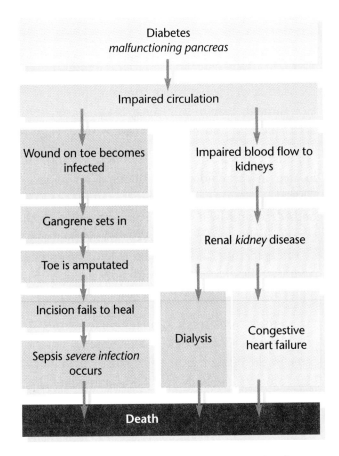

Diabetes
malfunctioning pancreas

↓

Impaired circulation

↓   ↓

Wound on toe becomes infected   Impaired blood flow to kidneys

↓

Gangrene sets in   Renal *kidney* disease

↓

Toe is amputated

↓   ↓   ↓

Incision fails to heal

Dialysis   Congestive heart failure

↓

Sepsis *severe infection* occurs

↓   ↓   ↓

Death

Fig. 9-1. A malfunctioning organ can lead to a chain reaction that ends in death.

3. Nervous (NERV-us)
4. Circulatory (SER-kyoo-la-tor-ee) or cardiovascular (kar-dee-oh-VAS-kyoo-lar)
5. Respiratory (RES-spir-a-tor-ee)
6. Urinary (YOOR-i-nayr-ee)
7. Digestive (di-JEST-iv) or gastrointestinal
8. Endocrine (EN-doh-krin)
9. Reproductive (ree-pro-DUK-tiv)
10. Immune (i-MYOON)
11. Lymphatic (lim-FAT-ik)

The body systems can be damaged by trauma, infection, genetics (birth defects or conditions that develop or worsen with time), or exposure to chemicals and toxins. Such damage can lead to disease that is acute or chronic. Both acute and chronic illnesses can cause disruption of the normal functions of the body, discomfort, disability, and even death. Chronic illnesses that gradually get worse with time are known as **progressive** or **degenerative** conditions.

Body systems are made up of organs. Organs are made up of **tissues**. Tissues are made up of groups of cells that perform a similar function. For example, in the circulatory system, the heart is one of the organs, and it is made up of tissues and cells. **Cells** are the building blocks of our bodies. Living cells divide, develop, and die, renewing the tissues and organs of our body systems (**Fig. 9-2**).

this book we divide the human body into eleven body systems.

1. Integumentary (in-teg-you-MEN-tar-ee), or skin
2. Musculoskeletal (mus-kyoo-lo-SKEL-e-tal)

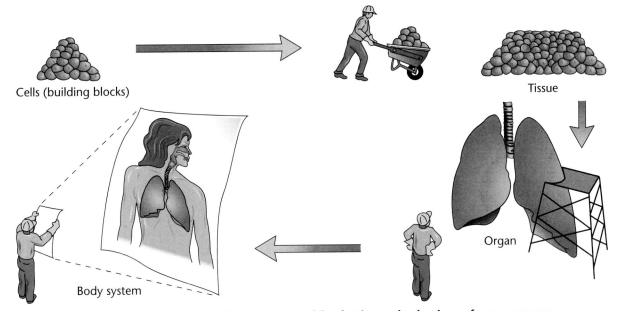

Cells (building blocks)

Tissue

Organ

Body system

Fig. 9-2. Cells are the building blocks of body tissue; body tissue forms organs; and organs make up body systems.

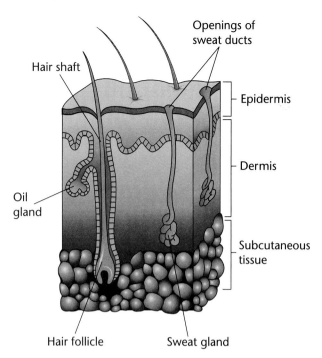

Fig. 9-3. Cross-section showing details of integumentary system.

Hair shaft
Openings of sweat ducts
Epidermis
Dermis
Oil gland
Subcutaneous tissue
Hair follicle
Sweat gland

❑ 1. The Integumentary System

The largest organ and system in the body is the skin, a natural protective covering or integument (in-TEG-you-ment). Skin prevents injury to internal organs and protects the body against entry of bacterial organisms. It prevents the loss of excessive amounts of water, which is essential to life. Skin is made up of tissues and **glands** (structures that secrete fluids).

The skin is also a **sense organ** that feels heat, cold, pain, touch, and pressure, and then tells the brain what it is feeling. Body temperature is also regulated in the skin, which has blood vessels that dilate (DYE-late, or widen) when the outside temperature is too high, bringing more blood to the body surface to cool it off during evaporation. The same blood vessels **constrict** (narrow) when the outside temperature is too cold. By restricting the amount of blood reaching the skin, the blood vessels help the body retain heat.

The blood vessels, called capillaries (KAP-il-ayr-ees), are located in the **dermis,** the inner layer of skin. The dermis also contains nerves, **sweat glands, oil glands,** and hair roots. Sweat glands help regulate body temperature by secreting **sweat,** a fluid that contains mostly water, but also salt and a small amount of waste products. Sweat comes to the body surface through **pores,** or tiny openings in the skin, and cools the body as it evaporates. Oil glands in the dermis secrete oil, which comes to the skin surface through hair follicles (FOL-i-kuls, or roots). Oil keeps the skin and hair soft (**Fig. 9-3**).

No blood vessels and only a few nerve endings are located in the **epidermis,** or outer layer of skin. Thinner than the dermis, the epidermis contains both dead and living cells. The dead cells, which are eventually sloughed off (worn off), began deeper in the epidermis and were pushed to the surface as other cells divided. The epidermis also contains pigment cells that give the skin its color.

Hair grows from roots located in the dermis. It grows through hair follicles that extend upward through the epidermis to the outside of the body. Hair protects the body from heat and cold. Hair inside the nose and ears also protects the body from particles and germs trying to enter the body.

Common Disorders of the Integumentary System

Pressure sores. A common illness of the integumentary system is **pressure sores,** or decubitus (dee-KYOO-bi-tus) **ulcers** (**Fig. 9-4**). Pressure sores occur when the skin deteriorates (breaks up) from pressure and **shearing** (pressure from sliding skin across another surface). Eventually blood does not circulate properly and sores or ulcers form, swell, and may become infected.

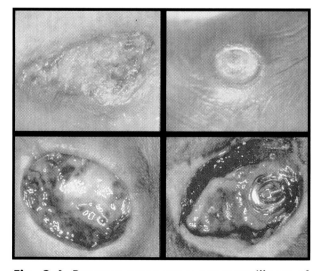

Fig. 9-4. Pressure sores are a common illness of the integumentary system.

Pressure sores usually occur in areas of the body where bone is close to the skin, with little fat or muscle for padding. Common sites for pressure sores are the heels, elbows, and sacrum, or lower part of the spinal column (**Fig. 9-5**). When a client is confined to bed for long periods of time and is unable to move, pressure on a body part reduces circulation of blood to the area. As a consequence, the skin in that region receives less oxygen and nutrients, and cells and tissue begin to break down. Pressure sores can become large and deep, affecting muscle and requiring skin grafts. The sores or ulcers can also become infected.

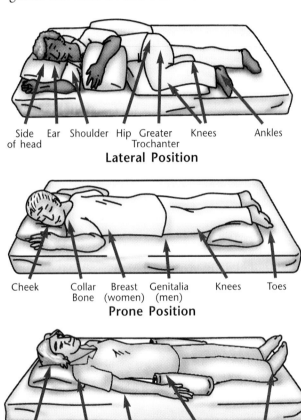

Fig. 9-5. Pressure sore danger zones.

Pressure sores can be prevented by good care: careful observation of the skin, frequent position changes, and good skin care, including regular bathing and lubricating dry skin. Other ways to prevent pressure sores include using devices such as special mattresses, egg crate mattress covers, sheepskin pads, and elbow and heel pads. These devices are designed to reduce pressure on areas at risk of developing pressure sores. Chapters 12 and 13 provide more information on position changes, skin care, and pressure sore prevention.

Observing and Reporting: Integumentary System

During daily care, the client's skin should be observed for changes that may indicate disease. Any of the following conditions can be signs of illness and should be reported to your supervisor immediately:

- rashes or scales
- bruising
- cuts, boils, sores, wounds, abrasions
- changes in color or moistness/dryness
- swelling
- scalp or hair changes
- skin that appears different from normal or that has changed

❑ 2. The Musculoskeletal System

Muscles, **bones**, **ligaments**, **tendons**, and cartilage (KAR-ti-lidj) give the body shape and structure. They work together as a system of pulleys and levers to allow the body to move.

Bones. The skeleton, or framework, of the human body has 206 bones. Bones are hard and rigid, but are made up of living cells. Blood vessels supply oxygen and nutrients to the bones just as they do to other tissues of the body. Besides allowing our bodies to move, another function of our bones is to protect our organs. For example, the skull protects the brain and the **vertebrae** (VERT-e-bray) protect the spinal cord.

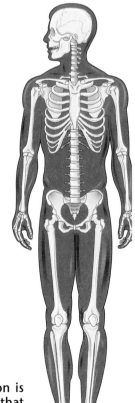

Fig. 9-6. The skeleton is composed of 206 bones that facilitate movement and protect organs.

Joints. Two bones meet at a joint. Different types of joints allow different types of movement.

1) The **ball and socket joint**, in which the round end of one bone fits into the hollow end of the other bone, makes movement possible in all directions. The hip and shoulder joints are examples.

2) The **hinge joint**, like the hinge of a door, permits movement in one direction only. The elbow and knee are hinge joints. They only bend in one direction.

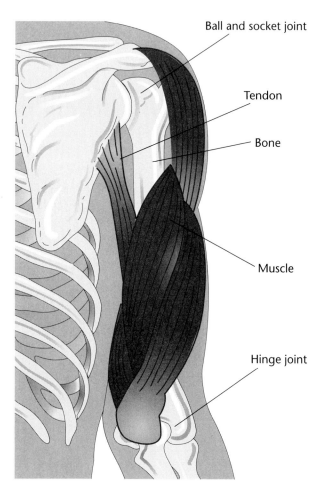

Fig. 9-7. Muscles are connected to bone by tendons. Bones meet at different types of joints, including the ball and socket joint and the hinge joint shown here.

Muscles. Muscles provide movement of body parts to maintain body posture and to produce body heat. Muscles can be **voluntary** or **involuntary**. Voluntary muscles are also called **skeletal muscles**. They are attached to bones and we can move them when we want. Examples of voluntary muscles are the arm (bicep and tricep) and leg (quadricep) muscles, which we consciously control. Involuntary muscles cannot be consciously controlled, but they act automatically to regulate the movement of our organs and blood vessels. Examples of involuntary muscles are the heart and the **diaphragm** (DYE-a-fram, the muscle that makes us breathe).

Activity and Mobility. The musculoskeletal system is directed by the nervous system to move the body to action. To stay healthy physically and mentally, the body must be mobile and active. Physical activity reduces tension and stress, improving a person's mental state. A good mental state can help prevent physical disease. Physical activity also promotes health and well-being in other ways. It improves the lungs' ability to take in oxygen. It improves circulation, increasing the amount of blood pumped to vital organs and other tissues, including the skin and muscles, and allowing body systems to work their best.

Inactivity and immobility can result in mental and physical problems, including loss of self-esteem, depression, pneumonia, urinary tract infection, constipation, blood clots, and dulling of the senses. Clients who are ill or elderly can develop muscle **atrophy** (AT-roh-fee) or **contractures** (kon-TRAK-churz) as a result. When atrophy occurs, the muscle wastes away, decreases in size, and becomes weak. When a contracture develops, the muscle shortens, becomes inflexible, and "freezes" in position, causing permanent disability of the limb.

Range of motion (ROM) exercises can help prevent these conditions. With ROM exercises, the joints are extended and flexed in the measured degrees of a circle (**Fig. 9-8**). Exercise increases circulation of blood, oxygen, and nutrients and improves muscle tone. Regardless of physical condition, all clients typically should have some form of exercise included in the care plan. Exercise can range from simple ROMs, to walking with assistance, to specific exercise ordered by the physician and monitored by a physical therapist on the care team.

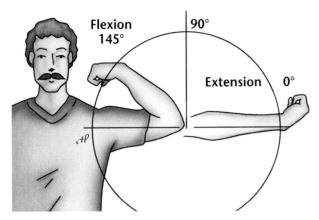

Fig. 9-8. A complete circle is 360°. Degrees of a circle are used to determine how far the client's joints flex or extend during ROM exercises.

When caring for clients with musculoskeletal problems, pay attention to activity orders in the client's care plan. Clients who need help in movement should be moved cautiously, and if limbs are moved, they should be supported at each joint. Clients who are confined to bed usually have orders in the care plan for ROM exercises to maintain muscle tone, improve circulation, and prevent joint stiffness. ROM exercises may be active (client does the exercises himself), or passive (aide moves the client's limbs and joints through the exercises). Chapter 15, Promoting Independence: Rehabilitation and Restorative Care, provides more information on ROM exercises.

Common Disorders of the Musculoskeletal System

A fracture (FRAKT-chur) is a broken bone. To treat fractures, bones are held immobile (by a cast if possible) until the bone can fuse itself back together. This process can take longer in elderly clients than in younger people.

Osteoporosis (os-tee-oh-poh-ROH-sis) is a disease that causes bones to become porous and brittle. Brittle bones can fracture easily, so home care aides must be very careful when helping clients with osteoporosis. Osteoporosis develops in varying degrees as persons age, but it occurs most commonly in women after menopause (MEN-oh-paws, or stopping of men-

strual periods). Osteoporosis can be prevented by adding extra calcium to the diet and exercising to strengthen bones. Signs and symptoms of osteoporosis include low back pain, stooped posture, and becoming shorter over time (**Fig. 9-9**).

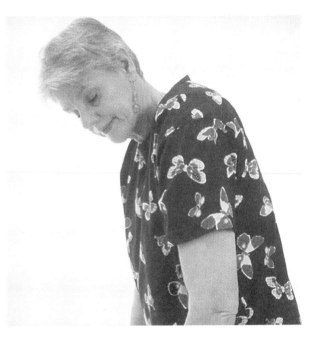

Fig. 9-9. Stooped posture is a common sign of osteoporosis.

Arthritis (ar-THRYE-tis) is inflammation, or swelling, of a joint. It can result in pain and difficulty with movement. Swelling can also cause muscle damage, making it difficult or impossible for the client to move, or reducing muscle strength. More information on caring for clients with arthritis is provided in Chapter 20, Common Chronic and Acute Conditions.

Observing and Reporting: Musculoskeletal System

Observe and report the following:

- changes in ability to perform routine movements and activities
- any changes in clients' ability to perform ROM exercises
- pain during movement
- any new or increased swelling of joints
- white, shiny, red, or hot areas over a joint

- bruising
- aches and pains clients report to you

❑ 3. The Nervous System

The nervous system is the control center and message center of the body. It controls and coordinates all body functions. The nervous system also senses and interprets information from the environment outside the human body.

The **neuron** (NEW-ron), or nerve cell, is the basic unit of the nervous system. Neurons transmit messages or sensations from the **receptors**, located in different parts of the body, through the **spinal cord**, to the brain (**Fig. 9-10**). For example, if your hand touches a hot stove, receptors in your hand transmit a message that travels through your neurons and spinal cord to your brain. The message is a sensation of heat. Your brain then reacts to the message, sending a message back to your hand to pull away from the stove. The brief time it takes for your brain to get the message that you have touched something hot, and to react, shows how quickly a healthy nervous system works. However, nerves are easily injured and they heal slowly. Disorders of the nervous system can be extremely debilitating.

The nervous system has two main parts: the **central nervous system (CNS)** and the peripheral (per-IF-er-al) **nervous system** (**Fig. 9-11**). The central nervous system is composed of the brain and spinal cord. The peripheral nervous system deals with the

periphery, or outer part of the body via the **nerves** that extend throughout the body.

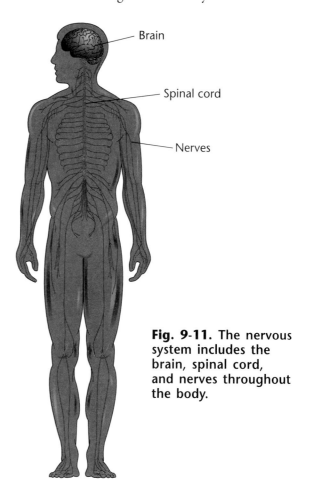

Fig. 9-11. The nervous system includes the brain, spinal cord, and nerves throughout the body.

The Central Nervous System. The brain is housed within the skull. The spinal cord is housed within the spinal column, extending from the brain into the trunk of the body. Both the brain and the spinal cord are covered by a protective membrane made up of three layers. Between two of these layers is the cerebrospinal (sir-ee-broh-SPYE-nal) **fluid**. This fluid circulates around the brain and spinal cord, providing a protective cushion against injuries.

The brain has three main sections: the cerebrum (sir-EE-brum), the cerebellum (sayr-e-BEL-um), and the **brainstem** (**Fig. 9-12**). The largest section of the human brain is the cerebrum. The outside layer of the cerebrum is called the cerebral cortex (sir-EE-bral KOR-tex), the part of the brain in which thinking, analysis, association of ideas, judgement, emotions, and memory occur. The cerebral cortex also

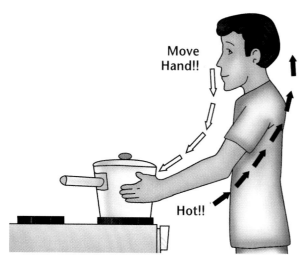

Fig. 9-10. Neurons pass messages from receptors to the brain and back again.

directs speech and emotional response; interprets messages from the eyes, ears, nose, tongue, and skin; and controls voluntary muscle movement.

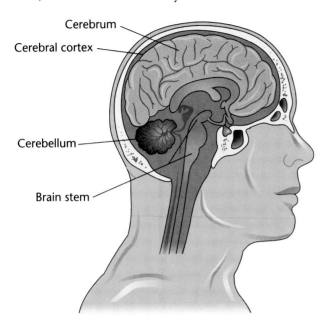

Cerebrum

Cerebral cortex

Cerebellum

Brain stem

Fig. 9-12. The three main sections of the brain are the cerebrum, the brainstem, and the cerebellum.

The cerebrum is divided into two halves, the right and the left hemispheres (HEM-is-fears). The right hemisphere controls movement and function in the left side of the body. The left hemisphere controls movement and function in the right side of the body. Any illness or injury to the right hemisphere affects functions on the left side of the body. Illness or injury to the left hemisphere causes disruption of function on the right side.

The cerebellum controls balance and regulates the body's voluntary muscles, producing and coordinating smooth movements. Someone who has a problem in the cerebellum will be uncoordinated and show jerky movements and muscle weakness.

The cerebrum and cerebellum are connected to the spinal cord by the brainstem. The brainstem contains a kind of regulatory center that controls heart rate, breathing, swallowing, coughing, vomiting, and constriction or dilation of blood vessels.

The spinal cord is connected to the brain and is protected by the bones of the spinal column. Nerve pathways run through the spinal cord, conducting messages between the brain and the body.

Common Disorders of the Central Nervous System

Common illnesses of the central nervous system are dementias (dee-MEN-shee-ahs), including Alzheimer's (ALTZ-high-mers) **disease** and **Parkinson's disease; multiple** sclerosis (skle-ROH-sis); epilepsy (EP-i-lep-see); and cerebral palsy (SER-ee-bral PAL-zee).

Dementia is a general term that refers to changes in the brain that alter personality and impair the ability to think and remember. Dementia usually occurs in the elderly as a result of diminished blood supply to the brain or chemical changes that occur for unknown reasons.

Alzheimer's disease is an example of a dementia with an unknown cause. It cannot be cured, is irreversible, and gets progressively worse. Alzheimer's disease can affect middle adults as well as the elderly. More information on caring for clients with Alzheimer's disease can be found in Chapter 20, Common Chronic and Acute Conditions.

Parkinson's disease, another illness that commonly occurs in the elderly, causes a section of the brain to degenerate slowly and progressively. However, mental function is not impaired in the early stages. Symptoms of Parkinson's disease include tremors (shaking) that may be most noticeable when the person tries to complete a task like picking up a glass full of water. A person with Parkinson's disease may also rub together the finger and thumb of one hand in a motion called "pill rolling." Other signs and symptoms include a mask-like facial expression, slurred or monotone speech, drooling, muscle stiffness and weakness, slow movements, stooped posture, and a shuffling **gait,** or walk. As the disease progresses, the person may become confused and forgetful.

Multiple sclerosis (MS) usually affects young and middle adults. When a person has MS, the myelin

(MYE-e-lin) **sheath** that covers the nerves, spinal cord, and white matter of the brain breaks down over time. Without the myelin sheath, the nerves cannot conduct impulses to and from the brain in a normal way. The first symptoms of MS typically occur in the early twenties and thirties. Signs and symptoms include blurred vision, tremors, poor balance, difficulty walking, weakness, numbness and tingling, dizziness, poor coordination, incontinence, and behavior changes. Clients with MS can eventually develop blindness, muscle contractures, respiratory distress, and **quadriplegia** (kwad-ri-PLEE-jee-a), or loss of function in the arms, trunk, and legs.

Epilepsy is an illness of the brain that produces seizures. Epileptic seizures can range from mild tremors or brief blackouts to violent convulsions lasting several minutes. We do not know what causes most cases of epilepsy; however, the disease can sometimes be caused by excessive alcohol intake, substance abuse, brain tumors, or injuries.

Cerebral palsy is the result of an injury to the cerebrum that occurs during pregnancy or the birth process. The resulting brain damage causes a loss of muscle control, poor coordination, problems with balance, and difficulty in speaking.

Head and spinal cord injuries commonly occur in teenagers and young adults because of risk-taking behaviors common in those age groups. Diving, gymnastics, or other sports injuries, and car and motorcycle accidents are common causes of these injuries. Head injuries can cause permanent brain damage. The extent of spinal cord injuries depends on the force of the impact and where on the spinal cord the injury is located. The higher the site of injury in the spinal cord, the greater the loss of function. People with head and spinal cord injuries may have **paraplegia** (payr- a-PLEE-jee-a) and be unable to move or use their legs. Head and spinal cord injuries may also cause quadriplegia, in which the person is unable to use his legs, trunk, and arms.

Observing and reporting: Central Nervous System

Observe your clients carefully and report any of the following signs and symptoms:

▶ fatigue or pain with movement or exercise
▶ shaking or trembling
▶ inability to speak clearly
▶ inability to move one side of body
▶ disturbance or change in vision or hearing
▶ changes in eating patterns or fluid intake
▶ difficulty swallowing
▶ bowel and bladder changes
▶ depression or mood changes
▶ memory loss or confusion
▶ violent behavior
▶ any unusual or unexplained change in behavior
▶ decreased ability to perform ADLs

The Nervous System: Sense Organs

The eyes, ears, nose, tongue, and skin are the body's major sense organs. They are considered part of the central nervous system because they contain receptors that receive impulses from the environment and relay these impulses to nerves. Changes in the sense organs occur as we age. These changes are discussed later in this chapter and throughout the book. The sense organs and common disorders are described in the next few pages.

The eye, which is approximately an inch in diameter, is located in a bony socket in the skull. The bony socket protects the eye, which is surrounded

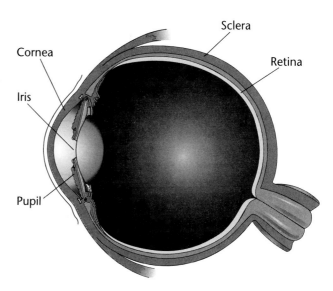

Fig. 9-13. The parts of the eye.

by muscles that control its movements (**Fig. 9-13**). The outer part of the eye is called the sclera (SKLAYR-a). The sclera appears white, except in front, where it is called the cornea (KORN-ee-a). The cornea is actually clear, but it appears colored because it lies over the iris (EYE-ris), which is the colored part of the eye. The pupil (PYOO-pil), or black circle in the center of the iris, dilates (widens) or constricts (narrows) to adjust the amount of light that enters the eye. Inside the back of the eye is the retina (RET-in-a), which contains cells that respond to light and send a message to the brain, where the picture is interpreted so you can "see."

The ear is a sense organ that provides balance and hearing. It is divided into three parts: the **external ear**, the **middle ear**, and the **inner ear** (**Fig. 9-14**). The external ear is the funnel-shaped outer part, sometimes called the auricle (OR-i-kul) or pinna (PIN-na), that guides sound waves into the auditory (AW-di-tor-ee) **canal**. This canal is approximately one-inch long and contains many glands that secrete cerumen (se-ROO-men), or earwax. Cerumen and hair in the ear protect the ear from foreign substances. The **eardrum**, which is also called the tympanic (tim-PAN-ik) **membrane**, separates the external ear from the middle ear.

The middle ear consists of the eustachian (you-STAY-kee-an) **tube** and three ossicles (OSS-i-kuls), small bones that amplify sound transmitted by the eardrum. The ossicles transmit sound to the inner ear. The eustachian tube, which connects the middle ear to the throat, functions to allow air into the middle ear to equalize pressure on the tympanic membrane. The inner ear contains fluid that carries sound waves from the middle ear to the auditory nerve, which then transmits the impulse to the brain. The inner ear also contains structures that help in maintaining balance.

Common Disorders of the Eyes and Ears

Cataracts (KAT-a-rakts), milky or cloudy spots that develop in the eye, are common in the elderly. Cataracts eventually impair vision and can affect one or both eyes. They can be surgically removed, and an artificial lens is usually implanted. After cataract surgery, clients must avoid bending over, sneezing, or falling for several days. Glaucoma (glaw-KOH-ma) is a condition in which the fluid inside the eyeball is unable to drain. Pressure inside the eye increases and causes damage that often leads to blindness. Glaucoma is less common than cataracts.

Otitis media (oh-TYE-tis MEE-dee-a) is an infection of the middle ear that can be caused by a variety

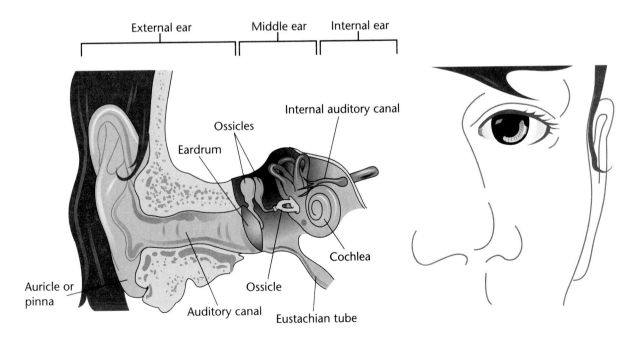

Fig. 9-14. The external ear, middle ear, and inner ear are the three main divisions of the ear.

of microorganisms. Middle ear infection occurs commonly in children, especially some bottle-fed babies, as the result of respiratory infections and accumulation of fluid in the ear. **Deafness** is partial or complete loss of hearing. It can occur as the result of heredity, disease, or injury. Vertigo (VER-ti-goh), or dizziness, is usually the result of an inner ear disturbance, but it can also be caused by diseases of the brain. In the elderly, the aging process commonly causes loss of hearing, as well as impaired vision, smell, and taste.

Observing and reporting: Eye and Ear

Report any of the following observations about your clients to your supervisor immediately:

▶ changes in vision or hearing

▶ signs of infection

▶ dizziness

▶ client complaints of pain in eyes or ears

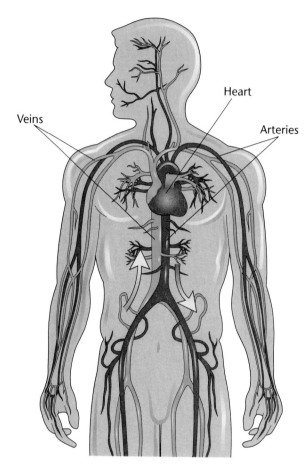

Fig. 9-15. The heart, blood vessels, and blood are the main components of the circulatory system.

Veins

Heart

Arteries

❑ 4. The Circulatory or Cardiovascular System

The circulatory system is made up of the heart, blood vessels, and blood (**Fig. 9-15**). The heart pumps blood through the blood vessels to the cells. The blood carries food, oxygen, and other substances that are essential for the cells to function properly.

The circulatory system performs the following major functions:

▶ supplying food, oxygen, and hormones to cells

▶ producing and supplying antibodies and other infection-fighting blood cells

▶ removing waste products from cells

▶ controlling body temperature: blood vessels in the skin constrict to keep heat in the body and dilate to release heat and cool the body

A healthy cardiovascular system is essential for life. Cells, tissues, and organs need adequate circulation to function well. If circulation is reduced, cells do not receive adequate oxygen and nutrients, waste products of cell metabolism are not removed, and organs become diseased.

Blood contains blood cells and **plasma**. Plasma carries many substances, including blood cells, nutrients, and waste products. Analyzing the following components in blood samples can help identify illness and infection.

Red blood cells carry oxygen from the lungs to all parts of the body. Red blood cells are produced by bone marrow (MAR-oh), a substance found inside our hollow bones. Iron, found in bone marrow and red blood cells, is essential to our blood, and gives it its red color. Red blood cells function for a short time, then die and are filtered out of the blood by the liver and spleen. Iron in our diets allows our bodies to produce new red blood cells.

White blood cells defend the body against foreign substances, such as bacteria and viruses. When the body becomes aware of these invaders, white blood cells rush to the site of infection and multiply rapidly. The bone marrow, spleen, and thymus gland produce white blood cells.

Platelets are also carried by the blood. They cause the blood to clot, preventing excess bleeding. Platelets are also produced by the bone marrow.

The heart is the pump of the circulatory system. The heart is a muscle located in the middle lower chest, pointing to the left side. The heart muscle is made up of three layers: the **peri-cardium** (payr-i-KAR-dee-um), the outer sac; the **myocardium** (mye-oh-KAR-dee-um), a thick, muscular, middle layer; and the **endocardium** (en-doh-KAR-dee-um), an inner layer that lines the chambers of the heart.

The interior of the heart is divided into four chambers (**Fig. 9-16**). The two upper chambers, called **atria** (AY-tree-a) or the left atrium and right atrium, receive blood. The two lower chambers or **ventricles** (VEN-tri-kuls) pump blood. The right atrium receives blood from the veins. This blood, containing carbon dioxide, then flows into the right ventricle, where it is pumped to the blood vessels in the lungs, and carbon dioxide is exchanged for oxygen. The heart's left atrium receives the oxygen-saturated blood, which then flows into the left ventricle where it is pumped through the arteries to all parts of the body. Two valves, one located between the right atrium and right ventricle and the other between the left atrium and left ventricle, allow the blood to flow in only one direction.

The heart functions in two phases: 1) the resting phase or **diastole** (dye-AS-toh-lee), when the chambers fill with blood, and 2) the contracting phase or **systole** (SIS-toh-lee), when the ventricles pump blood through the blood vessels. When a person's blood pressure is taken, the numbers measure these two phases.

Three types of **blood vessels** are found in the body: arteries (AR-ter-ees), capillaries (KAP-i-layr-ees), and veins (vayns).

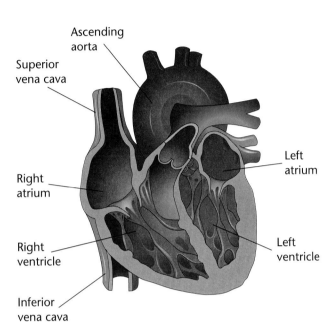

Fig. 9-16. The four chambers of the heart connect to the body's largest blood vessels.

Labels: Ascending aorta; Superior vena cava; Right atrium; Right ventricle; Inferior vena cava; Left atrium; Left ventricle

Arteries carry oxygen-rich blood away from the heart. The blood is pumped from the left ventricle, through the aorta (ay-OR-ta), the largest artery, and then through other arteries that branch off from it, including the coronary (KOR-oh-nayr-ee) **arteries** that carry blood to the heart itself (**Fig. 9-16**).

Capillaries are tiny blood vessels that receive blood from the arteries. Nutrients, oxygen, and other substances in the blood pass from the cap-illaries to the cells. Waste products, including car-bon dioxide, pass from the cells into the capillaries.

Veins carry the blood containing waste products from the capillaries back to the heart. Near the heart, the veins branch together to form the two largest veins, the inferior vena cava (in-FEER-ee-or VEE-na KAY-va) and the superior vena cava (soo-PEER-ee-or VEE-na KAY-va), which empty into the right atrium of the heart (**Fig. 9-16**). The inferior vena cava carries blood from the legs and trunk. The superior vena cava carries blood from the arms, head, and neck.

Common Disorders of the Cardiovascular System

Atherosclerosis (ath-er-oh-skle-ROH-sis) is a disease process in which fat is deposited between the inner and middle layers of the blood vessels. Numerous fat deposits eventually harden and cause the walls of the blood vessels to become less flexible. These hardened deposits prevent blood from flowing as it should to certain parts of the body, causing all kinds of physical changes. Clots form around the fat deposits, making it even more difficult for blood to flow to the organs. This is especially serious when blood flow is reduced to the heart or the brain. Clots can also detach and flow to another area, where they block other blood vessels, thus interfering with the blood supply to the area that vessel nourishes.

Myocardial infarction (MI) (mye-oh-KAR-dee-al in-FARK-shun), or **heart attack**, occurs when the heart muscle itself does not receive enough oxygen because blood vessels are blocked. Someone having an MI, or heart attack, will experience shortness of breath and a crushing, vise-like pain in the center of the chest. This pain may extend or radiate down the left arm or to the neck region. Early in a heart attack, the discomfort may be dismissed as indigestion. The pain may also be felt in the abdomen, causing it to be mistaken for a gallbladder attack. Myocardial infarction is a life-threatening condition, but early medical intervention improves the chances of survival. Clients who recover from an MI have permanent heart damage, but most can resume their activities with some restrictions. Chapter 7, Emergency Care and Disaster Preparation, provides information on what to do if you suspect a client is having an MI.

Angina pectoris (an-JYE-na PEK-tor-is) is a condition that causes temporary constriction of a coronary artery. This condition sometimes occurs in clients who have **coronary artery disease**. Angina is a squeezing pain or feeling of pressure in the chest, left arm, or jaw. The spasm of the vessel temporarily restricts blood flow and oxygen to the heart. Angina can be a warning sign of an impending heart attack. It can be brought on by cold or stress and can be treated with medication.

A cerebrovascular (se-ree-broh-VAS-kyoo-lar) **accident (CVA)**, or **stroke,** occurs when blood supply to a part of the brain suddenly decreases as the result of a blocked or burst blood vessel. A CVA can cause sudden **paresis** (weakness) or **paralysis** (immobility) of certain parts of the body. Paresis

and paralysis usually affect one side of the body. Depending on the region of the brain that has been damaged, other functions of the body may be impaired, including the ability to speak and swallow. The location and the extent of injury to the brain determines whether the effects of a stroke are temporary or permanent. Rehabilitation therapy improves the outcome for many clients who have had a CVA.

Hypertension (high-per-TEN-shun) or **high blood pressure** affects a large percentage of people, and is generally thought to be caused by heredity and poor circulation resulting from hardening of the arteries. Hypertension is especially common in smokers, people with hyperlipidemia (high-per-lip-id-EE-mee-a, or high cholesterol), middle adults, and African Americans. Hypertension is difficult to detect, because there are no external signs in the early stages. Late stage symptoms include shortness of breath, swelling of extremities, discoloration of lips and nailbeds, chest pains and palpitations, fatigue, and headache. If untreated, hypertension can cause injury to the heart, brain, and kidneys. You should report a client's elevated blood pressure and complaints of headaches and dizziness immediately to a supervisor. Hypertension is often treated by encouraging weight loss and exercise, reducing salt in the diet, and prescribing medication.

Congestive heart failure can result from years of untreated hypertension, myocardial infarction, infection, and other illnesses. Congestive heart failure occurs when the heart is no longer able to pump effectively, preventing the normal fluid exchange between organs, especially the liver and lungs. Fluid backs up in the tissues of these organs causing congestion or swelling. Excessive fluids in these organs can cause shortness of breath, weight gain, and swollen ankles. These symptoms should be reported to a supervisor immediately.

Peripheral vascular disease is a disease in which the extremities (legs, feet, arms, or hands) receive a reduced blood supply because of atherosclerotic changes in the blood vessels that supply the extremities. The legs, feet, arms, and hands feel cool or cold, nailbeds become ashen or blue from insufficient circulation, swelling occurs in the hands and feet, and clients may develop ulcers of the legs and feet that can become infected.

Observing and Reporting:
Cardiovascular System

Report to your supervisor:

▶ changes in pulse rate
▶ weakness, fatigue
▶ loss of ability to perform activities of daily living (ADLs)
▶ swelling of hands and feet
▶ pale or blue appearance of hands, feet, or lips
▶ chest pain
▶ weight gain
▶ shortness of breath, changes in breathing patterns, inability to "catch their breath"
▶ severe headache
▶ inactivity (which can lead to circulatory problems)

❑ 5. The Respiratory System

The respiratory system of the body has two functions: 1) it brings oxygen into the body, and 2) it eliminates carbon dioxide produced as the body uses oxygen. Respiration (res-pir-AY-shun), the body taking in oxygen and removing carbon dioxide, involves breathing in [inspiration (in-spir-AY-shun)], and breathing out [expiration (ex-pir-AY-shun)]. This process is accomplished by the lungs (Fig. 9-17).

As the lungs inhale, the air is pulled in through the nose

and into the pharynx (FAYR-inks), a tubular passageway for both food and air. From the pharynx, air passes into the larynx (LAYR-inks) or voice box, which is located at the beginning of the trachea (TRAY-kee-a), commonly known as the windpipe. The trachea divides into two branches at its lower portion, the right bronchus (BRONG-kus) and the **left bronchus**, or the bronchi (BRONG-kye). Each bronchus leads into each lung and then subdivides into bronchioles (BRONG-kee-ohls). These smaller airways subdivide further until they end in alveoli (al-VEE-oh-lye), tiny, one-cell sacs that appear in grape-like clusters. Blood is supplied to the alveoli by capillaries. Oxygen and carbon dioxide are exchanged between the alveoli and capillaries.

Oxygen-saturated blood then circulates through the capillaries and venules (VEN-yools) of the lung, into the pulmonary vein (PUL-moh-nayr-ee vayn) and left side of the heart. The carbon dioxide is exhaled through the alveoli into the bronchioles and bronchi

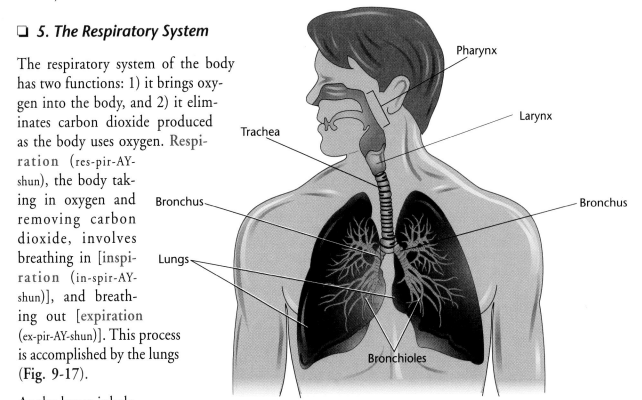

Fig. 9-17. The respiratory process begins with inspiration through the nose or mouth. The air then travels through the trachea and into the lungs via the bronchi, which then branch into bronchioles.

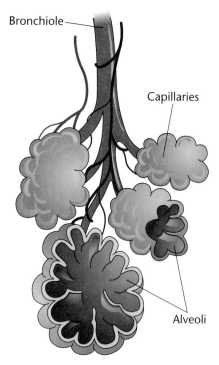

Bronchiole

Capillaries

Alveoli

Fig. 9-18. Once in the lungs, air travels from the bronchi into smaller bronchioles and finally, into the alveoli. Oxygen and carbon dioxide are exchanged between the alveoli and the capillaries that supply them with blood. Carbon dioxide travels out of the body during expiration.

of the lungs, the trachea, through the larynx, the pharynx, and out the nose and mouth.

The numerous sacs or alveoli located in the lungs create a spongy appearance. Each lung also appears to be divided into segments. These segments are called lobes; the left lung has two lobes and the right lung has three. Each lung is covered by the pleura (PLOOR-a), a membrane with two layers, one attached to the chest wall and one attached to the surface of the lung. The space between the layers is filled with a thin fluid that lubricates the layers, preventing them from rubbing together during breathing.

Common Disorders of the Respiratory System

Some diseases of the respiratory system that you may encounter as a home care aide include asthma (AZ-ma), **upper respiratory infection**, bronchitis (brong-KYE-tis), pneumonia (new-MOH-nee-a), emphysema (em-fi-SEE-ma), **lung cancer**, and tuberculosis (too-ber-kyoo-LOH-sis).

Asthma is a chronic inflammatory disease. It occurs when the respiratory system is hyper-reactive (that is, it reacts quickly and strongly) to irritants, infection, cold air, or to **allergens** such as pollen and dust. Strenuous exercise and stress can also bring on asthma attacks in some people. The bronchi become irritated and constrict, making it difficult to breathe. As a response to irritation and inflammation, the mucous membrane produces thick mucus that further inhibits respiration. As a result, air is trapped in the lungs, producing coughing and wheezing.

Upper respiratory infection (URI), commonly called a cold, is the result of a bacterial or viral infection of the nose, sinuses, and throat. Symptoms vary, depending on the region infected and the type of organism, but usually include nasal discharge, sneezing, sore throat, fever, and fatigue. For most people, a URI is a condition that can be dealt with by the body's immune system and by rest, fluids, and antibiotics if the infection is bacterial. However, people with chronic respiratory disease may develop complications and must be carefully observed.

Bronchitis is an irritation and inflammation of the lining of the bronchi. **Acute bronchitis** is usually caused by infection, beginning with an upper respiratory infection that spreads to the lungs. As in the nose, the mucous membrane lining the bronchi responds to an invasion of microorganisms by producing mucous to wash them away. Mucus, dead cells, and other fluid eventually produce a discharge that results in a productive cough. **Chronic bronchitis** is caused by airborne irritants, such as cigarette smoke, car exhaust, allergens, and other pollutants.

Pneumonia occurs lower in the respiratory tract than bronchitis and can be caused by a bacterial, viral, or fungal infection. Acute inflammation occurs in a portion of lung tissue, and the affected person develops a fever, chills, cough, chest pains, and rapid pulse. In the later stages, a thick discharge is produced by the mucous membrane. The discharge blocks alveoli and prevents the efficient exchange of oxygen and carbon dioxide. Older adults and persons with chronic illnesses are susceptible to complications, and recovery may take longer.

Emphysema is a chronic disease of the lungs that usually develops as the result of chronic bronchitis and smoking. The walls of the alveoli stretch out to the point that they deteriorate and cease to function properly (**Fig. 9-19**). People with emphysema have difficulty breathing. Other symptoms include coughing, breathlessness, and a rapid heart beat.

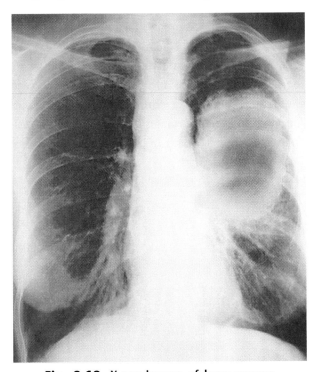

Fig. 9-19. X-ray image of lung cancer.

Lung cancer involves the development of abnormal cells or tumors in the lungs. Symptoms of lung cancer include chronic cough, shortness of breath, and bloody sputum (**Fig. 9-19**).

Tuberculosis is a highly infectious (contagious) lung disease. Symptoms include coughing, shortness of breath, and bloody sputum. Chapter 5, Infection Control and Standard Precautions, includes more information about tuberculosis.

Observing and Reporting: Respiratory System

It is very important that people with acute or chronic upper respiratory conditions are not exposed to cigarette smoke or polluted air. When caring for a client with an upper respiratory condition, you may need to assist the client with deep breathing exer-

cises or coughing routines. You will also observe respirations and remind the client to take medications. People who have difficulty breathing will usually be more comfortable sitting up than lying down. Clients with severe breathing difficulties may be placed on oxygen to give relief and assist in breathing higher oxygen levels.

Home care aides should report to a supervisor the following signs and symptoms:

- change in respiratory rate
- shallow breathing or breathing through pursed lips
- coughing or wheezing
- nasal congestion or discharge
- sore throat, difficulty swallowing, or swollen tonsils
- the need to sit after mild exertion
- the need to rest on two pillows
- pale or bluish color of the lips and extremities
- pain in the chest area
- discolored sputum (green, yellow, blood-tinged, or grey)

Because the respiratory and circulatory systems work together to supply oxygen to the body, failure of one system often means there will be damage to the other.

❑ 6. The Urinary System

The urinary system has two vital functions:

1. Through urine, it eliminates waste products created by the cells, much as the lungs remove carbon dioxide from the blood.

2. It maintains the water balance in the body.

The **kidneys** are located in the upper part of the abdominal cavity on each side of the spine (**Fig. 9-20**). These two bean-shaped organs are protected by the muscles of the back and the lower part of the rib cage. When blood flows through the kidneys, waste products from the cells and excess water are filtered out. Necessary water and substances are reabsorbed into the bloodstream, while waste and the remaining fluid form urine. The body must maintain a proper **fluid balance** between water absorbed in the body and waste fluids that are released from the body. Home care aides may play an important role in helping clients maintain fluid balance by monitoring or measuring **intake** of fresh fluids and **output** of waste fluids. You will learn more about measuring and documenting fluid intake and output in Chapter 13, Performing Basic Nursing Skills.

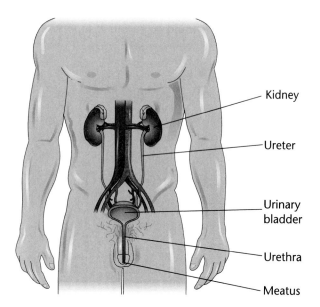

Fig. 9-20. The urinary system consists of two kidneys and their ureters, the bladder, the urethra, and the meatus.

Each kidney has a **ureter** (you-RE-ter) approximately ten to twelve inches long, which is attached to the **bladder.** Urine flows through the ureters to the bladder, a muscular sac in the lower part of the abdomen. Urine flows from the bladder through the **urethra** (you-REE-thra) and passes out of the body through the **meatus** (mee-A-tus), the opening at the end of the urethra. In the female, the meatus is located in the genital area just in front of the opening of the **vagina** (va-JYE-na, see reproductive system description, below). In the male, the meatus is located at the end of the **penis** (PEE-nis, see reproductive system description, below).

Common Disorders of the Urinary Tract

Illnesses of the urinary tract that home care aides may encounter include **urinary tract infection (UTI)**, **kidney stones**, **nephritis** (ne-FRYE-tis), **renovascular hypertension** (ree-noh-VAS- kyoo-lar high-per-

TEN-shun), and **chronic kidney failure**.

UTI causes inflammation of the bladder and the ureters, resulting in a painful burning sensation during urination and the frequent feeling of needing to urinate. Urinary tract infection or **cystitis** (sis-TYE-tis, also inflammation of the bladder) may be caused by bacterial infection. Certain situations, such as confinement to bed, cause urine to stay in the bladder too long, providing an ideal environment for bacteria to grow. Cystitis is more common in women, because the urethra is much shorter in women (three to four inches) than in men (seven to eight inches) (**Fig.** 9-21). To avoid infection, women should wipe the **perineal** (payr-i-NEE-al) area from front to back after bladder and bowel elimination. Report to your supervisor if a client urinates frequently and in small quantities, and if the urine is cloudy.

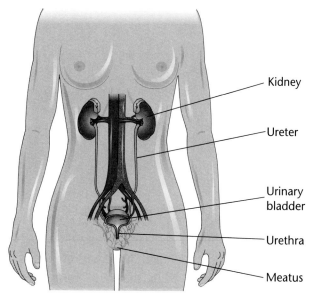

Fig. 9-21. The female urethra is shorter than the male urethra. Because of this, the female bladder is more likely to become infected by bacteria traveling up the urethra.

Calculi (KAL-kyoo-lye), or **kidney stones,** form when urine crystallizes in the kidneys. Kidney stones can block the kidneys and ureters, causing severe pain. Kidney stones can be caused by some of the same conditions that cause cystitis, or they can be the result of a vitamin deficiency, mineral imbalance, structural abnormalities of the urinary tract, or infection.

Nephritis is an inflammation of the kidneys that interferes with the filtering of waste products from the blood. It can affect all age groups, but it is more common in children. Nephritis may appear after an infection of the throat or skin. Signs and symptoms include a decrease in urine output, urine becoming a rusty color, and a burning feeling during urination. A person with nephritis often has a swollen face, eyelids, and hands because she is retaining fluid. Children and young adults usually recover without continuing problems. Older people can develop a chronic form of nephritis.

Renovascular hypertension is a condition in which a blockage of arteries in the kidneys causes high blood pressure. The most common cause of renovascular hypertension is atherosclerosis of the **renal** (REE-nal) arteries.

Chronic kidney failure, or **uremia** (you-REE-mee-a), occurs because the kidneys become unable to eliminate certain waste products from the body. This disease can develop as the result of chronic urinary tract infections, nephritis, or diabetes. Excessive salt in the diet can also cause damage to the kidneys. Over time, the disease gradually becomes worse, affecting all parts of the body. **Kidney dialysis** (dye-AL-i-sis), an artificial means of removing the body's waste products, can improve and extend life for several years (**Fig. 9-22**). Some clients may receive a kidney transplant. Unless treatment involves fluid restrictions, clients should be encouraged to drink plenty of fluids.

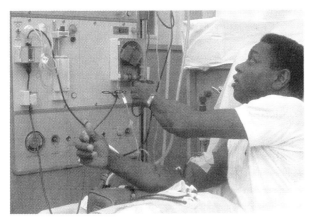

Fig. 9-22. A kidney dialysis machine removes the body's waste products.

Benign prostatic hypertrophy (be-NINE pros-TAT-ik HIGH-per-troh-fee), an enlargement of the prostate gland, is an illness of the endocrine system that can affect a man's urinary tract. This condition causes frequent urination, dribbling of urine instead of a steady stream, and difficulty or hesitancy in starting the flow of urine. Urinary retention (urine remains in the bladder) may also occur, causing urinary tract infection. Urine can also back up into the ureters and kidney, causing damage to these organs. Benign prostatic hypertrophy can be treated with medications.

Observing and Reporting: The Urinary System

Watch for the following signs and report them to your supervisor:

▶ weight loss or gain
▶ swelling in the upper or lower extremities
▶ painful urination or burning during urination
▶ changes in the characteristics of urine, such as cloudiness, odor, or color
▶ changes in frequency and amount of urination
▶ swelling in the abdominal/bladder area
▶ client complaining that bladder feels full or painful
▶ incontinence/dribbling
▶ pain in the kidney or back/flank region
▶ inadequate fluid intake

❏ 7. The Gastrointestinal (GI) System

The **gastrointestinal system** has two functions:

1. **Digestion** is the process of preparing food physically and chemically so that it can be absorbed into the cells.

2. **Elimination** is the process of expelling solid wastes made up of the waste products of food that are not absorbed into the cells.

The GI system or **digestive system** is made up of the **alimentary** (al-i-MEN-tayr-ee) **canal** and the accessory digestive organs (**Fig. 9-23**). The alimentary canal or **GI tract** is a long passageway extending from the mouth to the **anus** (A-nus), the opening of the rectum. Food passes from the mouth through the **pharynx, esophagus** (e-SOF-a-gus), **stomach,** small intestine (where nutrients are absorbed from the food into the bloodstream), **large intestine**, and out of the body as solid waste. The **teeth, tongue,** salivary glands (SAL-i-vayr-ee glands), **liver, gall bladder,** and pancreas (PAN-kree-us) are the accessory organs to the process of digestion. They help prepare the food so it can be absorbed.

Food is first placed in the mouth, where the teeth chew the food by cutting it, then chopping and grinding it into smaller pieces that can be swallowed. Saliva (sa-LYE-va) secreted by the salivary glands moistens the food and begins chemical digestion. The tongue helps with chewing and swallowing by pushing the food around between the teeth and then into the pharynx.

The **pharynx,** located at the back of the mouth and extending into the throat, is a muscular structure that contracts with swallowing and pushes the food into the esophagus. The muscles of the **esophagus** then move the food into the stomach through involuntary contractions called peristalsis (payr-i-STAL-sis).

The **stomach,** a muscular pouch located in the upper left part of the abdominal cavity, provides physical digestion by stirring and churning the food to break it down into smaller particles. The glands in the stomach lining also aid in digestion by secreting gastric juices that chemically break down food. As a result of the stomach's actions, food is turned into a semi-liquid substance called chyme (KYME). Peristalsis continues in the stomach, pushing the chyme into the small intestine.

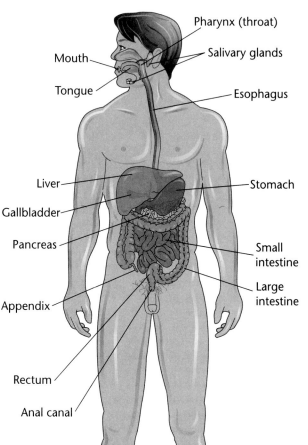

Fig. 9-23. The gastrointestinal tract consists of all the organs needed to digest food and process waste.

Labels: Pharynx (throat), Mouth, Salivary glands, Tongue, Esophagus, Liver, Stomach, Gallbladder, Pancreas, Small intestine, Large intestine, Appendix, Rectum, Anal canal

The small intestine is approximately twenty feet long. Here enzymes secreted by the liver and the pancreas finish digesting the chyme. **Bile,** a green liquid produced by the liver, is stored in the **gallbladder** and released into the small intestine. Bile helps break down dietary fat. The liver converts fats and sugars into glucose (GLOO-kohs), a sugar that can be carried to cells by the blood. The liver also stores glucose. The pancreas produces insulin (IN-soo-lin), an enzyme that regulates the body's conversion of sugar into glucose.

The chyme is moved by peristalsis through the small intestine, where villi (VIL-eye), tiny projections lining the small intestine, absorb the digested food into the capillaries.

Peristalsis moves the chyme that has not been digested through the **large intestine.** In the large intestine, which is also called the **large bowel** or **colon,** most of the water in the chyme is absorbed. What remains is feces (FEE-seez), a semisolid material comprising water, solid waste material, bacteria, and mucus. Feces passes by peristalsis through the rectum (REK-tum), the lower end of the colon, and moves out of the body through the rectal opening or anus (AY-nus).

Common Disorders of the Gastrointestinal System

Disorders of the gastrointestinal tract that you may encounter in your clients include **heartburn, gastric reflux,** nausea (NAWS-ee-a) and **vomiting,** peptic ulcers (PEP-tik UL-sers), constipation (kon-sti-PAY-shun), diarrhea (dye-a-REE-a), hepatitis (hep-a-TYE-tis), colitis (koh-LYE-tis), and **hemorrhoids** (HEM-a-royds).

Heartburn is a common condition that occurs frequently as people age. It is the result of a weakening of the **sphincter** (SFINK-ter) muscle which joins the esophagus and the stomach. When healthy and strong, this muscle prevents the leaking of stomach acid and other contents back into the esophagus. Stomach acid causes a burning sensation, commonly called heartburn, in the esophagus. If heartburn occurs frequently and remains untreated, it can cause scarring or **ulceration** (ul-ser-AY-shun).

Gastric reflux occurs when stomach contents pass through the esophagus into the lungs. This problem often occurs during sleep, when the horizontal body position helps the stomach contents travel up into the esophagus. If it occurs frequently, aspiration into the lungs is a serious problem that can cause deterioration of lung tissue leading to asthma, pneumonia, and even death.

Heartburn and gastric reflux must be reported to your supervisor. These conditions are usually treated with medications. Make your clients comfortable by having the evening meal served three to four hours before bedtime. Provide an extra pillow so the body is more upright during sleep. Do not allow client to lay down until at least half an hour after eating. Serving the largest meal of the day at lunchtime, serving several meals of small portions throughout the day, and reducing fast foods, fatty foods, and spicy foods in the diet may also help.

Nausea and vomiting occurs with many gastrointestinal disorders. Although it can be a sign of something as simple as the flu, it can also be a sign of more serious problems. Nausea and vomiting should always be reported to a supervisor. Vomiting may be of special concern if you are monitoring a client's fluid balance. Vomitus must be included as part of the client's output. Chapter 14, Performing Basic Health Care Skills, provides more information on measuring intake and output.

Peptic ulcers are raw sores in the stomach (a gastric ulcer) or the small intestine [a duodenal (doo-oh-DEE-nal) ulcer]. A dull or gnawing pain occurs one to three hours after eating, accompanied by belch-

ing or vomiting. The pain is temporarily relieved by food, antacids, and medications. Ulcers are caused by excessive acid production, which commonly results from heredity, stress, or infection. Clients with peptic ulcers should avoid smoking and drinking too much alcohol and caffeine, which increase the production of gastric acid. Peptic ulcers may cause bleeding. Feces, or bowel movements, may appear black and tarry because of the bleeding.

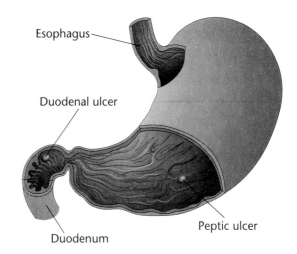

Fig. 9-24. Ulcers can occur in the stomach (peptic) or the duodenum (duodenal).

Constipation is the difficult and often painful elimination of a hard, dry stool (bowel movement). Constipation occurs when the feces moves too slowly through the intestine as the result of decreased fluid intake, poor diet, inactivity, medications, aging, certain diseases, or ignoring the urge to eliminate. Treatment often includes increasing the amount of fiber eaten, increasing the activity level, and possibly medication.

Diarrhea is frequent elimination of liquid or semi-liquid feces. The stool moves through the large intestine so quickly that fluid is not absorbed before elimination. Abdominal cramps, urgency, nausea, and vomiting can accompany diarrhea, depending on the cause. Bacterial and viral infections, microorganisms in food and water, irritating foods, and certain medications can cause diarrhea. Treatment of diarrhea usually involves medication to slow peristalsis and a change of diet. A diet of **bananas, rice, apples,** and **tea/toast** (BRAT diet) is often recommended when diarrhea is a problem, particularly for children.

Hepatitis, an inflammation of the liver, is caused by a virus. It begins with symptoms that resemble the flu (fever, fatigue, nausea, vomiting) but eventually **jaundice** (JAWN-dis) appears. Jaundice is a condition in which the skin and body fluids appear yellow. Different types of hepatitis have different causes. The virus causing hepatitis A is carried in food. Hepatitis B is contracted through blood or needles that are contaminated with the virus, or by sexual contact with an infected person. Hepatitis C is also transmitted through blood and possibly sexual intercourse.

Hepatitis B and C can lead to cirrhosis and liver cancer. Good nutrition and rest are important in the treatment of hepatitis because they can help repair damaged tissues and maintain health in other systems. Because hepatitis is an infectious disease, following standard precautions when caring for all clients offers the best protection for you and your clients.

Ulcerative colitis (UL-ser-a-tiv koh-LYE-tis) is a chronic inflammatory disease of the large intestine that usually occurs in young adults. It is characterized by periodic episodes of cramping diarrhea, with pain occurring to one side of the lower abdomen, and loss of appetite. Ulcerative colitis is a serious illness that can cause intestinal bleeding and death if left untreated. Medications can relieve symptoms such as diarrhea and abdominal cramps, but they cannot cure ulcerative colitis. Surgical treatment may include a **colostomy** (koh-LOS-toh-mee), which is the diversion of waste to an artificial opening (stoma) through the abdomen. All bowels are diverted through the stoma instead of the anus. Information on caring for a client with a colostomy can be found in Chapter 13, Performing Basic Nursing Skills.

Colitis or **irritable bowel syndrome** has symptoms similar to but milder than those of ulcerative colitis. Colitis can usually be controlled by diet or a combination of diet and medications.

Colorectal (koh-loh-REK-tal) **cancer** is cancer of the gastrointestinal tract. Signs and symptoms include changes in normal bowel patterns, cramps, abdominal pain, and rectal bleeding. Colorectal cancer must be treated surgically.

Hemorrhoids are enlarged veins in the rectum that may also be visible outside the anus. Rectal itching, burning, pain, and bleeding are signs and symptoms of hemorrhoids. The care plan for clients with hemorrhoids may include medication to keep the feces soft, and compresses or sitz baths to relieve pain and itching. Chapter 13, Performing Basic Home Care Skills, provides more information on applying compresses and giving sitz baths. Surgery may be necessary to correct hemorrhoids in some clients. When cleaning the anus, be very careful to avoid causing pain and bleeding from hemorrhoids.

Observing and Reporting: The Gastrointestinal System

Observe your clients for signs and symptoms that indicate changes in the gastrointestinal system, including:

- difficulty swallowing or chewing (including denture problems or mouth sores)
- fecal incontinence (losing control of bowels)
- weight gain/weight loss
- anorexia (loss of appetite)
- abdominal pain and cramping
- diarrhea
- nausea and vomiting (especially vomitus that looks like coffee grounds)
- constipation
- flatulence
- hiccoughs, belching
- abnormal colored stool (bloody, black, or hard)
- heartburn
- poor nutritional intake

Any of these signs should be reported to your supervisor, especially if they persist.

8. The Endocrine System

The endocrine system is made up of glands that secrete **hormones**. Hormones are chemical substances that control many of the organs and body systems. They are carried in the blood to the various organs, where they perform the following functions:

- maintaining homeostasis
- influencing growth and development

- regulating levels of sugar in the blood
- regulating levels of calcium in the bones
- determining how fast cells burn food for energy

The function of the endocrine system is to secrete hormones that regulate essential body processes.

The **pituitary** (pi-TOO-i-tayr-ee) **gland** is located behind the eyes at the base of the brain, and is the "master" gland of the body. It is called the master gland because it secretes key hormones that cause other glands to produce other hormones.

Hormones secreted by the pituitary gland include the following:

- growth hormone, which regulates growth and development
- antidiuretic (an-tee-dye-you-RET-ik) hormone, or ADH, which controls the balance of fluids in the body
- oxytocin (ok-se-TOH-sin), which causes the **uterus** (YOU-ter-us, see reproductive system) to contract during and after childbirth

The **pituitary**, the master gland, produces hormones that regulate the **thyroid gland** (THIGH- royd gland) and the **adrenal** (a-DREE-nal) **glands** (Fig. 9-25).

The **thyroid gland** is located in the neck in front of the larynx. It produces thyroid hormone, which regulates **metabolism** (me-TAB-oh-lizm), the burning of food for heat and energy.

The **parathyroid glands** (payr-a-THIGH-royd glands) secrete a hormone that regulates the body's use of calcium. Nerves and muscles require calcium to function smoothly; therefore, a deficiency of this hormone can cause severe muscle contractions and

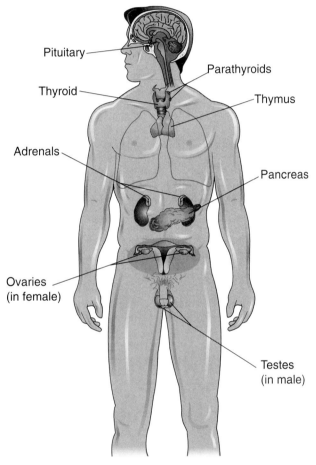

Fig. 9-25. The endocrine system includes organs that produce hormones that regulate body processes.

Labels: Pituitary, Thyroid, Adrenals, Ovaries (in female), Parathyroids, Thymus, Pancreas, Testes (in male)

spasms that can be fatal if untreated.

The **pancreas**, a gland located in the upper mid-section of the abdomen, secretes insulin, a hormone that regulates the amount of sugar (glucose) available to the cells for metabolism. Sugar cannot be absorbed by the cells without insulin.

Two **adrenal** glands located at the tops of the kidneys produce hormones that are essential to life. These hormones are important because they help the body: 1) regulate carbohydrate (kar-boh-HIGH-drayt) metabolism, 2) control the body's reaction to inflammation and stress, and 3) regulate salt and water absorption in the kidneys.

The adrenal glands also produce the hormone **adrenaline** (a-DREN-a-lin) or **epinephrine** (ep-i-NEF-rin), which regulates muscle power, heart rate, blood pressure, and energy levels during stressful situations or emergencies.

Gonads (GOH-nadz), or sex glands, produce hormones that regulate the body's ability to reproduce. The **testes** (TES-teez) in the male secrete **testosterone** (tes-TOS-te-rohn). The **ovaries** (O-var-ees) in the female secrete **estrogen** (ES-troh-jen) and **progesterone** (proh-JES-te-rohn).

Common Disorders of the Endocrine System

Thyroid disorders and **diabetes** (dye-a-BEE-teez) are common problems of the endocrine system that you may encounter among your clients.

Hyperthyroidism (high-per-THIGH-royd-ism). When the thyroid produces too much thyroid hormone, the cells burn too much food, speeding up the body processes. Weight loss, nervousness, and hyperactivity occur. Hyperthyroidism is usually treated with medication. Occasionally, part of the thyroid is surgically removed.

Hypothyroidism (high-poh-THIGH-royd-ism). When the thyroid produces too little thyroid hormone, the body processes slow down. As a result, weight gain and physical and mental sluggishness result. Other symptoms are often ignored because they are similar to some normal signs of aging: hoarseness, dry skin, deafness, muscle cramps, weakness of the hands, unsteady walking, and constipation. Hypothyroidism is sometimes treated with medication.

Diabetes Mellitus (mel-EYE-tus). When the pancreas produces too little insulin, sugar builds up in the blood and cannot get to the cells, making it difficult for the body to process carbohydrates, fats, and proteins. Diabetes is a chronic disease that has two forms: Type I, or insulin dependent diabetes mellitus (IDDM); and Type II, or non-insulin dependent diabetes mellitus (NIDDM). Type I, or juvenile diabetes, usually appears in childhood but can appear later in life. Type II, also known as late-onset diabetes, occurs in people who are 40 to 60 years old. Diabetes can be inherited. Aging and obesity are also risk factors for diabetes.

Signs and symptoms of diabetes include increased thirst and urine production, hunger, and weight loss. Urine tests show the presence of sugar in the urine. Blood tests indicate a high level of sugar in the blood.

The care plan for a client with diabetes depends on the severity of the disease. Mild forms can usually be managed by diet alone or by diet and oral medications. Other cases may require insulin injections in addition to diet restrictions. Meals for clients with diabetes must be served on time, and clients must eat all foods served. Good skin care is important, especially for the feet. Clients with diabetes are susceptible to skin infections that heal slowly. Foot and leg wounds can be very serious.

If not controlled, diabetes can affect other organ systems. Uncontrolled diabetes can lead to any of the following health problems:

- blindness
- diseases of the kidney
- diseases of the nerves
- diseases of the circulatory system, including stroke, heart attack, and slow healing
- frequent infections
- gangrene, which can lead to amputation of an affected body part

Clients with diabetes can go into **insulin shock** if they get too much insulin. A **diabetic coma** can occur if a client with diabetes does not receive enough insulin. Both insulin shock and diabetic coma can cause death. You will learn more about diabetes, insulin shock, and diabetic coma in Chapter 20, Common Chronic and Acute Conditions.

Observing and Reporting: Endocrine System

Many endocrine illnesses can be treated with hormone supplements. These supplements must be given very precisely. For example, too much insulin administered to a diabetic can cause the sudden onset of insulin shock. You should observe clients with endocrine disorders carefully. Report any of the following signs and symptoms to your supervisor:

- headache*
- weakness*
- blurred vision*
- dizziness*
- hunger*
- irritability*
- sweating*
- change in "normal" behavior*
- weight gain/weight loss

- loss of appetite/ increased appetite
- increased thirst
- frequent urination
- dry skin
- excessive perspiration
- sluggishness or fatigue
- hyperactivity
- * indicates signs and symptoms that should be reported *immediately.*

❑ 9. The Reproductive System

The reproductive system is made up of the reproductive organs, which are different in men and women. The function of the reproductive system is to allow human beings to **reproduce** or create new human life. Reproduction begins when a male and a female sex cell come together to form a potential new human. These sex cells are formed in the male and female sex glands, called the **gonads**.

The Male Reproductive System

In the male, the sex glands or gonads are the **testes** or **testicles**. The two oval glands are located outside the body in the scrotum (SCROH-tum), a sac made of skin and muscle that is suspended between the thighs. The testes produce the male sex cells, called **sperm**, and **testosterone**, the male hormone that is necessary for the reproductive organs to function properly. Testosterone is also responsible for the development of male **secondary sex characteristics.** Secondary sex characteristics include facial hair; pubic (PYOO-bik) and axillary (AK-sil-ayr-ee, or underarm) hair; hair on the chest, legs, and arms; deepening of the voice; and increase in neck and shoulder size.

Sperm travel from the testes through a coiled tube, the epididymis (ep-i-DID-i-mis) through another tube called the vas deferens (vas DEF-er-enz). Sperm then pass into the seminal vesicle (SEM-i-nal VES-i-kul) where semen (SEE-men) is produced. Semen is the fluid that carries sperm out of the body. The ducts coming from each seminal vesicle unite to form

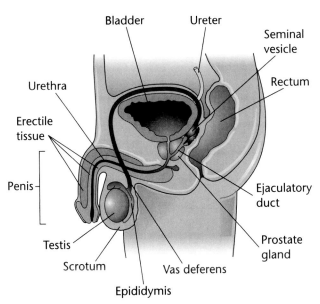

Fig. 9-26. Male reproductive system.

the ejaculatory (ee-JAK-you-la-tor-ee) **ducts**, which pass through the doughnut-shaped prostate gland (PROS-tayt gland) where more fluid is added to the semen. In the prostate, the ejaculatory ducts join the urethra, the tube through which both urine and semen pass. The urethra continues through the **penis**, the other sex organ located outside the body, in front of the scrotum. The penis is composed of erectile (ee-REK-tyle) tissue that becomes filled with blood during sexual excitement. As the penis fills with blood, it becomes enlarged and erect and can enter the **vagina**, the female reproductive tract, where semen containing sperm is released.

The Female Reproductive System

In the human female, the gonads are two oval glands called the ovaries (OH-var-ees). There are two ovaries, one located on each side of the **uterus**. The ovaries produce the female sex cells or eggs, ova (OH-va). They secrete the female hormones, estrogen and progesterone. Each month from puberty (PYOO-ber-tee),(when a female begins having menstrual periods), to menopause (men-o-paas), (when a female stops having menstrual periods), an **egg** is released from an ovary. This reproductive cycle is maintained by **estrogen** and **progesterone**, which are also responsible for the development of **female secondary sex characteristics,** such as increased breast size, wider and rounder hips, axillary and pubic hair, and a slightly deeper voice.

Each ovary has a fallopian (fal-LOH-pee-an) **tube** that is attached to the uterus. Once an egg is released from an ovary, it travels through the fallopian tube to the uterus, a hollow, pear-shaped, muscular organ located within the pelvis, behind the bladder and in front of the rectum. If sexual intercourse takes place while the egg is in the fallopian tube, the egg may be **fertilized** by sperm in the fallopian tube. The fertilized egg then travels down into the uterus, and implants in the endometrium (en-doh-MEE-tree-um), the lining of the uterus. Stimulated by hormones, the endometrium builds up during the menstrual cycle and has many blood vessels supplying it for the growth and nourishment of an embryo (EM-bree-oh). If the egg is not fertilized, the hormones decrease, and the blood supply to the endometrium diminishes. The endometrium then breaks up and sloughs off, a process called **menstruation** (MEN-stroo-ay-shun).

The main section of the uterus is the **fundus**. This is the section where a baby develops after the fertilized egg is implanted. The narrow neck of the uterus extending into the vagina is the **cervix** (SIR-vix). The cervix has an opening through which menstrual fluid can pass and semen can enter the vagina. The vagina is the muscular canal that opens to the outside of the body. The external vaginal opening is partially closed by the **hymen** membrane. The vagina is kept moist by secretions from glands in the vaginal walls. The vagina receives the penis during sexual intercourse, and it serves as the **birth canal**. The baby passes through the cervix, which is made thin by pressure from the baby's head during contractions. Once the cervix opens, the baby can then move out through the vagina.

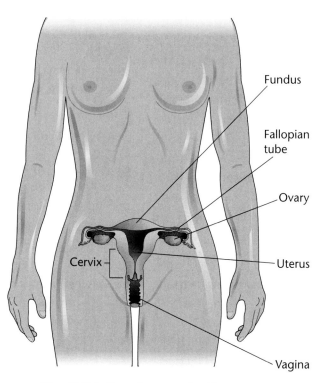

Fig. 9-27. Female reproductive system.

Labels: Fundus, Fallopian tube, Ovary, Uterus, Vagina, Cervix

Common Disorders of the Reproductive System

Diseases of the reproductive system include cancers of the breast, prostate, and ovaries. Chapter 20, Common Chronic and Acute Conditions, provides more information on caring for clients with cancer. **Vaginitis** (vaj-i-NYE-tis) and the sexually transmitted diseases **chlamydia** (kla-MID-ee- a), **gonorrhea** (gon-oh-REE-a), **syphilis** (SIF-i-lis), and **herpes** infection (HER-peez) are other common disorders of the reproductive system.

Vaginitis, an infection of the vagina, may be caused by a bacteria, protozoa (one-celled animals), or fungus (yeast). It may also be the result of hormonal changes in vaginal secretions after menopause. Women who have vaginitis have a white vaginal discharge, accompanied by itching and burning.

Benign prostatic hypertrophy is a fairly common disorder that occurs in men as they age. The prostate becomes enlarged and causes pressure on the urethra. The pressure on the urethra leads to urinary problems described earlier in this chapter (see discussion of the urinary system). Benign prostatic hypertrophy is treatable with medications or surgery. A test is also available to screen for cancer of the prostate. As men age, they are at increased risk for prostate cancer, which is usually slow growing and responsive to treatment if detected early.

Sexually Transmitted Diseases (STDs)

Sexually transmitted diseases, also called venereal (ven-EER-ee-al) diseases, are passed through sexual contact with an infected person. Sexual contact that can transmit these diseases includes not only sexual intercourse, but also contact of the mouth with the genitals or anus, and contact of the hands to the genitals. Using latex condoms during sexual contact can reduce the chances of being infected or passing on some STDs. The human immunodeficiency virus (HIV) and autoimmune deficiency syndrome (AIDS) and some kinds of hepatitis are sexually transmitted. HIV/AIDS is discussed in detail in Chapter 5, Infection Control and Standard Precautions. Other STDs are discussed below. STDs are very common, and they can have serious health consequences. Clients may be unaware of or embarrassed by symptoms that indicate an STD.

Chlamydia infection is caused by organisms introduced into the mucous membranes of the reproductive tract. Chlamydia infection of the reproductive tract can cause serious infection, including pelvic inflammatory disease (PID) in women. PID can lead to sterility. Symptoms of chlamydia infection include yellow or white discharge from the penis or vagina and a burning sensation during urination. Chlamydia is treated with antibiotics.

Syphilis can be treated effectively in the early stages, but, if left untreated, can cause brain damage, mental illness, and even death. Babies born to mothers infected with syphilis may be born blind or with other serious birth defects. Syphilis is easier to detect in men than in women, due to open sores called **chancres** (KAYN-kers) that develop on the penis soon after infection. However, the chancres are painless and can go unnoticed. If untreated, the infection progresses to the heart, brain, and other vital organs. Common symptoms at this stage include rash, sore throat, or fever. When detected, syphilis can be treated with penicillin or other antibiotics. The sooner the disease is treated, the better the person's chances of preventing long-term consequences and avoiding infection of sexual partners.

Gonorrhea, like syphilis, can be treated with antibiotics and is easier to detect in men than in women. If untreated, gonorrhea can cause sterility in both men and women. A baby born to a woman infected with gonorrhea can suffer permanent damage to the eyes. For this reason, all babies' eyes are treated with eyedrops shortly after birth to kill any infection.

Most women infected with gonorrhea show no early symptoms, making it easy for women to spread the disease without even knowing they are infected. Men infected with gonorrhea will typically show a greeenish or yellowish discharge from the penis within a week after infection. Burning during urination is another common symptom in men.

Herpes simplex II, unlike the other STDs discussed here, is caused by a virus and therefore cannot be treated with antibiotics. Once infected with the herpes virus, a person cannot be cured and may suffer repeated outbreaks of the disease for the rest of his life. A herpes outbreak includes burning, painful, red sores on the genitals that heal in about two weeks. The sores are infectious, but a person with herpes virus can spread the infection even when sores are not present.

Some people infected with herpes never experience repeated outbreaks, or the later episodes may not be as painful as the initial outbreak. Recently an antiviral drug has been used with some success to lessen the severity of herpes outbreaks. Babies born to women infected with herpes simplex II can be infected during birth, so pregnant women experiencing a herpes outbreak are usually delivered by **cesarian** (se-SAYR-ee-an) **section**, or **C-section**.

Observing and Reporting: Reproductive System

Report any of the following signs to your supervisor:

▶ discomfort or difficulty with urination

▶ discharge from the penis or vagina

▶ swelling of the genitals

▶ changes in menstruation

▶ blood in urine or stool

▶ breast changes, including size, shape, lumps, or discharge from the nipple

▶ presence of sores on the genitals

▶ client reports of impotence, or inability of male to have sexual intercourse

▶ client reports of painful intercourse

❑ 10. The Immune System

The function of the immune system is to protect the body from disease-causing bacteria, viruses, and organisms. The immune system protects the body in two ways: 1) through nonspecific immunity, which protects the body from disease in general, and 2) through specific immunity, which protects against a particular disease that is invading the body at a given time.

Nonspecific Immunity. To protect itself against disease in general, the body has several mechanisms.

▶ **Anatomic** (an-a-TOM-ik) **barriers**, which include the skin and the mucous membranes, provide a physical barrier to keep foreign materials — bacteria, viruses, or organisms — from invading the body. Saliva, tears, and mucus secretions also help protect the body by washing away substances.

▶ **Physiologic** (fi-see-oh-LA-jik) **barriers** include body temperature and acidity of certain organs. Most organisms that cause disease cannot survive high temperatures or high acidity. When the body senses foreign organisms, it can raise its temperature (by running a fever) to kill off the invaders. Acidity of organs like the stomach keeps bacteria from growing there.

▶ **Inflammatory response** refers to the body's ability to react to infection by inflammation or swelling of an infected area. When inflammation occurs, it indicates that the body has sent extra disease-fighting cells and extra blood to the infected area to combat the infection.

Specific Immunity. To protect itself against specific diseases or disease-causing germs, the body is capable of generating different types of cells that will combat a huge range of different invaders. Once it has successfully eliminated a particular invader, the immune system keeps a record of the invasion in the form of **antibodies**. Antibodies are carried within cells and prevent a disease from threatening the body a second time.

Acquired immunity is a kind of specific immunity that the body acquires either by fighting an infection or by **vaccination** (vak-sin-AY-shun). For example, you can acquire immunity to a disease like the measles in two ways: 1) you get the measles, and your body forms antibodies to the disease to make sure you won't get it again; or 2) you get a vaccine for the measles, which causes your body to produce the same antibodies to protect you from the disease.

Common Disorders of the Immune System

The immune system disorder that you will encounter most frequently as a home care aide is AIDS. AIDS is an example of immune system failure. It is caused by a massive infection of the immune system by HIV. The virus invades the body, multiplies, and disables the cells of the immune system so that they cannot protect the body from disease. People with AIDS usually die of pneumonia or other infections that their bodies are unable to fight. You will learn more about caring for clients with AIDS in Chapter 20, Common Chronic and Acute Conditions.

Other immune system diseases you may see are forms of cancer. **Lymphoma** (lim-FOH-ma) is cancer of the **lymphatic** (lim-FAT-ik) system. The lymphatic system is a network of tubes and nodes throughout the body that carry a colorless, watery fluid called **lymph** (limf). Lymph contains infection-fighting cells. One specific form of lymphoma is **Hodgkins Disease**. Treatment for lymphomas may include radiation therapy or chemotherapy. Chapter 20, Common Chronic and Acute Conditions, provides more information on caring for clients with cancer.

Observing and Reporting: Immune System

Symptoms of immune system weakness or failure include recurring infections (such as pneumonia, diarrhea, and fevers), swelling of the lymph nodes, and increased fatigue. Report any of these signs to your supervisor. Some clients may have weakened immune systems due to certain cancer treatments or other diseases. These clients must not be exposed to bacteria or viruses that their bodies are not prepared to fight. Particular care should be taken to be sure that the home environment is clean and that the chance of infection is minimized.

❑ *11. The Lymphatic System*

The function of the lymphatic system is to remove excess fluids and waste products from the body's tissues and to help the immune system fight infection. Closely related to both the immune system and the circulatory systems, the lymphatic system consists of lymph vessels and lymph capillaries in which a fluid called **lymph** circulates (**Fig. 9-28**). Lymph is a clear yellowish fluid that carries disease-fighting cells called lymphocytes (LIM-foh-sytes).

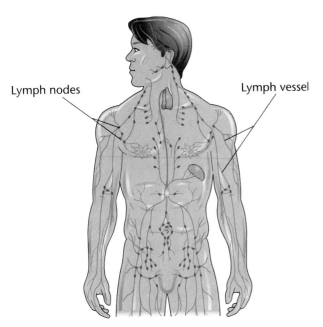

Lymph nodes

Lymph vessel

Fig. 9-28. Lymph nodes are located throughout the body.

When the body is fighting an infection, swelling may occur in the **lymph nodes**, oval-shaped bodies that can be as small as a pinhead or as large as an almond. Located in the neck, groin, and armpits, the lymph nodes filter out germs and waste products carried from the tissues by the lymph fluid. After lymph fluid has been purified in the lymph nodes, it flows into the bloodstream.

Unlike the circulatory system, in which the heart functions as a pump to move the blood, the lymph system has no pump. Lymph fluid is circulated by muscle activity, massage, and breathing. A sore muscle may feel better if you rub it, because the rubbing action helps the lymph fluid circulate, carrying waste products away from the tired muscle.

Summary

The human body is a complicated piece of machinery. Even for physicians and nurses with years of education and experience, remembering every sign and symptom of every disease is very difficult. Just the few signs and symptoms mentioned in this chapter may seem overwhelming. This is why it is so important to note and report any *change* in your client. From the color of a patch of skin, to changes in a client's abilities, to differences in a client's attitude—your observations could reveal important signs of a significant problem! Home care aides, because they may see clients much more often than other health care providers, are in the best position to observe and report changes in a client's health and well being. Make noticing these changes a mission!

> **"From the color of a patch of skin, to changes in a client's abilities, to differences in a client's attitude—your observations could reveal important signs of a significant problem! Make noticing these changes a mission!"**

Chapter 10

Understanding Human Development and Aging

Part 1
Human Development and Age-Related Disorders

Throughout their lives, people change physically and psychologically. Physical changes occur in the body; psychological changes occur in the mind and in the person's behavior. As a home care aide, you will care for clients of all ages. For this reason, it is important that you learn about the ways people change during the different stages of life. These changes are called human growth and development.

Everyone will go through the same stages of development during their lives, but no two people will follow the exact same pattern or rate of development. Each client must be treated as an individual and a whole person who is growing and developing rather than someone who is merely ill or disabled.

Two learning objectives apply to each stage of human development discussed in Part 1 of this chapter:

❑ 1. Describe major characteristics of each stage of human development

❑ 2. Identify disorders common to each age group

Infancy, Birth to Twelve Months

Infants grow and develop at an incredible rate. In one year a baby moves from total dependence on the caregiver to the relative independence of moving around, communicating basic needs, and feeding himself.

By satisfying the basic biological and psychological needs of infants, caregivers set the stage for future growth and development. Physical and emotional well-being are intimately connected throughout life, but especially in infancy. For example, when an infant is held and fed, not only is the need for food met, but the infant's needs for love and security are met as well.

In order to develop into a healthy and confident child, a baby must have his basic physical and emotional needs met consistently. Ideally, the same one or two caregivers or parents should care for the baby. Responding to an infant's cries and meeting his needs forms a bond based on trust and a feeling of security in the child. Without trust and security, infants become anxious and fearful.

Physical development in infancy moves from the head down. For example, infants gain control over the muscles of the neck before they are able to control the muscles in their shoulders. Control over muscles in the trunk area, such as the shoulder, develops before control of the extremities. This head-to-toe sequence should be respected when caring for infants. For example, newborns must be supported at the shoulders, head, and neck, and babies who cannot sit or crawl should not be encouraged to stand or walk.

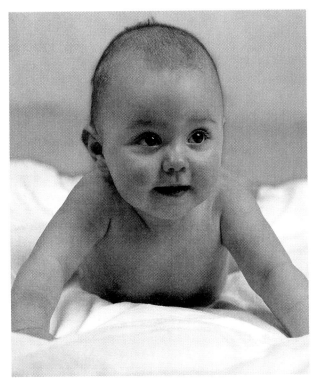

Fig. 10-1. Infant's physical development moves from the head down.

Common Disorders: Infancy

Some disorders of infancy are the result of prematurity, low birth weight, or birth defects. Others are caused by viruses or bacteria. As a home care aide you may be assigned to care for babies with any of the following disorders:

Prematurity. Babies who are born before 37 weeks gestation (more than three weeks before the due date) are considered premature. These babies may weigh from one to six pounds, depending on how early they are born. Often, premature babies will remain in the hospital for some time after birth. At home, premature babies may need special care, including medication, heart monitoring, and frequent feedings to ensure weight gain.

Low birth weight. Babies born at full term but weighing less than five pounds are called low birth weight babies. Low birth weight babies can have many of the same problems premature babies have, and they are cared for in much the same way as premature babies.

Birth defects. The term birth defects is very general, including many different conditions that affect an infant from birth. Some birth defects are inherited from parents, others are caused by injury or disease during pregnancy. Some of the conditions you may see include the following:

▶ **Cerebral palsy** is the result of an injury to the cerebrum (part of the brain) that occurs during pregnancy or the birth process. The resulting brain damage causes a loss of muscle control, poor coordination, problems with balance, and difficulty in speaking.

▶ **Cystic fibrosis** is a disorder of the respiratory and digestive systems. Although there is no cure, special care delays death.

▶ **Down's syndrome** is a chromosomal disorder that causes mental retardation and a characteristic appearance that includes a small skull, a flattened nose, short fingers, and a wider space between the first two fingers of each hand and the first two toes of each foot. Some babies with Down's syndrome can grow up to live independently.

Viral or bacterial infections can cause fever, runny nose, coughing, rash, vomiting, diarrhea, or secondary infections of the sinuses or ears. Some babies have a tendency to contract these infections. Bacterial infections can be treated with antibiotics. Viral infections are treated with extra rest, fluids, and sometimes over-the-counter medications for cough or congestion.

Finally, you should be aware of **sudden infant death syndrome (SIDS)** or crib death. SIDS babies stop breathing and die for no known reason while asleep. Doctors do not know how to prevent SIDS, but studies have shown that putting the baby to sleep on its back or side can reduce the chances of SIDS. Because SIDS is more common among premature or low birth weight babies, these infants often wear apnea (AP-nee-a) **monitors** to alert parents if breathing stops. Another factor that may contribute to SIDS is second-hand smoke. Parents and caregivers should never smoke around infants or children.

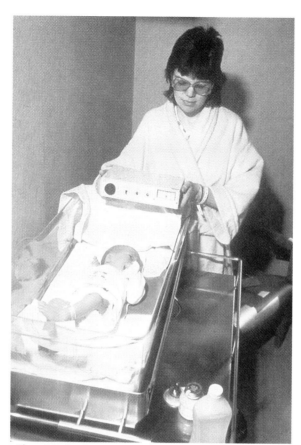

Fig. 10-2. Apnea monitors are often used in the home for premature or low birth weight babies.

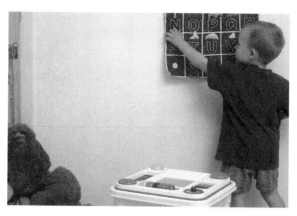

Fig. 10-3. Toddlers' rooms should be child proofed and electrical outlets should be plugged.

gain independence. One part of this independence is new control over their bodies. Toddlers learn to speak, gain coordination of their limbs, and control over their bladders and bowels.

Toddlers assert their new independence by exploring further and further from the caregiver. **Child proofing**, putting away or locking up poisons and removing other hazards, such as sharp objects or unsteady furniture, is essential to keep toddlers safe.

Psychologically, toddlers learn that they are individuals, separate from their parents. Children this age may try to control their parents. They may try to get what they want by throwing tantrums, whining, or refusing to cooperate. This is a key time for parents to establish rules and standards. If these limits are consistently applied, toddlers will eventually learn to live by them.

Childhood

The Toddler Period, Ages One to Three

During the toddler years, children who began life completely dependent on their parents or caregivers

The Preschool Years, Ages Three to Six

Children in their preschool years develop skills that will help them become more independent and have social relationships. They develop a vocabulary and language skills, and learn to play cooperatively in groups. Children in this age group become more physically coordinated, and learn to care for them-

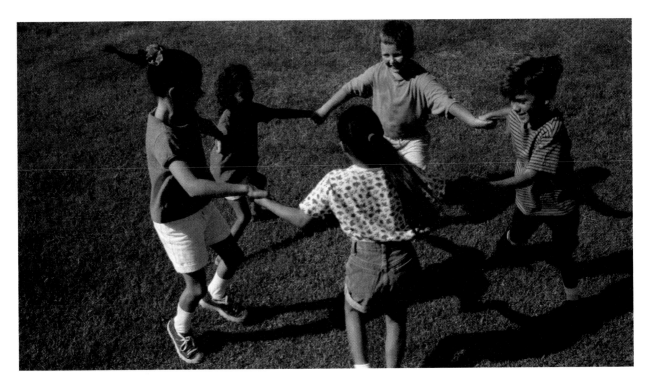

Fig. 10-4. Preschool children playing cooperatively.

selves. They also develop ways of relating to family members, and they learn to distinguish right from wrong.

School-Age Children, Ages Six to Twelve

From ages six to about eight years, children's development is centered around cognitive (KOG-ni-tiv) **development** (developing thinking and learning skills), and social development. As children enter school, they also explore the environment around them and relate to other children through games, peer groups, and classroom activities. In these years, children learn to get along with each other. They also begin to behave in a way that is common among their sex, and they develop a conscience, morals, and self-esteem.

Between eight and twelve years of age, children begin to display more physical and psychological maturity.

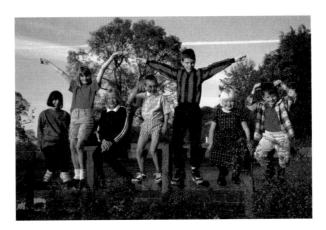

Fig. 10-5. School-age children on a field trip.

Their bodies change as they make the transition to adolescence. Girls display more change in these years as breasts bud and hips become broader, with fat pads forming. Boys' genitals become more mature.

Children in late childhood learn to behave morally and ethically and to understand male and female differences. Friendships with children of the same sex are important. Children become curious about sex and share information. They begin to question the authority of parents and other adults and to see weaknesses and imperfections in the adults they know.

Common Disorders: Childhood

Children born with birth defects may continue to be affected during childhood or may learn to manage their conditions. Other childhood disorders that you may see as a home care aide include the following:

Chicken pox. Chicken pox is a highly contagious, viral illness that strikes nearly all children. It generally has no serious effects for healthy children, but in adults or in anyone with a weakened immune system it can have more serious consequences. A new vaccine against chicken pox may gradually eliminate this disease.

Infections caused by viruses or bacteria. Children, as well as infants, may be susceptible to colds, flu, or other infections. As discussed above, bacterial infections can be treated with antibiotics. Viral infections are treated with extra rest, fluids, and over-the-counter medications for cough or congestion.

Leukemia (loo-KEE-mee-a). A form of cancer, leukemia refers to the inability of the body's white blood cells to fight disease. Children with leukemia may be susceptible to infections and other disorders.

Chemotherapy can be used to fight this disease. You will learn more about caring for clients with cancer in Chapter 20, Common Chronic and Acute Conditions.

Child abuse. The term child abuse refers to physical, emotional, and sexual mistreatment of children, as well as neglect and maltreatment. **Physical abuse** includes hitting, kicking, burning, or intentionally causing injury to a child. **Emotional abuse** includes withholding affection, constantly or severely criticizing, or ridiculing a child. **Sexual abuse** includes engaging in or allowing another person to engage in a sexual act with a child. **Neglect** and **maltreatment** include not providing adequate food, clothing, or support; allowing children to use alcohol or drugs; leaving children alone; or exposing them to danger. You will learn more about the signs and symptoms of child abuse in Chapter 19, Caring for New Mothers, Infants and Children.

Fig. 10-6. Commonly accepted vaccination schedule

United States, January–December 1998

Vaccines are listed under the routinely recommended ages. Bars indicate range of acceptable ages for immunization. Catch-up immunization should be done during any visit when feasible. Shaded ovals indicate vaccines to be assessed and given if necessary during the early adolescent visit.

Age / Vaccine	Birth	1 mo.	2 mos.	4 mos.	6 mos.	12 mos.	15 mos.	18 mos.	4–6 yrs.	11–12 yrs.	14–16 yrs.
Hepatitis B[2,3]	Hep B[1]	Hep B[2]	Hep B[2]		Hep B[3]					Hep B[3]	
Diphtheria, Tetanus, Pertussis[4]			DTaP or DTP	DTaP or DTP	DTaP or DTP		DTaP or DTP[4]		DTaP or DTP	Td	
H Influenzae type b[2]			Hib	Hib	Hib		Hib				
Polio[2]			Polio[2]	Polio	Polio[2]				Polio		
Measles, Mumps, Rubella[7]						MMR			MMR[7]	MMR[7]	
Varicella[2]							Var			Var[4]	

Measles, mumps, rubella, diphtheria, smallpox, whooping cough, polio. These diseases, once common in childhood, can all be prevented now with vaccinations. According to the American Academy of Pediatrics, infants and children should be vaccinated according to the schedule in **Fig. 10-6.**

Adolescence

Puberty

Puberty (PYOO-ber-tee) is the stage of growth when secondary sex characteristics appear and reproductive organs begin to function due to the secretion of the reproductive hormones. The onset of puberty occurs between the ages of ten and sixteen for girls and twelve and fourteen for boys.

In girls, puberty begins with menstruation (men-stroo-ay-shun). Secondary sex characteristics also appear: breasts increase in size, pubic and axillary hair appears, hips become wider and rounder, and the voice deepens slightly. In boys, puberty occurs when the genitals have matured to the degree that nocturnal emissions (nok-TER-nal ee-MIH-shuns) occur. A nocturnal emission (sometimes called a "wet dream") occurs during sleep, when the penis becomes erect and emits semen. Secondary sex characteristics develop: hair appears in the pubic and axillary regions and on the face. The voice becomes deeper and the size of the neck and shoulders increases.

Adolescence, Ages Twelve to Eighteen

Many teenagers have a difficult time adapting to the rapid changes that occur in their bodies after puberty. Because peer acceptance is important to them and because they see images of perfection in the media, adolescents (ad-o-LES-ents) may be afraid that they are unattractive or even abnormal. Girls worry about being overweight and may think their breasts or hips are too large or too small. Boys may be concerned about their size, clumsiness, height, or genital size.

This concern for body image and peer acceptance, combined with changing hormones that influence moods, can cause adolescents to swing from one mood to another. Conflicting pressures develop as they remain dependent on their parents and yet need to express themselves socially and sexually. The long process of becoming independent from parents reaches a climax during adolescence. Eventually, most teenagers gain more control over their emotions, more acceptance of who they are, and more confidence in themselves.

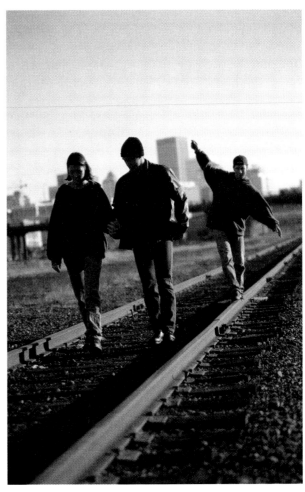

Fig. 10-7. Adolescence is a time of exploring independence and adapting to change.

Social interaction between members of the opposite sex becomes very important in adolescence. Sexual activity may begin in these years, and teenagers sometimes make decisions without considering the consequences. Adolescents often feel that they are immortal or that nothing can hurt them. This mistaken belief can cause reckless behavior leading to car accidents, drug abuse, pregnancy, or sexually transmitted diseases.

Common Disorders: Adolescence

Eating disorders. As their bodies change, adolescents, especially girls, may develop an obsession with being thin. Anorexia (an-or-EX-ee-a) is a disease in which a person does not eat or exercises excessively to lose weight. A person with bulimia (byoo-LIM-ee-a) **binges**, eating huge amounts of foods or very fattening foods, and then **purges** or eliminates the food by vomiting, using laxatives or exercising excessively. Eating disorders can be serious and even life-threatening for adolescents as well as adults, and must be treated with therapy and in some cases, hospitalization.

Sexually transmitted diseases (STDs). Teenagers can contract STDs such as chlamydia (kla-MID-ee-a), herpes (HER-peez), and AIDS if they are sexually active. If teenagers are sexually active, only condoms offer some protection from sexually transmitted diseases. The signs and symptoms, means of transmission, and treatments for sexually transmitted diseases are discussed in Chapter 9, The Human Body in Health and Disease.

Teenage pregnancy. Girls who are sexually active and do not use birth control, or do not use it properly, can become pregnant. Teenage pregnancy can have terrible consequences for adolescents, their families, and the babies born to teenage parents. Teenagers should understand that they can avoid pregnancy by using birth control or by abstaining from (not having) sexual intercourse. Teenagers who choose to be sexually active should know what birth control methods are available and understand the importance of proper use.

Teenagers who do become pregnant will find that pregnancy puts a great deal of stress on their bodies. Adolescent girls are still children, their bodies are still developing, and in most cases they are not physically ready to bear a child. It is common for teenage mothers to give birth to premature or low birth weight babies.

Aside from the physical stress of pregnancy, adolescents are typically not ready for the emotional and financial demands of parenthood. Many teenage mothers remain single mothers and begin a cycle of poverty that they are unable to escape. Children of teenage mothers are more likely to grow up poor and with fewer social and educational advantages.

Depression and suicide. Because of the many physical and emotional changes they are experiencing, adolescents may become depressed and even attempt suicide. Parents, teachers, and friends should watch for the signs of depression, including withdrawal, loss of appetite, weight gain or loss, sleep problems, moodiness, and apathy. Teenagers who are depressed should see a doctor, counselor, therapist, minister, or other trusted adult who can get them the help they need.

Trauma or accidental injury. Adolescents can sustain trauma (TRAW-ma), or severe injury, to the head or spinal cord in car accidents or sports injuries. These injuries can be temporarily or permanently disabling or even fatal.

Adulthood

Young Adulthood, Ages Eighteen to Forty

By the age of eighteen, most young adults have stopped growing. Psychological and social development continues, however. The developmental tasks of these years include selecting an appropriate education and an occupation or career, selecting a mate, learning to live with a mate or others, raising children, and developing a satisfying sex life.

Middle Adulthood: Forty to Sixty-five Years

In general, people in middle adulthood are more comfortable and stable than they were in previous stages. Many of their major life decisions have already been made. In the early years of middle adulthood people sometimes experience a "mid-life crisis," or a period of unrest centered around an unconscious desire for change and fulfillment of unmet goals.

Middle adults who are parents must deal with an "empty nest" by adjusting to children leaving home to lead their own lives. The supportive role of parenting continues in this stage, however, as children establish independent identities. In addition, middle adults may also be called on to provide sup-

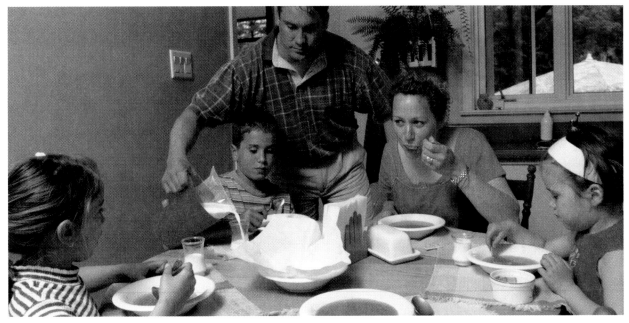

Fig. 10-8. Young adulthood often involves raising a family while managing a career.

port and care for their own parents who may be in poor health, in need of assistance, or dying.

Physical changes related to aging also occur in middle adulthood. Most adults in this age group become aware of these changes when they begin to have difficulty maintaining their weight or notice a decrease in strength and energy. Metabolism and other body functions slow down, wrinkles and grey hair appear, and vision and hearing loss may begin. Women experience menopause (MEN-o-paws), the end of menstruation, which occurs when the ovaries stop secreting hormones. Many diseases and illnesses can develop in these years, and these disorders can become chronic and life threatening.

If healthy eating habits and exercise are not already adopted, middle adults should try to make these habits a part of their lives. Proper diet, including low fat and high fiber food choices, helps maintain body weight, and may protect against heart disease and even cancer. Exercise has many of the same benefits, and can also help lower blood pressure, relieve stress, and provide more energy. People who smoke should make every effort to stop. Adopting a healthy lifestyle in the middle adult years can make life better now and prevent frailty and other health problems in later adulthood.

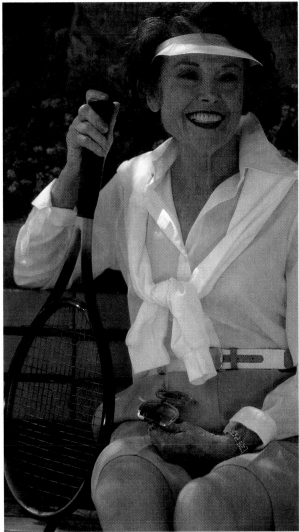

Fig. 10-9. Exercise and a good diet are as important in middle adulthood as any time of life.

Late Adulthood: Sixty-five Years and Older

Late adulthood is a time of many changes, physically, psychologically, and socially. Persons in late adulthood must adjust to the effects of aging, including the loss of physical strength and health, the death of loved ones, retirement, and preparation for their own death. Although the developmental tasks of this age appear to deal entirely with loss, the solutions to these problems often involve new relationships, friendships, and interests.

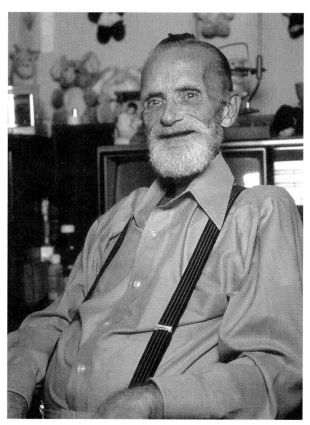

Fig. 10-10. New friendships and interests can help ease some of the transitions of late adulthood.

Because so many of the people receiving home care are older adults, in the rest of this chapter you will learn more about aging and the needs of elderly clients.

Common Disorders: Adulthood

The disorders a home care aide is most likely to see (AIDS, arthritis, Alzheimer's disease, cancer, diabetes, and stroke) are discussed in Chapter 20, Com-

mon Chronic and Acute Conditions. All of the common disorders of adulthood listed below are discussed in Chapter 9, The Human Body in Health and Disease:

- AIDS
- Alzheimer's Disease
- Angina pectoris
- Arthritis
- Asthma
- Atherosclerosis
- Benign prostatic hypertrophy
- Bronchitis
- Cancer
- Cataracts
- Chronic kidney failure, or uremia
- Congestive heart failure
- Deafness
- Diabetes
- Emphysema
- Epilepsy
- Heart attack, or myocardial infarction (MI)
- Hepatitis
- Hypertension
- Kidney stones, or calculi
- Multiple sclerosis
- Osteoporosis
- Parkinson's Disease
- Peripheral vascular disease
- Pneumonia
- Renovascular hypertension
- Stroke, or cerebrovascular accident (CVA)
- Thyroid disorders
- Tuberculosis
- Ulcerative colitis
- Urinary tract infection (UTI), or cystitis

Part 2
Normal and Abnormal Changes of Aging

❑ 3. Distinguish between fact (what is true) and fallacy (what is not true) about the aging process

We are all aging throughout our lives, since we are always getting older. But when we talk about the process of aging, we are usually referring to later adulthood, ages 65 and older, and the health changes that occur in those years.

Because later adulthood covers an age range of as many as 25 to 35 years, people in this age category can have very different capabilities, depending on their health. Some 70-year-old people still enjoy active sports, while others are not active. Many 85-year-old people can still live alone, though others may live with family members or in long-term care facilities. Generalizations or stereotypes about older people are often false, and they create prejudices against the elderly that are as unfair as prejudices against racial, ethnic, or religious groups.

On television or in the movies older people are often shown as helpless, lonely, disabled, slow, forgetful, dependent, or inactive. However, research indicates that most older people are active and engaged in work, volunteer activities, learning programs, and exercise regimens. Aging is a normal process, not a disease. Most older people live independent lives and are able to manage without assistance.

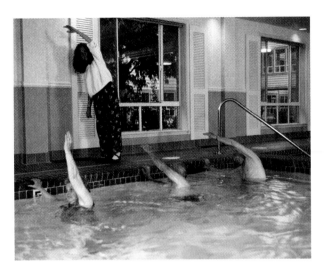

Fig. 10-11. Many older people are active in work, volunteer activities, learning programs, and exercise regimens.

As a home care aide you are likely to spend much of your time working with elderly clients. You must be able to distinguish between what is true about aging and what is not true. While older adults do go through many physical, psychological, and social changes as they age, normal changes of aging do not mean an older person must become dependent, ill, or inactive. Learning to separate normal changes of aging from signs of illness or disability will allow you to work most effectively with your elderly clients.

For most older adults, **the challenge of aging is the need to adjust to change.** As personal, physical, social, and work lives change, older adults must become more flexible. Being able to adjust to change, as well as maintaining good physical health, will help older adults continue to live independently and happily.

❏ 4. Discuss normal changes of aging and list guidelines for appropriate care

Aging is a continuous process from conception to death. Each person ages in a unique way, influenced by genetics and lifestyle. Although we cannot choose our genetic makeup, we can choose the lifestyle we lead. Habits of diet, exercise, attitude, social and physical activities, and health maintenance affect our well-being later in life.

Some of your older clients will need assistance in performing activities of daily living (ADLs). Clients who are chronically ill and need a lot of help still benefit from living at home. As a home care aide, you perform an important role in letting older clients stay in familiar surroundings while getting the help they need. Remembering the changes that occur in the elderly will help you provide the right care for your elderly clients. Over the next several pages, you will learn about normal and abnormal changes of aging in each body system.

Integumentary system

Changes: Skin is thinner, drier, and more fragile. Much of the fatty layer beneath the skin is lost. Texture of hair may change. Nails are harder and more brittle. Reduced circulation to the skin can cause dryness, itching, and irritation.

Care:

▸ Dry skin can become more irritated and itchy if your elderly clients take tub baths too often. Older adults perspire less and do not need to bathe as often. Most elderly people generally need a complete bath only twice a week, with sponge baths every day.

Special moisturizing lotions can help relieve dry skin. Be gentle when assisting clients with personal care; elderly clients' skin can be fragile and tear easily.

Hair also becomes drier and needs to be shampooed less often. Brush dry hair to stimulate and distribute the natural oils.

Musculoskeletal system

Changes. Muscles are not as strong as they once were. Bones may become more brittle. Joints may stiffen and become painful. Illness, poor balance, or difficulty walking may discourage some clients from moving about, changing position, or performing activities.

Care:

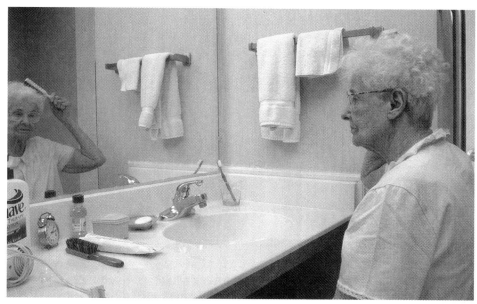

Fig. 10-12. Brushing hair helps stimulate and distribute natural oils.

To prevent further loss of physical and mental capacities, encourage clients to perform ADLs and range of motion (ROM) exercises that they are capable of within the guidelines of the care plan. You will learn how to assist with ROM exercises in Chapter 15, Promoting Independence: Rehabilitation and Restorative Care. Encourage clients to eat in the kitchen and walk to the bathroom, for example, until these activities are no longer possible. Encourage clients to make decisions and dress themselves, with assistance if necessary, no matter how long it takes.

To prevent or slow osteoporosis (os-tee-oh-po-RO-sis), the condition that is responsible for fragile bones, clients should be encouraged to walk and do other light exercise. Exercise can strengthen the bones as well as muscles.

Nervous system

Changes in mental function. As we age, we lose some of our ability to think logically and quickly. How much ability we lose depends on the indi-

vidual. Aging can also affect concentration and memory. Elderly clients may experience memory loss of recent events. This short-term memory loss may cause anxiety in older clients. Long-term memory, or memory for past events usually remains sharp, and many elderly people enjoy **reminiscing**, or talk-

ing about the past. As we age, maturity and long experience in life give us a different perspective on the past. By reminiscing, we can review our lives and resolve longstanding problems.

Care:

You may be able to help your clients with memory loss by suggesting they make lists or write notes about things they want to remember. Placing a calendar or clock nearby may help the client remain oriented.

If your clients enjoy reminiscing, take an interest in their past experiences by asking to see photos or hear stories.

Older people are still able to learn and enjoy new activities, although they sometimes do not learn as quickly as younger adults. Finding new hobbies or activities can be very beneficial for older clients.

Changes in vision, hearing, taste, and smell. The failing vision of many elderly clients may make reading or other activities difficult or impossible. Fail-

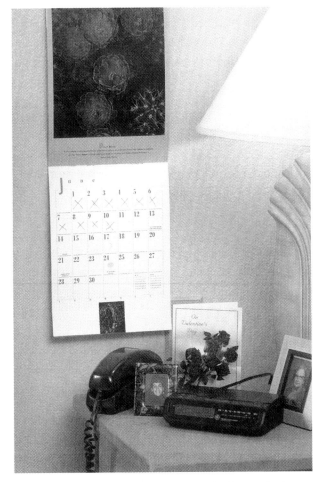

Fig. 10-13. A calendar and a clock can help a client remain oriented. Show interest if your client likes to reminisce about the past.

ing hearing may make it frustrating for older adults to try to communicate. Weakened sense of smell, taste, and touch may present dangers for older adults.

Care:

- Many books and some magazines are available printed in large type. "Talking books" or books on tape are available at libraries and bookstores.

- Keep clients' eyeglasses clean. Bright colors and good light will also help clients with poor eyesight. Sometimes the eyes of the elderly do not adapt quickly to glare or to changes from light to dark. If glare is a problem, encourage clients to wear sunglasses outdoors. When going into another room, be sure the lights are on before your client enters.

- If your client is having trouble hearing, speak in a low-pitched voice. For some people, low-pitched sounds are easier to hear. You may also need to

repeat words to help the client understand them. Some clients need hearing aids and should be encouraged to use them. Excess cerumen (se-ROO-men) or earwax can make hearing difficult. If you suspect excess earwax, tell your supervisor. A nurse can treat this problem.

- If a client has difficulty hearing, face him or her and speak slowly, simply, and clearly. Be careful not to overdo this. Don't assume that all your elderly clients are hard of hearing. Speaking loudly or oversimplifying your speech when it is not necessary can make clients feel they are being treated like children.

- Because we lose taste buds as we age, older people often cannot taste as well. Decreased sense of smell may contribute to the altered sense of taste. Make sure the food in the house is fresh, because older clients may not be able to smell or taste that food is spoiled. Older clients should always have smoke and carbon monoxide detectors in their homes, particularly since they may not smell leaking gas or smoke.

- The sense of touch is also affected by aging. Be careful with hot drinks and hot bath water. Clients sometimes cannot tell if something is too hot for them. The elderly client who is confined to bed may not feel uncomfortable, but because of decreased circulation and dry skin, he or she is at risk for developing **pressure sores** (sometimes called decubitus ulcers) or bedsores. The sense of pain may also be diminished in the elderly. As always, be alert to changes in your clients' health.

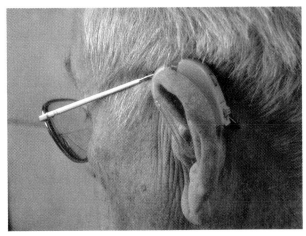

Fig. 10-14. Senses, such as vision and hearing, may be weakened or may fail with age.

Disorientation, or confusion about time and place, may occur in new surroundings or as a result of infection or medication. Disorientation is *not* a normal part of aging. Disorientation caused by medication is called **drug intoxication**. Many elderly people take one or more kinds of medication. Taking the wrong amount or combination of medications can cause disorientation.

Care:

▷ As with all changes in your clients' health, always report any observations you make about decreased senses. Disorientation may be a sign and symptom of an illness.

▷ Techniques for working with confused clients can be found in Chapter 20, Common Chronic and Acute Conditions.

Circulatory system

Changes in the efficiency of the heart. As we age, our hearts pump less efficiently. Increased activity places greater demand on the heart, which it may not be able to meet. Older people may need more rest to reduce demand on the heart. They may not be able to walk long distances, climb stairs, or exert themselves.

Care:

▷ Moderate exercise is necessary and helpful. Walking, stretching, and even lifting light weights can help older people maintain strength and mobility.

▷ Active or passive ROM exercises are important for clients who cannot get out of bed. Your clients' care plans will specify what kinds of exercise or activity they should be doing. Abilities can vary a great deal from client to client.

▷ Clients with heart conditions, particularly heart failure, must avoid vigorous activity or exercise, including carrying heavy objects. Some clients may experience dizziness when they stand up too quickly. Encourage clients to rise slowly and to stand still for a few moments, supporting themselves by holding on to a chair or other piece of furniture.

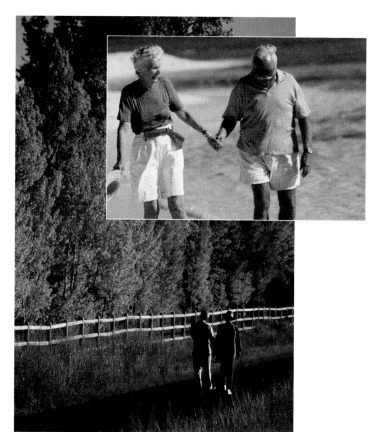

Fig. 10-15. Moderate exercise can help older adults maintain strength and mobility.

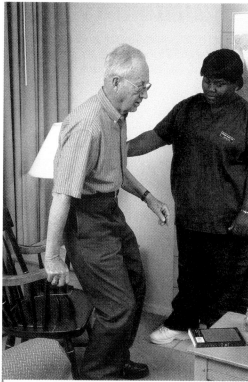

Fig. 10-16. An older adult may need to rise slowly and stand still for a moment to keep from getting dizzy.

Changes in circulation and sensitivity to hot and cold. Less efficient circulation of blood in older people causes older adults to be more sensitive to the cold.

Care:

▹ Houses may need to be kept at a higher temperature than normally preferred, and older clients may need to wear layers of clothing to keep warm. Some elderly clients who are concerned about the cost of heating may actually lower the thermostat to a dangerous level.

▹ Poor circulation in the extremities causes the feet to feel cold. Be sure your client wears slippers or shoes and socks.

▹ Do not use hot water bottles or heating pads. Poor circulation causes dry skin that is fragile and can burn easily. In addition, because of the dulled sense of pain mentioned previously, an older person may not realize he or she is being burned until it is too late.

Respiratory system

Shortness of breath. As the body ages, the lungs have fewer alveoli in which oxygen/carbon dioxide exchange can take place. Shortness of breath is a common problem for older adults. Older clients may also have a harder time coughing up mucus.

Care:

▹ You may need to provide frequent rest periods when assisting a client with ADLs.

▹ Follow the care plan carefully for exercise and activity instructions. As noted above in guidelines associated with the circulatory system, moderate exercise is helpful, but overdoing it can be very dangerous for an older adult. If you have a question about the activity level specified in the care plan, talk to your supervisor.

Urinary system

Urine elimination. The bladder is not able to hold the same amount of urine as it did when clients were younger. Older clients may need to urinate more frequently. Many elderly persons awaken several times during the night to urinate.

Care:

▹ Clients should always drink plenty of fluids during the day. However, some clients should reduce fluids in the evening to avoid frequent trips to the bathroom at night.

Incontinence (in KON-ti-nens) is the inability to control the bladder. Incontinence is *not* a normal part of aging. For clients who are incontinent, the care plan may specify bladder training or the client may wear incontinence pads or briefs.

Care:

▹ Always report incontinence. It may be a sign and symptom of an illness.

▹ Cleanliness and good skin care are important for clients who are incontinent.

▹ Some clients may have urinary catheters (YOUR-i-nayr-ee KATH-e-ters), or tubes that run from the bladder to a bag outside the body. You will be instructed on what care to give and how to perform it for clients with urinary catheters.

Digestive system

Poor nutrition. Older people who cannot get around easily or who live alone may skip meals or eat foods that are not nutritious. A dulled sense of taste, often made worse by side effects of medications, may result in a poor appetite.

Care:

▹ You may be assigned to shop for and prepare meals. Chapters 22 and 23 provide more information on nutrition and meal preparation.

▹ Older people may have trouble chewing (because of loose dentures, dental problems, or gum disease) and may require soft foods.

▹ Decreased saliva production not only affects the ability to chew, but also places older clients at risk of choking. Provide plenty of fluids with meals.

Changes in digestion and bowel elimination. Digestion takes longer and is less efficient in older adults. Many older adults have trouble with **indigestion**, or an upset stomach. Body waste moves more slowly through the intestines, and **constipation**, the inability to have a bowel movement, may occur.

Care:

- Some clients need to eat several small meals a day or have the large meal in the middle of the day.

- Clients should be encouraged to drink plenty of fluids to keep bowel movements moist.

- Clients should eat a diet that contains fiber.

Dehydration is a condition that results from inadequate fluid in the body. It is *not* a normal sign of aging; however many older people do not feel thirsty and may not be aware that they are dehydrated. Dehydration can cause constipation, weight loss, dry skin, infection, dizziness and weakness, and other illnesses that require medical attention.

Care:

- Encourage clients to drink an adequate amount of fluids each day.

- Several medical conditions and medications can affect a client's hydration status, so always check with your supervisor before increasing a client's fluid intake.

- You may be assigned to measure fluid intake and output. Measure and document carefully to ensure that the client's fluid balance is healthy. You will learn how to monitor fluid balance in Chapter 13, Performing Basic Health Care Skills.

Endocrine system

Changes: Levels of reproductive hormones are lower. Pancreas function lessens, which may lead to diabetes for some clients.

Care:

- Older clients may need to take insulin or eat certain foods to regulate blood sugar. The client's doctor or nurse will teach the client what to do. Any special instructions on care you are to give will be included in the care plan.

Reproductive system

Changes in genitals. Genital areas may become dry and uncomfortable. In males, the prostate gland increases in size. In females, fatty tissue in the breasts may diminish, and mucous secretions in the vagina decrease. Though the reproductive organs change, sexual needs and desires do not necessarily change.

Care:

- Avoiding too many hot baths can help prevent discomfort in the genital area.

- Despite changes in the reproductive organs, older adults remain sexual beings. Allow your clients as much privacy as you can while still providing good care. Do not make any assumptions or generalizations about the sexual feelings of older adults.

- Do report any behavior that makes you uncomfortable or that seems inappropriate. Inappropriate behavior is *not* a normal sign of aging, and could be a sign of illness.

Immune system

Weakened immunity. As we age, our immune system gradually weakens. It also may take longer to recover from an illness. Bone marrow activity (which produces white blood cells that fight infections) decreases as we age. Changes in the respiratory system's protective surface may also result in increased respiratory infections. Many elderly people develop anemia, especially iron-deficiency anemia, due to poor nutrition and less efficient use of nutrients by the body. While anemia is common, it is *not* a normal sign of aging. Report any signs and symptoms of anemia, including weakness, fainting, light-headedness, and headache.

Care:

- Vaccines against common infections, such as influenza (flu), are very important for older adults.

- Helping the client maintain good nutrition can help him stay healthy (See care tips under digestive system. Chapters 22 and 23 provide more information on nutrition and meal preparation).

Lymphatic system

The number and size of lymph nodes is reduced. Along with the changes in the immune system, these changes result in the body being less able to contract a fever to fight infection.

Care:

▷ An older adult fighting an infection may not experience a fever. Even a slight temperature increase may be an indication that the person is fighting an infection. Taking accurate vital signs is very important, especially with older adults. You will learn how to take vital signs in Chapter 13.

Psychological

Some forgetfulness is a normal part of aging, but constant memory lapses or forgetting basic information such as family members' names are *not* normal changes of aging.

Care:

Any of the following signs should be reported to your supervisor immediately, as they may indicate illness:

▷ disorientation, or change in ability to remember who they are, what month or season of the year it is, or other basic facts

▷ difficulty concentrating

▷ depression

▷ dementia, or a loss of mental abilities that interferes with ADLs

▷ confusion

▷ suicidal thoughts

▷ insomnia (inability to sleep)

Depression is very common among the elderly, but it is *not* a normal sign of aging. Elderly persons may not admit feelings of depression to themselves or others. According to the National Center for Health Statistics, the elderly are at higher risk for suicide than all other age groups. Report any signs of depression in your clients to your supervisor. In many cases, depression may be successfully treated.

Care:

▷ Observing and reporting signs and symptoms is the best way to help a client who may be suffering from depression. Signs and symptoms of depression include **anorexia**, or loss of appetite; **insomnia**, or difficulty sleeping; acting moody or withdrawn; and other changes in appearance, speech, movement, and behavior. Sleep disorders and emotional changes, such as hopelessness, anxiety, apathy (lack of interest), agitation, restlessness, and demanding or violent behavior, are particularly important to report.

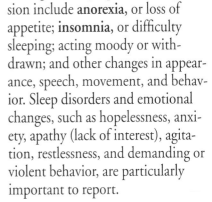

Depression is common among the elderly, but is not a normal sign of aging.

Lifestyle Changes. Aging brings many social, physical, and mental changes. Friends, colleagues, and relatives die; physical strength and stamina diminish; and fears of illness, injury, and death may increase. Retirement causes changes in what and how much people do each day. Living arrangements may also change. These changes require adjustment, which can become more difficult as people age.

Care:

▷ You can help your clients adjust to change by listening to them and caring about their feelings.

▷ Ensuring that clients are safe is another way you help them adapt to their changing lifestyles. Chapter 6, Safety and Body Mechanics describes how to help make clients' homes safe for them.

Part 3
Psychological and Social Needs of the Elderly

The psychological and social needs of older adults are the same as for younger people. The needs for love and affection, acceptance by others, and interaction with other people do not go away with age. Chapter 8, Basic Human Needs: Supporting

Physical, Psychological, and Social Health, discusses the basic psychological and social needs of humans.

❑ 5. Identify attitudes and living habits that promote good mental and physical health for older adults

Staying active, maintaining self-esteem, and living independently can promote good physical and mental health for older adults. You can encourage your clients in these attitudes and habits in the following ways.

Encourage your clients to pursue activities they enjoy and can succeed in. Many older people enjoy reading, playing checkers, playing cards, doing crafts, or enjoying music. Working with others on charity or community service projects can allow older people to share their knowledge and experience. Senior centers or community centers offer classes, hobby groups, and field trips that some older clients may enjoy. Many older people are involved in activities through a church or synagogue. You can encourage even your homebound Medicare clients to participate in activities by asking them about what they are doing, admiring their work, or even participating yourself in games or crafts when time permits.

Help clients develop a routine for the day. Structuring the day around meals, activities, rest, and self-care can help fight depression and give older people a sense of purpose. Older people who don't have a routine may simply stay in bed or become bored and lonely.

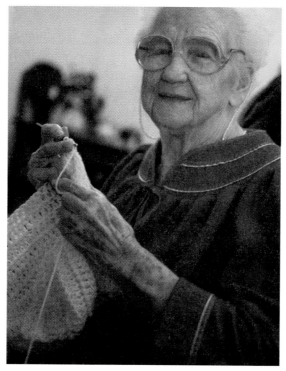

Fig. 10-17. Continuing to participate in activities they enjoy promotes good mental and physical health for older adults.

Encourage self-care. Your clients should do as much for themselves as they possibly can. You won't be helping a client by giving her a bath if that is something she can do for herself. **Your job is to assist with or perform activities the client cannot do alone.** The more your clients can care for themselves, the better they will feel about themselves. Follow the care plan, and keep in touch with your supervisor about changes in the client's abilities.

Help your clients be well groomed. Appearance affects the way we feel about ourselves. Help

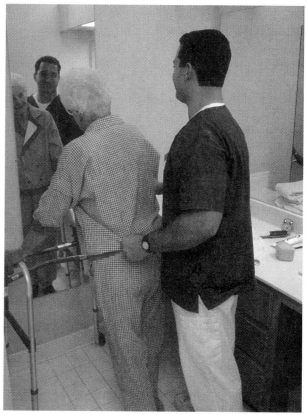

Fig. 10-18. A well-groomed appearance helps people of all ages feel good about themselves.

or work if he or she seems to want this. Knock before you enter the room, even if the door is open. Remember that clients may not want to talk all the time. When visitors come by or call, let your client visit undisturbed and do not try to participate in the conversation. Treat visitors respectfully and make them feel welcome. Even if an unannounced visit disrupts your schedule, remember how important social contact is and try to be flexible.

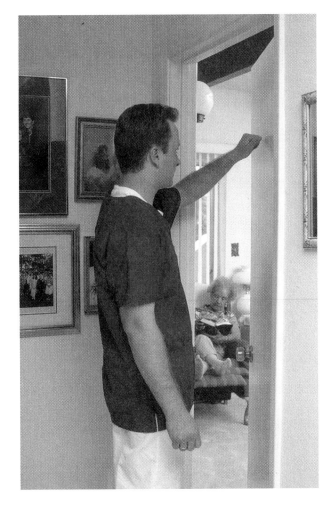

Fig. 10-19. Having respect for your clients' privacy is one way you can help them feel they are still in control of their lives.

your clients style hair, dress neatly, use cosmetics, or shave.

Address your clients respectfully. Your elderly clients will probably be older than you, so do not call them by their first names unless they ask you to. Use your clients' last names with whatever title they prefer (Mr., Ms., Miss, Mrs., or Dr.). Speak to them with respect. Ask for their opinions and let them make their own decisions as much as possible. The more independent and capable they feel the more independent and capable they will be. Never treat a client like a child or talk about a client as if he or she were not there.

Respect the needs for privacy and for social interaction. Let your client be alone to read, study, pray,

---

Part 4
Abuse and Neglect of the Elderly

❏ **6. List ways to recognize and report elder abuse and neglect**

In the past ten years the health care community has become aware of the problem of elder abuse and neglect. In 1991, it was estimated that between 1.5 million and 2 million cases of elder abuse occur in the United States each year. As the elderly population grows, this problem may become worse.

Elderly people may be abused intentionally or unintentionally, through ignorance, inexperience, or inability to care for them. People who abuse elders may mistreat them physically, psychologically, verbally, financially, and/or materially. They may deprive them of their rights or they may neglect them by failing to provide food, clothing, shelter, or medical care. Some older adults may also become self-abusive or neglect their own needs.

As a home care aide working with elderly clients, you will be in an excellent position to observe and report abuse or neglect. Home care aides have an ethical responsibility to observe for signs of elder abuse and report suspected cases to a supervisor. In many states, reporting abuse is also a legal responsibility. Give your supervisor as much information as possible so the supervisor can contact the appropriate members of the health care team. Take this responsibility seriously and help end this disturbing trend.

❑ 7. Identify community resources available to help the elderly

Government and private agencies exist in most areas to serve the needs of the elderly. These agencies may have counselors to work with victims of abuse or neglect, and other programs to protect senior citizens' rights and contribute to their quality of life. Look in the phone book under community services, senior citizens, or elder services. Local churches or synagogues may also have programs for seniors. Be familiar with programs available in your area, or refer clients or families to your supervisor or a social worker.

Signs of elder abuse

▶ Old and new bruises, contusions and welts

▶ Scars

▶ Fractures, dislocation

▶ Burns of unusual shape and in unusual locations

▶ Scalp tenderness and patches of missing hair

▶ Swelling in the face, broken teeth, nasal discharge

▶ Bruises, bleeding, or discharge from the vaginal area

▶ Withdrawal or apathy

▶ Agitation

▶ Low self-esteem

▶ Client or family reports of questionable care

▶ Fear, vigilance, apprehension

▶ Mood changes, confusion, disorientation

▶ Weight loss

▶ Pill counts not changing

▶ Living conditions that are unsafe, unclean, or inadequate

▶ Private conversations are not allowed, or the family member/caregiver is present during all conversations

Chapter 11

Dying, Death and Hospice

Part 1
Death and Dying

❑ **1. Discuss the stages of dying**

Death can occur suddenly and without warning, or it can be expected. Older people, or people with **terminal illnesses**, may have time to prepare for death. A terminal illness is a disease or condition that will eventually cause death. Preparing for death is a process that involves the dying person's emotions and behavior.

Dr. Elizabeth Kubler-Ross researched and wrote about the process of dying. Her book, *On Death and Dying*, published in 1970, describes five stages that dying people and their families or friends may experience before death. These five stages are described below. Not all clients will go through all the stages. Some may stay in one stage until death occurs. Clients may move back and forth between stages during the process.

Denial. People in the denial stage may refuse to believe they are dying. They often believe a mistake has been made. They may talk about the future and avoid any discussion about their illnesses. This stage may last a few hours, days, or longer. Some people are still in the denial stage at the time of death. This is the "No. Not me." stage.

Anger. Once they start to face the possibility of their death, people with terminal illnesses become angry that they are the ones who are dying. They may be angry because they believe they are too young or because they have always been "good" or taken care of themselves. They are still not ready to accept the idea of their death. Anger is a normal and healthy reaction. The caregiver must learn not to take anger personally. This is the "Why me?" stage.

Bargaining. Once people have begun to believe that they really are dying, they may make promises to God or somehow try to bargain for their recovery. They may promise to do something special or change their lives if they are allowed to recover or live longer. This is the "Yes me, but..." stage.

Depression. As they become physically weaker and symptoms of the progressing illness become more pronounced, people who are dying may become deeply sad or depressed. They mourn for their lives and may talk about all the things they are leaving behind. They may cry or withdraw into silence or be unable to perform even simple activities. They need physical and emotional support from skilled health care providers and family members. At this stage, they will need to be able to review their lives and their feelings. It is important for you to listen and be understanding with clients in this stage of death.

Acceptance. Some people who are dying are eventually able to accept death and prepare for it. They may make plans for their last days or for the ceremonies that may follow. At this stage, people who are dying may seem emotionally detached.

❑ 2. Describe the grief process

Just as dealing with dying is a process with different stages, dealing with grief after the death of a relative or friend is a process as well. People may have several feelings at once or they may pass through different stages of grief at different times. As with dying, grieving is an individual process and no two people will grieve in exactly the same way. Clergy, counselors, or social workers can provide help for people who are grieving. Family members or friends may have any of the following reactions to the death of a loved one.

Shock. Even when a client has lived a long time with a terminal illness and death was expected, family members and friends may still be shocked after death occurs. Many of us do not know what to expect after the death of a relative or friend and may be surprised by our feelings, even when we knew death was coming.

Denial. Sometimes we want to believe that everything will quickly return to normal after a death. We want to believe that we do not have many feelings to cope with. Denying or refusing to believe we are grieving can help people deal with the hours or days after a death. But eventually we must face our feelings. Grief can be so overwhelming for some

people that they may take years to face their feelings. Professional help can be very valuable.

Anger. Although it is hard to admit it, many of us feel angry after a death. We may be angry at ourselves, at God, at the doctors, or even at the person who died. There is nothing wrong with feeling anger as part of grief.

Guilt. It is very common for families, friends, and even caregivers to feel guilty after a death. We may wish we had done more for the dying person, or we may simply feel that he or she did not deserve to die any more than we did. We may feel guilty that we are still living.

Regret. Often we have regrets about what we did or did not do for the dying person. We may regret things we said or did not say to a person who has died. Many people carry regrets with them for years.

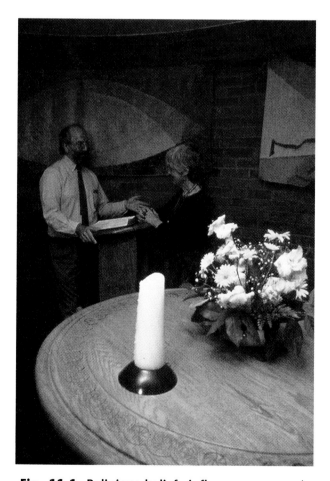

Fig. 11-1. Religious beliefs influence a person's feelings about death.

Sadness. Feeling depressed or down is very common after a death. We may cry or feel emotionally unstable. We may suffer headaches or insomnia when we cannot express our sadness.

Loneliness. Missing someone who has died is very normal and can bring up other feelings, such as sadness or regret. Many things may remind us of the person who died. The memories may be painful at first. With time, we usually feel less lonely and memories are more positive and less painful.

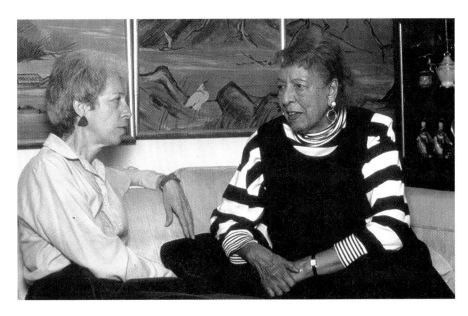

Fig. 11-2. Cultural practices affect the way a family grieves.

❑ 3. Discuss how feelings and attitudes about death differ among people

Death is a very sensitive topic. Many people find it hard to discuss death. Our feelings and attitudes about death can be influenced by many factors.

Experience with death. Someone who been through the deaths of other friends or relatives may have a different understanding of death than someone who has never experienced the death of someone close.

Personality type. Open, expressive people may have an easier time talking about and coping with death than people who are very reserved or quiet. Expressing feelings is a way of working through fears and concerns. For quiet persons, keeping a diary and writing down feelings may help.

Religious beliefs. Religious practices and beliefs can influence the experience with death, including the process of dying, rituals at the time of death, burial or cremation practices, services held after death, and mourning customs. For example, some Catholics do not believe in cremation. Orthodox Jews may not believe in viewing the body after death, and thus bury their dead within

a day after death. Beliefs about what happens to people after death can also influence the process of grief. People who believe in an afterlife, such as heaven, may be comforted by this belief. Home care aides who understand their clients' religious and spiritual beliefs can be very supportive to the family and friends.

Cultural background. The practices we grow up with will affect how we deal with death. Different cultural groups may have different practices associated with death and grieving. In some groups, friends and neighbors provide meals and other services for the family of the person who has died, but may say very little about the person's death. In other cultures, talking about and remembering the person who has died may be a way of comforting family and friends.

❑ 4. Recognize and report common signs of approaching death

Death can be sudden or gradual. Certain physical changes occur that can be recognized as signs and symptoms of approaching death. Changes occur in the circulatory system that affect the vital signs and skin color. The central nervous system shows signs of deterioration that may include disorientation, confusion, and reduced reflexes and responsiveness.

Vision, taste, and touch usually diminish; however, hearing is often present until death occurs.

Signs of Approaching Death

▶ Blurred vision that gradually fails

▶ Unfocused eyes that seem to stare without seeing anything

▶ Impaired speech

▶ Diminished sense of touch

▶ Loss of movement, muscle tone, and feeling, beginning in the feet and spreading upward

▶ Rising body temperature or below normal temperature

▶ Decreasing blood pressure

▶ Weak pulse that is abnormally slow or rapid

▶ Slow, irregular respirations or rapid, shallow respirations

▶ Cold, pale skin

▶ Mottling, spotting, or blotching of skin caused by poor circulation

▶ Perspiration

▶ Incontinence

▶ Disorientation or confusion

❑ 5. Discuss guidelines for providing care for a dying client

As always, you will follow the care plan when caring for a client who is dying. However, keep the following guidelines in mind to help you make the client as comfortable as possible.

Diminished Senses. As vision fails in clients who are dying, they naturally turn toward light. They may fear the dark. Keep the room softly lighted and without glare. Because they cannot see well but may still be able to hear, dying clients should be told about any procedures that are being done or what is happening in the room.

Speaking may become difficult for the dying client, but hearing usually remains until death occurs. Therefore, talk to the client in a normal voice, but do not expect an answer. Ask few questions and only those that require a simple yes or no. Encourage family to speak to the client, but to avoid subjects that are disturbing. Anticipate the client's needs by observing body language.

Care of the Eyes, Nose, and Mouth. Mucous secretions in the eyes, nose, and mouth may collect and become uncomfortable. Mouth care should be given frequently. As the client drinks less fluids and the mouth becomes dry, you will have to provide mouth care without assistance from the client. The skin around the eyes can be bathed with normal saline solution. A lubricant may be applied lightly to the nose if irritation and crusting occur.

Elimination. Bowel incontinence or constipation may occur. Enemas may be ordered for constipation, and medications and special diet for diarrhea. **Foley catheters**, special tubes that are inserted into the bladder for urinary drainage, may be used for urinary incontinence or to help drain urine if urinary retention is a problem. Waterproof pads or disposable pads may be used. Clients should be kept clean and dry.

Skin Care. Clients who are perspiring should be bathed often, and sheets and clothes should be changed for their comfort. Skin care to prevent pressure sores is important, especially for clients who are immobile or incontinent.

Comfort. Pain relief is very important and clients may not be able to communicate that they are in pain. Observe your clients for signs of pain and report them. Clients can also be made comfortable with frequent changes of position, back massage, good skin care, frequent mouth care, and proper body alignment. This type of care is discussed more in Chapters 12 and 13. Because body temperature usually increases, many clients are more comfortable with light covers, even when the skin feels cool to touch. The client may perspire more.

Environment. Display favorite objects, photographs, cards, flowers, religious items, and mementos in places where the client can easily see them. They will provide comfort. Cover equipment that may be disturbing. Make sure the room is comfortable, appropriately lighted, and well ventilated.

Emotional and Spiritual Support. We often feel uncomfortable talking with those who are seriously ill or who are dying. We are afraid of saying something that would be upsetting or inappropriate. What most people who are dying need, however, are not words. In the early stages of death, they may need

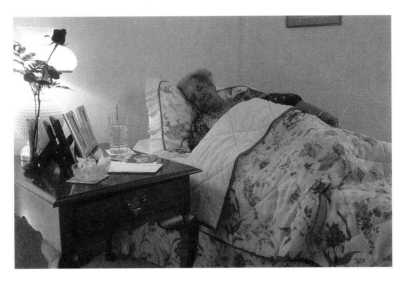

Fig. 11-3. A dying client's room should be softly lighted. Favorite objects displayed where the client can see them can provide comfort.

someone who will listen to them as they reflect on their lives or discuss their fears and concerns about dying. Later on they may simply need the quiet, reassuring, and loving presence of another person. Touch can be very important. Holding your client's hand as you sit quietly can be very comforting. Clients who are dying may also seek spiritual comfort from clergy members.

Guidelines for providing postmortem care

Postmortem care means care of the body after death. Be sensitive to the needs of the family after death occurs. Family members or friends may wish to sit by the bed to say goodbye. Be aware of religious practices that the family wants to observe. Home health agencies will also have different policies on what postmortem care a home care aide may give. Always follow your agency's policies and procedures, and only perform assigned tasks. Guidelines for postmortem care include the following:

Bathe the body as you would a client in bed. Be gentle to avoid bruising. Place drainage pads where needed, most often under the head and/or under the perineum (payr-i-NEE-um, or the area between the genitals and anus). Be sure to follow standard precautions.

Check with family members or friends about how to dress the client and whether to remove jewelry.

Do not remove any tubes or other apparatus. Either a nurse will do this or the funeral home will do it later.

Put dentures back in the mouth and close the mouth. You may need to place a rolled towel under the chin to support the closed mouth position.

Close the eyes carefully.

Position the body on the back, with legs straight, arms folded across the abdomen, and a small pillow under the head.

Strip the bed after body has been removed.

Open windows to air the room, as appropriate, and straighten up.

Arrange personal items carefully so they are not lost.

Document according to your agency's policy.

Ask family members or friends how you can be of help. If you are working with a hospice program or agency, you may be asked to answer the phone, make coffee or a meal, supervise children, or keep family members company. Do not leave the home until the client's body has been removed or until your supervisor says you may leave.

❑ 6. Define the goals of a hospice program

Hospice care is the term used for the special care that a dying person needs. Hospice care may be provided in a hospital, a special care facility, or in the home. A hospice can be any location where a person who is dying is treated with dignity by caregivers who are specially trained to provide for their physical, emotional, social, and spiritual needs.

In most of your assignments as a home care aide, the goals of care will focus on the client's recovery, or at least on helping the client to care for him or herself as much as possible. In hospice care, however, the goals of care are the comfort and dignity of the client. This is an important difference. You will need to adjust your mindset when caring for hospice clients, to focus on relieving their pain and making them comfortable, rather than on teaching them to care for themselves with an eye to recovery.

Besides pain relief, comfort, personal care, and emotional and spiritual support, clients who are dying also need to feel some independence for as long as possible. caregivers should allow clients to retain as much control over their lives as possible. Eventually, caregivers may have to meet all of the client's basic needs and perform the activities of daily living.

Family members or friends who are caregivers for the dying person will appreciate your help. You are providing them with the opportunity for a break. This kind of care is

sometimes referred to as respite (RES-pit) **care.** You must be aware of the feelings of family caregivers. Encourage them to take breaks and take care of themselves, but do not insist that they do so. Many will want to do all they can for their loved one during his or her last days. Do observe family care givers for signs of excessive stress, and report any signs to your supervisor. Your agency may be able to refer them to local support services.

❑ 7. Identify special skills and attitudes helpful in hospice work

As we have said, the most important attitude required for hospice work is the focus on providing comfort for the dying client, rather than on promoting wellness or recovery. Other attitudes and skills useful when providing hospice care include the following.

Be a good listener. It is hard to know what to say to someone who is dying or to his or her relatives and friends. Most often, people need someone to listen more than they need someone to tell them things. Review the listening skills discussed in Chapter 4. A good listener can be a great comfort in the home of someone who is dying. Recognize that some people will not want to confide in you, and never push someone to talk.

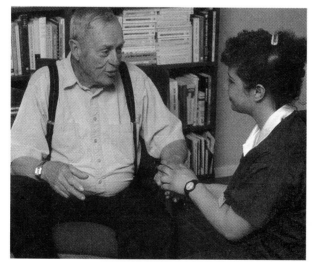

Fig. 11-4. Being a good listener can be a great help to a dying client and his or her family.

Respect privacy and independence. A dying client may be visited by relatives, friends, clergy, or others who have important goodbyes to say. Make it easy for these difficult visits to take place. Stay out of the way when you can and don't join in the conversation unless you are asked. Dying clients can hold on to some independence even when they need total care from you. Let the client make choices when possible, such as whether to bathe now or later, or what to eat or drink.

Be sensitive to individual needs. Different clients and families will have different needs. The more you can tune into what the client or family needs from you, the more helpful you will be. Some clients need a quiet, calm atmosphere and would prefer the least disruption possible. Others appreciate a cheery presence and might like you to make small talk or stay close by. If you are not sure what you can do to help, ask someone.

Be aware of your own feelings. Caring for people who are dying can be draining. Know your limits and respect them. Discuss your feelings of frustration or grief with your supervisor or another member of the health care team. Request a change of assignment when you need a break.

Be sure to follow the plan of care. Know who to call and when to call them.

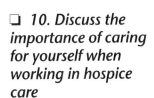

Fig. 11-5. As much as possible, give your client and his or her visitors the privacy they need.

may include physicians, nurses, social workers, counselors, home care aides, therapists, clergy, dietitians, and volunteers.

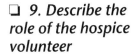

9. Describe the role of the hospice volunteer

According to the National Hospice Organization, of the 115,000 people providing hospice care in America, 95,000 are volunteers. Volunteers give more than 5 million hours of their time each year to helping people who are dying. Hospice volunteers go through a training program to prepare them for hospice work. Volunteers provide a variety of services, including caring for the home or family of a dying person, driving or doing errands, and providing emotional support.

10. Discuss the importance of caring for yourself when working in hospice care

As mentioned above, hospice care can be very draining physically and psychologically. caregivers must keep their own needs in mind and learn to take care of themselves while taking care of others. It is easy to get "burned out" when working in hospice care, especially if you ignore your own needs.

Recognize the stress. Just realizing how stressful it is to work with clients who are dying is a first step toward caring for yourself. Talking with a friend, spouse, or family member about your experiences at work can help you understand and work through your feelings.

8. Identify the members of the hospice team

Hospice care may be provided by any caregiver, but often specially trained nurses, social workers, and volunteers provide hospice care. The hospice team

Take good care of yourself. Eating right, exercising, and getting enough rest are ways of taking care of yourself physically. Remember to care for your emotional and spiritual health, too. Acknowledging and talking about your feelings and taking time out to do things for yourself, like reading a book, taking a bubble bath, or whatever you enjoy, are ways of caring for yourself emotionally. Your spiritual needs may be met by attending religious services, reading, praying, meditating, or just taking a quiet walk. Recognizing and meeting your own needs will allow you to do the best job of meeting other people's needs in your work.

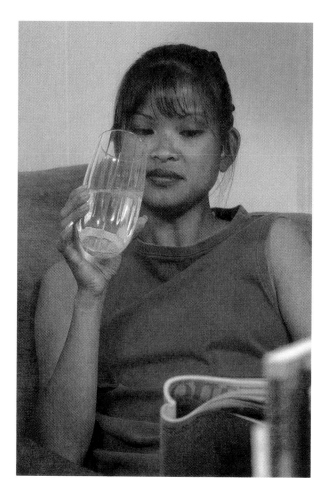

Fig. 11-6. Recognize the stress of caring for a dying client, and take good care of yourself.

Take a break when you need to. Taking a break can mean several different things. Finding ten minutes to sit down and relax or to stand up and stretch may be enough of a break in some situations. There may come a time when the demands of hospice care are too great and you need to request a change of assignment from your supervisor. Don't feel guilty about doing this when you need to.

SECTION IV
Developing Personal Care and Basic Health Care Skills

Chapter 12

Providing Safe and Comfortable Transfers, Ambulation, and Positioning

Part 1
Transfer and Ambulation

❑ 1. Explain the guidelines for lifting, holding, or transferring a client

Review the principles of body mechanics in Chapter 6. Always use good body mechanics when moving or positioning a client. Avoid lifting whenever possible. Instead, push, roll, slide, or pivot, so that you are not bearing the client's weight. Using good body mechanics helps protect both you and your clients.

Learning Objectives

In this chapter you will learn to:

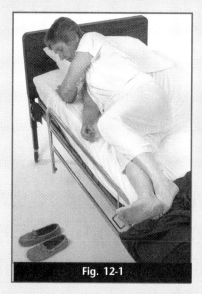

Fig. 12-1

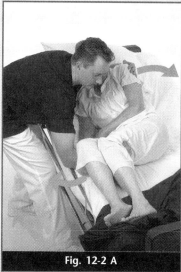

Fig. 12-2 A

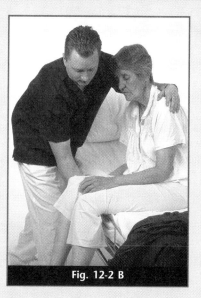

Fig. 12-2 B

1. Explain what you will do.

2. Provide privacy if the client desires it.

3. Wash your hands.

4. If the bed is adjustable, position it at a height that is comfortable for you.

5. Fanfold (fold into pleats) the top covers to the foot of the bed. Ask the client to roll onto her side, facing you. Assist as needed (Procedure 9 in this chapter describes how to help a client roll over).

6. Tell the client to reach across her chest with her top arm and place her hand on the edge of the bed near her opposite shoulder. Ask her to push down on that hand to raise her shoulders up while swinging her legs over the side of the bed (**Fig. 12-1**).

7. Always allow the client to do all she can for herself. However, if the client needs assistance, have her lie on her back propped up on pillows or with the head of the bed raised. With the client bending her knees and assisting as able, reach your arm under the client's neck and grasp her far shoulder. Slip your other arm under her knees and grasp her far knee. Stand with your legs about 12 inches apart, with one foot 6-8 inches in front of the other. Bend your knees and pull your body a quarter turn backward (**Fig. 12-2**). In a smooth movement, swing the client's knees toward you and over the side of the bed. The weight of the client's legs hanging down from the bed helps the client sit up.

8. Allow the client to sit on the edge of the bed to gain her balance.

This procedure is called **dangling**. It gives the client time to adjust to being in an upright position after lying down.

9. Put slippers on the client while she is dangling. Do not leave the client alone. If the client is dizzy for more than a minute, have her lie down again. Take her pulse and respirations and report to your supervisor according to your agency's policy (you will learn how to take vital signs in Chapter 14, Performing Basic Health Care Skills).

10. The care plan may direct you to allow the client to dangle for several minutes and then return her to lying down, or it may direct you to allow the client to dangle in preparation for walking or a transfer. Follow the instructions in the care plan.

11. Wash your hands after the client is safely back in bed or the transfer is completed.

12. Document the procedure and your observations. How did the client tolerate sitting up? Did the client become dizzy?

1. Explain what you will do.

2. Provide privacy if the client desires it.

3. Wash your hands.

4. Stand facing the head of the bed, with your legs about 12 inches apart and your knees bent. The foot that is further from the bed should be slightly ahead of the other foot (**Fig. 12-3**).

5. Place your arm under the client's armpit and grasp the client's shoulder. Have the client grasp your shoulder in the same manner. This hold is called the **arm lock** or **lock arm** (**Fig. 12-4**).

6. Reach under the client's head and place your other hand on the client's far shoulder. Have the client bend their knees. Bend your knees.

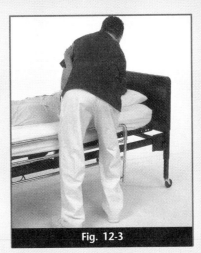

Fig. 12-3

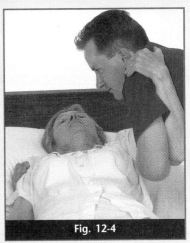

Fig. 12-4

7. At the count of three, rock yourself backward and pull the client to a sitting position. Use pillows or a bed rest to support the client in the sitting position.

8. Check the client for dizziness or weakness.

9. Wash your hands.

10. Document the procedure and any observations. Was the client able to help at all? Did the client become dizzy?

Before a client who has been lying down moves to a standing position, she should **dangle**, or sit up with her feet over the side of the bed for a moment to regain her equilibrium (ee-kwil-IH-bree-um), or balance. For some clients who are unable to walk, sitting up and dangling the legs for a few minutes may be ordered in the care plan.

If the client starts to fall, widen your stance and bring the client's body close to you to break the fall (**Fig. 12-5**). Bend your knees and support the client as you lower her to the floor. You may need to drop to the floor with the client to avoid injury to you or the client as you lower him or her to the floor. Do not try to reverse or stop a fall. You or the client can suffer worse injuries if you try to stop a fall than if you just break the fall.

If the client has fallen, call for help if a family member is around. Do not attempt to get the client up after the fall unless you are certain the client is not

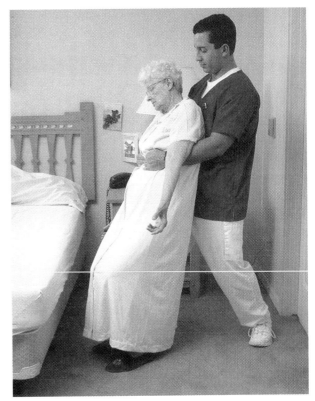

Fig. 12-5.

1. Explain what you will do.

2. Provide privacy if the client desires it.

3. Wash your hands.

4. Assist the client to a dangling position (see Procedure 1 in this chapter).

5. If the client is able, have her place her hands on the edge of the bed and push to standing, while you stay nearby to steady her or offer support if needed.

6. Always allow your client to do whatever she is able to do for herself. If the client is unable to stand without help, place one foot between the client's feet. If the client has a weak knee, brace it against your knee (**Fig. 12-6**).

7. Have the client place her stronger leg directly under herself.

8. Bending your knees and leaning forward, put both arms around the client's waist and

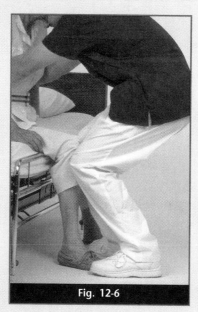

Fig. 12-6

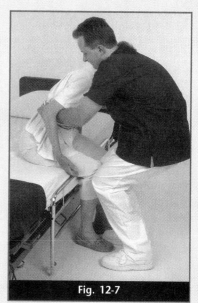

Fig. 12-7

hold her close to your center of gravity (**Fig. 12-7**).

9. Tell the client to lean forward, push down on the bed with her hands, and stand, on the count of three. When you start to count, begin to rock.

At three, rock your weight onto your back foot and assist the

client to a standing position.

10. Check the client for dizziness before you allow her to stand alone.

11. Wash your hands.

12. Document the procedure and any observations. How did the client tolerate standing? How much help did you offer?

injured. Many home health agencies do not allow a home care aide to help a client up after a fall until she has been evaluated by a nurse. Follow your agency's policies and procedures, and always call your supervisor if you are unsure of what to do after a fall. If you do help the client up, get her in bed, take vital signs, then report the fall to your supervisor.

Clients who have difficulty walking may use canes, walkers, or crutches to help themselves (**Fig. 12-8**). Understanding the purpose of each device will help you know how to use it properly. The purpose of a cane is to help with balance. A **straight cane** (a) is not designed to bear weight. A **quad cane** (b), with four rubber-tipped feet, is designed to bear a little weight. Clients using canes should be able to bear weight on both legs. If one leg is

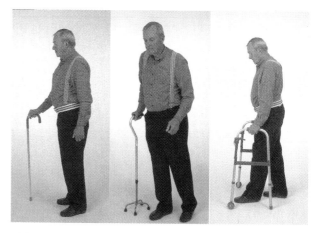

Fig. 12-8. Clients who have difficulty walking may use canes, walkers, or crutches to help themselves.

weaker, the cane should be held in the hand on the strong side.

Procedure 4: Using a transfer belt to assist with ambulation

Ambulation is walking. A client who is **ambulatory** is one who can get out of bed and walk. Many older clients are ambulatory, but need assistance to walk safely. Several tools, including transfer or gait belts, canes, walkers, and crutches, are available to assist with ambulation.

A **transfer belt**, or **gait belt**, is used to assist clients who are able to walk but are weak, unsteady, or uncoordinated (**Fig. 12-9**). The belt is made of canvas or other heavy material, sometimes has handles, and fits around the client's waist outside the clothing. The transfer belt is a safety device that gives you something firm to hold on to.

1. Explain what you will do.

2. Provide privacy if the client desires it.

3. Wash your hands.

4. Place the belt around the client's waist. Always apply the belt over clothing. *Never* place it next to skin.

5. Help the client stand up, as described in Procedure 3 of this chapter. Observe the client for strength and coordination.

6. Stand behind and to the side of the client as you hold on to the belt. If the client has a weaker side, stand on that side. Use the hand that is not holding the belt to offer support to the client on the weak side (**Fig. 12-10**).

7. Observe the client's strength while you walk together. Provide a chair if the client becomes dizzy or fatigued.

8. Return the client to the bed or chair and be sure they are positioned comfortably.

9. Wash your hands.

10. Document the procedure and your observations. How far did the client walk? How did the client appear or say he felt while walking? How much help did you give?

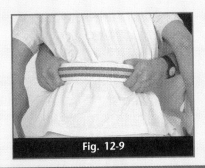
Fig. 12-9

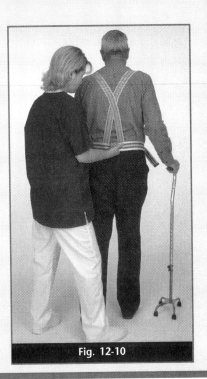
Fig. 12-10

Procedure 5: Assisting with ambulation for a client who uses a cane, walker, or crutches

1. Explain what you will do.

2. Wash your hands.

3. Make sure the client is wearing skid-resistant slippers or shoes.

4. Fasten the transfer belt around the client's waist.

5. Assist the client to a standing position.

6. Assist as necessary with ambulation.

a Cane: Client places cane about 12 inches in front of his stronger leg, brings weaker leg even with cane, and then brings stronger leg forward slightly ahead of cane (**Fig. 12-11**). Repeat.

b Walker: Client picks up or rolls the walker and places it about 12 inches in front of him. All four feet or wheels of the walker should be on the ground before client steps forward to the walker. The

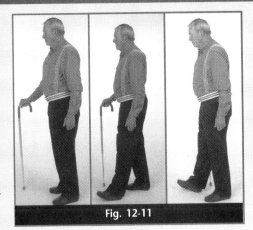
Fig. 12-11

Continued on page 146

Continued from page 145

walker should not be advanced again until the client has moved both feet forward and is in a steady position (**Fig. 12-12**). The client should never put his feet ahead of the walker.

c Crutches: Client should be fitted for crutches and taught to use

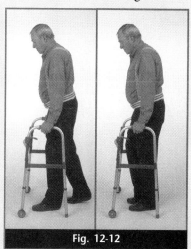

Fig. 12-12

them correctly by a physical therapist or nurse. The client may use the crutches several different ways, depending on what his weakness is. No matter how the client is using the crutches, weight should be on the client's hands and arms rather than on the underarm area. (**Fig. 12-13**).

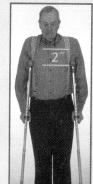

Fig. 12-13

7. Whether the client is using a cane, walker, or crutches, walk slightly behind the client, on the weak side if the client has one. Hold the transfer belt unless you think the client is steady

on his own.

8. Watch for obstacles in the client's path, and encourage the client to look ahead, rather than down at his feet.

9. Encourage the client to rest if fatigued. Allowing a client to become too fatigued increases the chance of a fall. Let the client set the pace, and discuss how far he plans to go based on the physician's orders.

10. Settle the client back into a safe and comfortable position after ambulation.

11. Wash your hands.

12. Document the procedure and your observations. How did the client feel or appear while walking? How far did the client walk? How much help did the client need?

1. Explain what you will do.

2. Assemble equipment, as applicable:

▶ robe and slippers

▶ transfer belt

▶ chair or wheelchair

▶ sheet or blanket

3. Provide privacy if the client desires it. Check the area to be certain it is uncluttered and safe.

4. Wash your hands.

5. Place the chair or wheelchair at the side of the bed on the client's **stronger** side. The chair should be at an angle slightly facing the client. If using a wheelchair, lock the brakes and rise or remove the foot and leg rests so they are not in the way.

Cover plastic seats with a bath blanket or a soft pillow.

6. Assist the client to the dangling position, as in Procedure 1.

7. Help the client stand up, as in Procedure 3.

8. Tell the client to take small steps in the direction of the chair while turning his back toward the chair. If more assistance is needed, have the client pivot on the foot that is farthest away from the chair. Always allow the

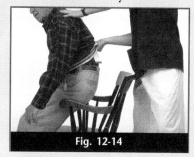

Fig. 12-14

client to do all he can for himself.

9. Have the client use one arm to grasp the arm of the chair. When the chair is touching the back of the client's legs, help the client lower himself into the chair (**Fig. 12-14**).

10. If using a wheelchair, lower the footrests and help the client place his feet on them. Check that the client is in good alignment. Place a lap robe, folded blanket, or sheet over the lap as appropriate.

11. Wash your hands.

12. Document the procedure and your observations. How did the client feel or appear during the transfer? How much assistance was required?

A slide board may be used to help transfer clients who are unable to bear weight on their legs. Slide boards can be used for almost any transfer that involves moving from one sitting or reclining position to another. For example, slide boards can be helpful for transfers from bed to chair, wheelchair to bathtub, or wheelchair to car.

1. Follow steps 1 through 6 of Procedure 6 for helping a client move from a bed to a chair.

2. Have the client lean away from transfer side to take the weight off her thigh. Place one end of the sliding board under the buttocks and thigh, taking care not to pinch the client's skin between the bed and the board. Place the other end of the sliding board on the surface to which the client is transferring (**Fig. 12-15**).

3. If the client is able, have her push up with her hands and scoot herself across the board. Stay close so you can provide support if needed. Always allow the client to do all she can for herself.

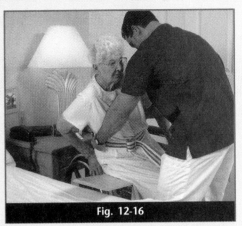

Fig. 12-16

4. If the client needs assistance, stand in front of her and put your knees in front and a little to the outside of her knees to keep them from buckling during the transfer. Make sure your back is straight.

5. Get as close to the client as possible and have her lean into you as you grasp the transfer belt from behind. Lean back with your knees bent. Using your legs rather than your back, pull the client up slightly and toward you to help her scoot across the

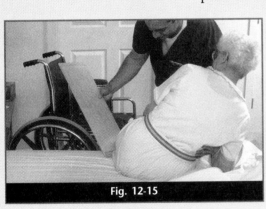

Fig. 12-15

board (**Fig. 12-16**).

6. Complete the transfer in two or three lifting and scooting movements. *Never* drag the client across the board. Friction from the client's skin dragging across the slide board can cause skin breakdown that can lead to pressure sores.

7. After the client is safely transferred, remove the sliding board. Make sure the client is positioned safely and comfortably.

8. Wash your hands.

9. Document the procedure and any observations. How did the client feel or appear during the transfer? How much assistance was required?

A **walker** (c) is used when the client can bear some weight on the legs. The walker provides excellent stability for clients who are unsteady or lack balance. The metal frame of the walker may have rubber-tipped feet and/or wheels. Crutches are used for clients who can bear no weight or limited weight on one leg. Some people use one crutch, and some use two.

Whichever device is being used, your role is to ensure safety. Stay near the person, on the weak side. Make sure the equipment is in proper condition. It must be sturdy, and it must have rubber tips or wheels on the bottom.

Guidelines: Assisting a client in using a wheelchair

▷ If your client uses a wheelchair of any kind, you must learn how it works. You should know how to apply and release the brake and how to operate the footrests.

The following is a basic procedure for transferring using a mechanical lift.

1. Explain what you will do. Ask someone to help you.

2. Assemble equipment:
- ▶ wheelchair or chair
- ▶ lifting partner, if available
- ▶ mechanical or hydraulic lift

3. Provide privacy if the client desires it.

4. Wash your hands.

5. Position wheelchair next to bed. Lock brakes.

6. Help the client turn to one side of the bed. Position the sling under the client, with the edge next to the client's back fanfolded if necessary, and the bottom of the sling even with the client's knees. Help the client roll back to the middle of the bed, and then spread out the fanfolded edge of the sling.

7. Roll the mechanical lift to bedside. Make sure the base is opened to its widest point, and push the base of the lift under the bed (**Fig. 12-17**).

8. Position the overhead bar directly over the client.

9. With the client lying on her back, attach one set of straps to each side of the sling, and one set of straps to the overhead bar. If available, have a lifting partner support the client at the head and shoulders and at the knees while the client is being lifted (**Fig. 12-18**). The client's arms should be folded across her chest. "S" hooks should face away from client.

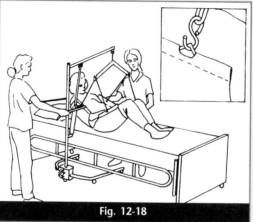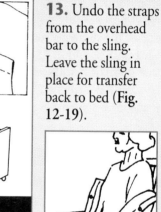

Fig. 12-18

10. Following manufacturer's instructions for operating the lift, raise the client two inches above the bed. Pause a moment

for the client to gain equilibrium.

11. If available, a lifting partner can help support and guide the client's body while you roll the lift so that the client is positioned over the chair or wheelchair.

12. Slowly lower the client into the chair or wheelchair. Push down gently on the client's knees to help the client into a sitting, rather than reclining position.

13. Undo the straps from the overhead bar to the sling. Leave the sling in place for transfer back to bed (**Fig. 12-19**).

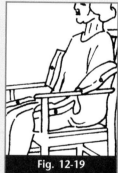

Fig. 12-19

14. Be sure the client is seated comfortably and correctly in the chair or wheelchair.

15. Wash your hands.

16. Document the procedure and any observations. How did the client tolerate the transfer? Were there any problems during the transfer? Did the equipment operate properly?

Fig. 12-17

To transfer to or from a wheelchair, the client must use the side or areas of the body that can bear weight to support and lift the side or areas that cannot bear weight. Clients who can bear no weight with their legs may use leg braces or an overhead trapeze to support themselves during transfers.

Your role in wheelchair transfers is to make sure the client is safe and comfortable. Ask the client how you can assist. Some clients may only want you to bring the chair to the bedside, while others may want you to be more involved. Always be sure the chair is as close as possible to the client and is locked in place. Use a transfer belt if you are going to assist in the transfer. Be sure the transfer is done slowly, allowing time for the client to rest. Check the client's alignment in the chair when the transfer is complete.

If the client needs to be moved back in the wheelchair, go to the back of the chair and reach forward and down under the client's arms. Ask the client to place his feet on the ground and push up. Pull the client up in the chair while the client pushes.

Some clients may have a mechanical lift in the home. If you are trained to do so, you may assist the client with many types of transfers using the mechanical or hydraulic lift. *Never* use equipment you have not been trained to use. You or your client could get hurt if you use lifting equipment improperly. There are many different types of mechanical lifts, so you must be trained on the specific lift you will be using.

**Part 2
Positioning**

❑ 2. Explain the guidelines for safely positioning a client in each of the five basic positions

Clients who spend a lot of time in bed often need help getting into comfortable positions. They also need to change positions periodically to avoid skin breakdown or pressure sores. **Positioning** means helping clients into positions that will be comfortable and healthy for them. Bed-bound clients should be repositioned every two hours. The position and time should be documented every time there is a change, so a 24-hour plan can be followed.

Which positions a client uses will depend on the diagnosis, the condition, and the client's preference. The client care plan will give specific positioning instructions. Remember, even immobile clients may not stay in the position you put them in, so recheck periodically. Always keep principles of body mechanics and alignment in mind when positioning clients. Also, check skin for blanching (turning white) or redness, especially around bony areas, each time you reposition a client.

The following are guidelines for positioning clients in the five basic body positions:

1. Supine (SUE-pine): In this position, the client lies flat on his back. To maintain correct body position, support the client's head and shoulders with a pillow. You may also use pillows or rolled towels or washcloths to support his arms (especially a weak or immobilized arm) or hands. Pillows or a footboard can be used to keep feet flexed slightly.

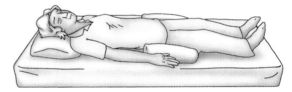

Fig. 12-20. A person in the supine position is lying flat on his or her back.

2. Lateral/Side: A client in the lateral position is lying on either side. There are many variations on the lateral, or side position. Pillows can be used to support the arm and leg on the upper side, the back, and the head. Ideally, the knee on the upper side of the body should be flexed, with the leg brought in front of the body and supported on a pillow. If the top leg cannot be brought

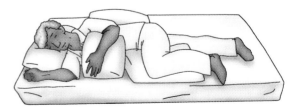

Fig. 12-21. A person in the lateral position is lying on his or her side.

forward and instead rests on the bottom leg, pillows should be used between the two legs to relieve pressure and avoid skin breakdown.

3. Prone: A client in the prone position is lying on the stomach, or front side of the body. This is not a comfortable position for many people, especially elderly people. Never leave a client in a prone position for very long, and always check the care plan before using the prone position. In this position, the arms are either at the sides or raised above the head. The head is turned to one side and a small pillow may be used under the head.

4. Fowler's: A client in the Fowler's position is in a semi-sitting position, with the head and shoulders elevated. The client's knees may be flexed and elevated using a pillow or rolled blanket as a support, and the feet may be flexed and supported using a footboard or other support. The spine should be straight. In a true Fowler's position (a) the upper body is raised to a point halfway between sitting straight up and lying flat. In a semi-Fowler's position (b) the upper body is not raised as high.

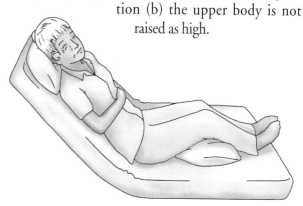

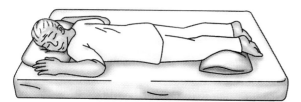

Fig. 12-22. A person lying in the prone position is lying on his or her stomach.

Fig. 12-23. A person lying in the Fowler's position is partially reclined.

Procedure 9: Turning a client in bed

1. Explain what you will do.

2. Provide privacy if the client desires it.

3. Wash your hands.

4. With the client in supine position and centered in the bed, stand at the side of the bed client will face. Place the client's near hand palm up under her hip.

5. Lift the client's far leg over her near leg, flexing the knee (**Fig. 12-25**).

6. Assume a good stance: your feet hip width apart, your knees bent, and one foot slightly in front of the other.

7. Grasp the client's far shoulder and far hip. Count to three, rocking your weight forward and back on each count. On three, roll the client onto her side (**Fig. 12-26**).

8. Use whatever pillows or supports are necessary to be sure the client is in a comfortable position, with good body alignment. Arrange the bed covers so that the client is comfortable.

9. Wash your hands.

10. Document the procedure and any observations.

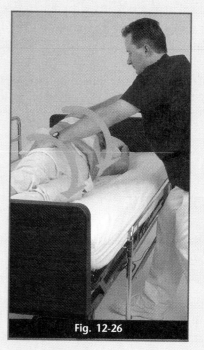

Fig. 12-26

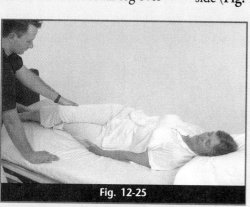

Fig. 12-25

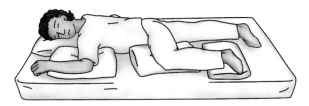

Fig. 12-24. A person lying in the Sims' position is lying on his or her side with one leg drawn up.

5. **Sims':** The Sims' position is a variation on the lateral, or side, position. The lower arm is behind the back and the upper knee is flexed and raised toward the chest, using a pillow as support.

Use the positions indicated in each client's care plan. If you have questions about how to position a client, ask your supervisor. In general, use positions that are natural and comfortable for the client. Always remember to check the skin for signs of irritation whenever you position or reposition a client.

Helping a client move up in bed not only helps the client feel more comfortable, but it also helps prevent skin irritation that can lead to pressure

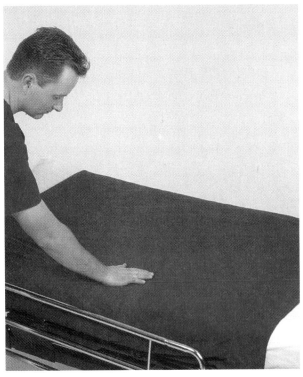

Fig. 12-27. A draw sheet is a special sheet (or a regular bed sheet folded in half) that is used to help move clients in bed without causing shearing on the skin.

Procedure 10: Moving a client up in bed

Always allow the client to do all she can for herself. Following is the procedure for clients who can help you move them up in bed.

1. Explain what you will do.

2. Provide privacy if the client desires it.

3. Wash your hands.

4. If the bed is adjustable, raise it to a height that is comfortable for you. If side rails are available, raise the rail on the far side of the bed. Remove the pillow and set it aside for later use.

5. Place one arm under the client's shoulders and the other under the client's buttocks.

6. Ask the client to bend her knees and push down on the mattress with her feet and hands on the count of three (**Fig. 12-28**).

7. Keeping your back straight and bending at the knees, help the client move toward the head of the mattress on the count of three. As always, allow the client to do all she can for herself.

8. Help the client into a comfortable position and arrange the pillow and blankets for her. If you raised an adjustable bed, be

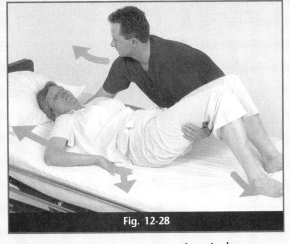

Fig. 12-28

sure to return it to its lowest position.

9. Wash your hands.

10. Document the procedure and any observations.

Continued on page 152

Continued from page 151

When the client cannot assist and there is no one else around to help you move her up in bed, take the following steps:

1. Follow steps 1 through 4 above.

2. Stand behind the head of the bed with your feet shoulder width apart and one foot slightly in front of the other.

3. Roll and grasp the top edge of the draw sheet.

4. With your knees bent and your back straight, rock your weight from the front foot to the back foot in one smooth motion (**Fig. 12-29**).

5. Help the client into a comfortable position and arrange the pillow and blankets for her. Unroll the draw sheet and leave it in place for the next repositioning. If you raised an adjustable bed, be sure to return it to its lowest position.

When you have help from another person, you can modify the procedure as follows:

1. Follow steps 1 through 4 from above.

2. Stand on the opposite side of the bed from your helper. Each of you should be turned slightly toward the head of the bed. For each of you, the foot that is closest to the head of the bed should be pointed that direction.

3. Roll the draw sheet up to the client's side, and have your helper do the same on his side of the bed. Grasp the sheet with your palms up, and have your helper do the same.

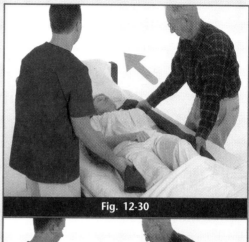

Fig. 12-30

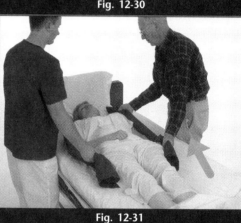

Fig. 12-31

4. Shift your weight to your back foot (the foot closer to the foot of the bed) and have your helper do the same (**Fig. 12-30**). On the count of three, you and your helper both shift your weight to your forward feet as you slide the draw sheet toward the head of the bed (**Fig. 12-31**).

5. Help the client into a comfortable position and arrange the pillow and blankets for her. Unroll the draw sheet and leave it in place for the next repositioning. If you raised an adjustable bed, be sure to return it to its lowest position.

6. Wash your hands.

7. Document the procedure and any observations.

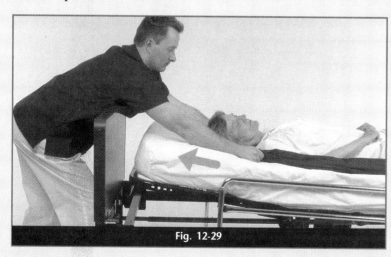

Fig. 12-29

6. Wash your hands.

7. Document the procedure and any observations.

Some clients' spinal columns must be kept in alignment. To turn these clients in bed, you will use a procedure called log rolling.

1. Explain what you will do.

2. Provide privacy if the client desires it.

3. Wash your hands.

4. If the bed is adjustable, raise it to a height that is comfortable for you.

5. Move the client to the side of the bed you are standing on. To do this, assume a good stance, with feet hip width apart, knees bent, and one foot slightly in front of the other. Slip your arms under the client's shoulders and move her toward you by rocking your weight backwards onto your back foot (**Fig. 12-32**). Keep your knees bent. Be

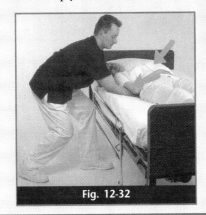

Fig. 12-32

careful not to slide the client across the sheets and cause **shearing** (pressure on the skin from sliding across another surface), which can lead to pressure sores.

6. Keeping the same good stance, slide your arms under the client's hips and shift them toward you, as you did her shoulders (**Fig. 12-33**). Make sure the client's head and legs are in alignment with her shoulders and hips before continuing with the procedure.

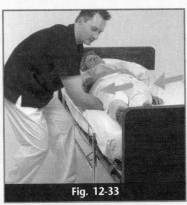

Fig. 12-33

7. If available, raise the side rail on the side of the bed the client is now closest to. If no side rail is available, be sure the client is safe and stable before moving to the next step.

8. Move to the other side of the bed and lower the side rail if there is one. Assume a good stance.

9. With your knees bent, grasp the client with one hand on the far hip and one on the far shoulder. Roll the client toward you onto her side (**Fig. 12-34**).

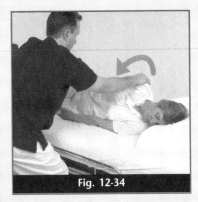

Fig. 12-34

10. Check the client's body alignment. Arrange pillows and covers for comfort. Raise the side rail if available and if necessary for client's safety. If you raised an adjustable bed, be sure to return it to its lowest position.

11. Wash your hands.

12. Document the procedure and any observations.

sores. You may have to help a client move up in bed by yourself, or you can use a helper if one is available. If the client is unable to assist you, use a **draw sheet** or **turning sheet**. A draw sheet is an extra sheet placed on top of the bottom sheet when the bed is made. It allows a caregiver to reposition the client without causing **shearing**, or friction and pressure on the skin from rubbing or dragging it across another surface (the bottom sheet).

Part 3
Comfort Measures

❑ *3. List three things you can do to help make your client comfortable*

There are several things you can do to provide for the comfort and safety of your client in and around the bed:

1. Explain what you will do.

2. Assemble supplies:

▶ body lotion

▶ towel

▶ cotton blanket

▶ gloves if client's skin is broken

3. Provide privacy if the client desires it.

4. Wash your hands.

5. If the bed is adjustable, position it at a comfortable working height, with the head of the bed flat.

6. Have the client lie in a prone position. If this is uncomfortable, have the client lie on his side. Cover the client with a cotton blanket, then fold back the bed covers. Expose the client's back to the middle of the buttocks. If the client is positioned on the side, place the towel on the bed along the length of his back. Back rubs can also be given with the client sitting up.

7. Pour the lotion on your hands and rub them together to spread it. You may want to warm the lotion and your hands first by immersing the lotion in warm water for five minutes and running your hands under warm water. Warn the client that the lotion may still feel cool. Always put the lotion on your hands rather than directly on the client's skin.

8. Place your hands on each side of the upper part of the buttocks and make long, smooth upward strokes with both hands along

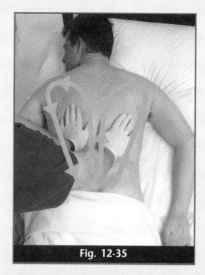
Fig. 12-35

each side of the spine, up to the shoulders (**Fig. 12-35**). Circle your hands outward and then move back along the outer edges of the back. At the buttocks, make another circle and move your hands back up to the shoulders. Without taking your hands from the client's skin, repeat this motion for three to five minutes.

9. Next, make kneading motions with the first two fingers and thumb of each hand. Place them at the base of the spine and move upward simultaneously along each side of the spine, applying downward pressure with the fingers and thumbs. Follow the same direction as with the long smooth

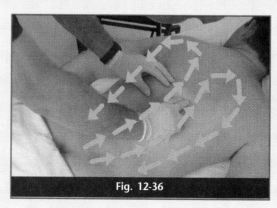
Fig. 12-36

strokes, circling at shoulders and buttocks (**Fig. 12-36**).

10. Finally, gently massage bony areas (spine, shoulder blades, hip bones) with circular motions of your fingertips. Gentle massage stimulates circulation and helps prevent skin damage. However, if any of these areas are red, massage *around* them rather than *on* them. The redness indicates that the skin is already irritated and fragile.

11. Let your client know when you are almost through. Finish with some long smooth strokes, like the ones you used at the beginning of the massage.

12. Dry the back if extra lotion remains on it. If appropriate, apply powder to the back to allow better movement against the sheets.

13. Remove the cotton blanket and towel.

14. Assist the client with getting dressed.

15. Help the client into a comfortable position.

16. Store the lotion and put dirty linens in the hamper.

17. Wash your hands.

18. Document the procedure and your observations. Did the client appear comfortable during the back rub? Did you observe any reddened areas, blanching, or broken skin?

- Have plenty of pillows available to provide support in the various positions.

- Use positioning devices (such as backrests, bed cradles and tables, footboards, and handrolls).

- Give back rubs for comfort and relaxation.

- Change positions frequently (every two hours) and as directed in the care plan.

- Always maintain the client's body alignment.

A back rub can help relax your client and make him or her more comfortable. Back rubs are often given after baths. Follow the instructions in the care plan for when to give back rubs and for how long.

Guidelines for using positioning devices

Many positioning devices are available to help make clients more comfortable. Some can be inexpensively made in the client's home. Check with your supervisor on the use of positioning devices for each client.

- Backrests can be made of pillows, cardboard or wood covered by pillows, or special wedge-shaped

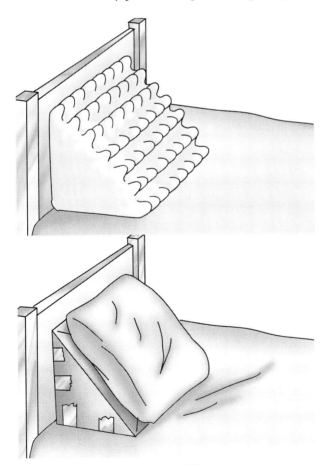

Fig. 12-37

foam pillows (**Fig. 12-37**).

- Bed cradles are used to keep the bed covers from pushing down on client's feet. Metal frames that work like a tent when the bed covers are over them can be purchased (**Fig. 12-38**). A cardboard

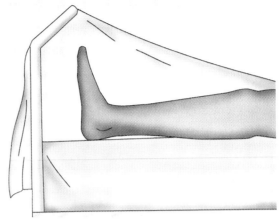

Fig. 12-38

box can be used as a bed cradle by placing the client's feet inside the box underneath the covers (**Fig. 12-39**).

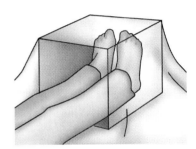

Fig. 12-39

- Bed tables are available commercially, or you can make one by cutting openings in each of the longer sides of a sturdy cardboard box (**Fig. 12-40**).

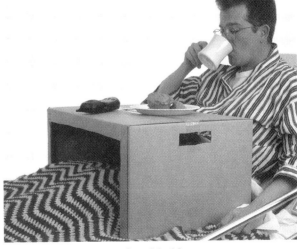

Fig. 12-40

Draw sheets or turning sheets may be placed under a client and used to help move clients who are unable to assist with turning in bed, lifting, or moving up in bed. Draw sheets also help prevent skin damage that can be caused by shearing. A regular bed sheet folded in half can be used as a draw sheet (**see Fig. 12-27**).

Footboards are padded boards placed against the client's feet to keep them flexed and prevent footdrop (**Fig. 12-41**). Rolled blankets or pillows can also be used as footboards.

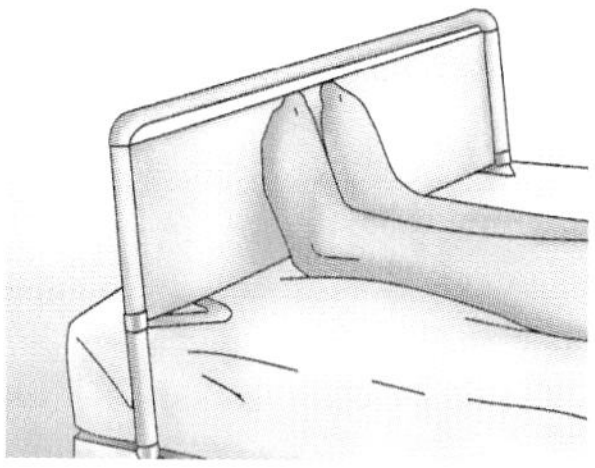

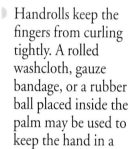

Fig. 12-41

Handrolls keep the fingers from curling tightly. A rolled washcloth, gauze bandage, or a rubber ball placed inside the palm may be used to keep the hand in a natural position (**Fig. 12-42**).

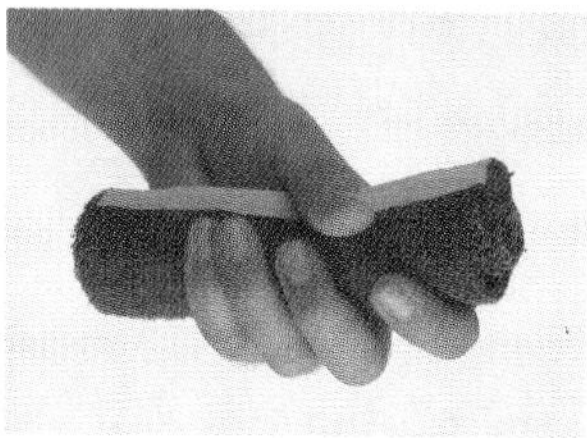

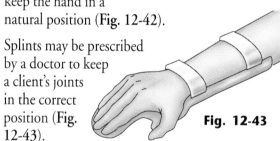

Fig. 12-42

Splints may be prescribed by a doctor to keep a client's joints in the correct position (**Fig. 12-43**).

Fig. 12-43

Trochanter rolls are used to keep the client's hips from turning outward. A rolled towel works well as an improvised trochanter roll (**Fig. 12-44**).

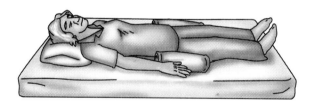

Fig. 12-44

Guidelines for the use of physical restraints

Throughout this book, we discuss ways to protect your clients' physical safety. For example, using side rails when available can prevent a client from rolling out of bed. Your supervisor may train you to use other devices to protect your clients in the home.

As discussed earlier in this book (Chapters 3 and 6), physical restraints, including vests and belts designed to restrict free movement, have been used in home care in the past. These restraints were intended to safeguard clients who wander, are violent, or are at risk of hurting themselves. However, because client abuse involving physical restraints became common, new laws restrict the use of restraints. In many states, restraints are illegal. In others, doctors must prescribe the use of restraints. Never use physical restraints unless a doctor has ordered it in the care plan and you have been trained in the use of the device. In some states, laws dictate the length of time restraints may remain in place (usually two hours), and they require that the restrained person be checked on periodically (usually at least every half hour).

Observing and Reporting: Physical Comfort and Safety

Your observations about your clients' physical comfort and safety can be very helpful to the care team. Report the following:

▶ how well clients tolerate positioning, transferring, and ambulation

▶ any signs of skin breakdown (blanching, redness, rashes, or broken skin)

▶ changes that could be made in the home environment to improve comfort or safety

Chapter 13

Providing Personal Care

Hygiene (HIGH-jeen) is the term used to describe practices (like bathing and brushing teeth) that we follow to keep our bodies clean and healthy. **Grooming** refers to practices like caring for fingernails and hair. Hygiene and grooming activities, as well as dressing, preparing meals, and eating, are called **activities of daily living (ADLs)**.

Some people who are ill may not have the energy to care for themselves. These clients may need assistance with their personal care, or they may need you to provide it for them entirely. You may be asked to provide any or all of the personal care, including bathing, perineal (payr-i-NEE-al) care [care of the perineum (payr-i-NEE-um), or area around and between the genitals and anus], mouth care, shampoo-

---

Learning Objectives

In this chapter you will learn to:

ing and combing the hair, nail care, shaving, dressing, and changing bed linens.

Some clients may never be able to care for themselves, but many clients will regain strength and be ready to take over their own personal care. An important part of your job as a home care aide is to help your clients be as independent as possible. This means teaching clients with disabilities to care for themselves, and encouraging other clients to get back into their old routines of self-care as soon as they have the strength. Promoting independence is an important aspect of care.

We all have routines for personal care and activities of daily living. We also have preferences for how they are to be done. These routines remain important to us even when we are elderly, sick, or disabled. Be aware of your client's individual differences and preferences concerning their personal care. Clients may prefer certain soaps or skin care products. They may choose to bathe in the morning or at night. It is important to ask clients about their routines and preferences.

Before you begin any procedure or task, explain to the client exactly what you will be doing. Ask if he or she would like to use the bathroom or bedpan first. Provide the client with privacy, and let him or her make as many decisions as possible about when, where, and how a procedure will be done. During the procedure, if the client appears tired, stop and take a short rest. After completing a procedure, always ask if the client would like anything else.

Providing or assisting with personal care gives you the opportunity to observe your client's skin, mental state, mobility, flexibility, comfort level, and ability to perform ADLs. For example, as you bathe a client, observe the skin for color, texture, temper-

ature, and whether it is dry or moist. Is it pale, yellow, ashen, or flushed? Are there blotches or a rash? Is there redness around bony areas (see Chapter 9, Fig. 9-5, pressure sore danger zones)? Is the skin dry and flaky?

Many clients will talk about any signs and symptoms they are experiencing during the time their personal care is administered. They may tell you that they have been itching or their skin feels dry. They may complain of numbness and tingling in a certain part of the body. Keep a small note pad in a pocket to jot down exactly how the client describes these symptoms, or make notes right away after the procedure. Remember to report these comments to your supervisor and then document them according to your agency's policies and procedures.

You should also observe the client's mental and emotional state at this time. Is the client depressed or confused? Can the client concentrate on the activity or hold a conversation? Is the client short of breath when moving or performing care? Does the client tremble or shake? Is the client having trouble using certain muscles or joints? You must focus on *changes* from the client's normal state. Is there a change in behavior, level of activity, skin color, movement, or anything else?

You may not know every sign and symptom of every possible illness, but you are in the *best* position to observe, report, and document any small change in your client. No matter what care task is assigned to you, performing the task is only half the job. For example, when bathing a client, you should take time to observe changes in the client's skin, changes in his ability to move, reach, or help himself, and

Historical Note

Much of the care you are learning to give was once performed by licensed nurses. Nurses receive years of education and experience to detect and assess signs and symptoms of many potential illnesses and health problems. As it becomes more common to delegate the care tasks you are learning, nurses lose an opportunity to personally discover early signs of illness or disease. Your role is to make certain small, subtle changes in a client's status do not go unnoticed.

changes in his willingness to help himself.

After you have finished a procedure, check the client's room. Is it a comfortable temperature? Is it well-ventilated, but free from drafts? Does the client have an easy way to signal for help? Does the room have good lighting? Are there electrical cords or other objects in the walkways? Is the room cluttered and unsafe? Also, make certain your client does not smoke in bed.

❏ 2. Explain guidelines for assisting with bathing

Bathing promotes good health and well-being by removing the perspiration, dirt, oil, and dead skin cells that accumulate on the skin. Taking a bath or having a bed bath can also be relaxing. For clients who are bed bound, the bed bath is an excellent time for moving extremities and increasing body movement and circulation. However, you should never give a client a tub bath unless you are assigned to do so in the care plan. Many home health agencies have rules against home care aides helping clients into the bathtub. These rules are for the safety of the client as well as the home care aide. Follow your agency's policies and procedures.

Many people prefer a daily bath or shower, but this is not really necessary. The face, hands, **axillae** (AK-sil-eye, or underarms), and perineum should be washed every day, but a complete bath or shower can be taken every other day or even less frequently. Older skin produces less perspiration and oil. Elderly people whose skin is dry and fragile should bathe only once or twice a week to prevent further dryness. When bathing older clients, be careful not to wash the skin too vigorously.

Before bathing any client or assisting with bathing, make sure the temperature of the room is warm enough. Remove any loose rugs that do not have slip-resistant, rubber backings. Be familiar with available safety and assistive devices (see below). Never leave an elderly person or young child alone while in the bathtub. Never use bath oils. They make the tub slippery and can cause a fall.

Wearing gloves is recommended whenever assisting clients with bathing. However, some home health agencies only require that you wear gloves for perineal care or if broken skin is present. As always, follow your agency's policies and procedures.

Guidelines for using assistive devices in bathing

Assistive devices, such as a transfer belt or lift, tub chair, and safety bars, can make bathing easier and safer, both for the client and for you. An **occupational therapist** (OT) may be used to teach you and the client transfer techniques for getting safely in and out of the bathtub. Occupational therapists help clients improve their abilities to perform ADLs.

Transfer belts attach around a client's waist for safety during transfers or ambulation. A transfer belt can make it easier for you to help the client lower him or herself into the tub and raise him or herself out of the tub. **Mechanical lifts** are another way to transfer a client from bed to wheelchair or tub chair and back. More information on using transfer belts and mechanical lifts can be found in Chapter 12.

A **tub chair, shower chair, or bath bench** is a sturdy chair or bench designed to be placed in a bathtub. It is designed to be water resistant and slip resistant. The chair or bench enables a client, who is unable to get down into a tub or too weak to stand in a shower, to bathe in the tub rather than in bed. **Safety bars/grab bars** are often installed in and near the tub and toilet to allow the client something to hold on to while changing position.

You will not find the same adaptive equipment in each client's home. Become familiar with the tools you have to work with. Learn how to use them before trying to assist the client. Report any need for equipment to your supervisor.

> Noticing and reporting change is perhaps the most important part of your job!

Procedure 1: Helping the client transfer to the bathtub

You may have to adapt this procedure to work with your clients' different strength levels.

1. Explain what you will do.

2. Assemble equipment:

- chair
- transfer belt, if appropriate
- shirt or robe to wear under transfer belt
- slide board, if appropriate
- tub chair
- bath supplies (as listed in Procedure 2)
- disposable gloves

3. Wash your hands.

4. Help the client to the bathroom. Chapter 12 includes instructions for assisting clients with ambulation or transfers.

5. Provide privacy for the client.

6. Seat the client in a chair facing the bathtub and centered between the grab bars. If using a wheelchair, lock brakes and raise footrests (**Fig. 13-1**).

Fig. 13-1

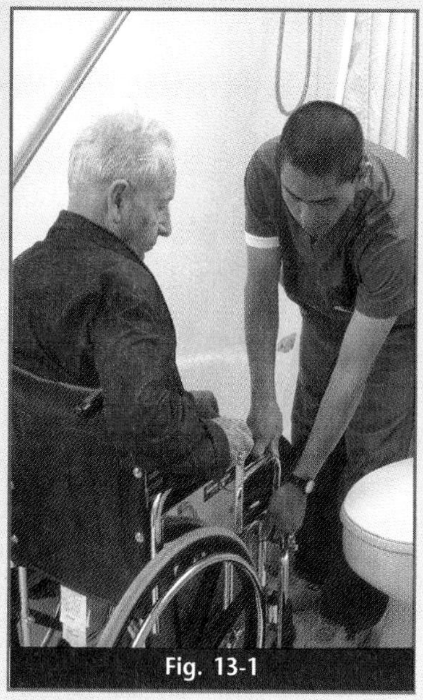

7. Ask the client to place one leg at a time over the sides of the tub.

8. Have client hold onto the grab bars or the edge of the tub to bring himself to a sitting position on the edge of the tub (**Fig. 13-2**). A slide board may also be used to help the client move from the chair to the tub. Procedure 7 in Chapter 12 explains how to assist in transfers using a slide board.

Fig. 13-2

9. Help the client lower himself into the tub or onto the tub chair while holding onto the edge of the tub or grab bars (**Fig. 13-3**). If necessary, you can assist by holding him around the waist or by having him wear a transfer belt. If using a transfer belt to get in and out of the tub, the client will need to wear a shirt or robe while transferring, so the belt is not placed directly against his skin.

10. Reverse this procedure to help the client out of the tub when the bath is over. If the client has trouble getting out of the tub, help him to his hands and knees. From that position, he can use the grab bar or the edge of the tub to help pull himself up. You can also help by putting the transfer belt back on the client (over a robe).

Fig. 13-3

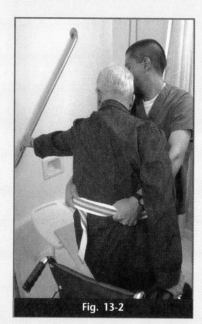

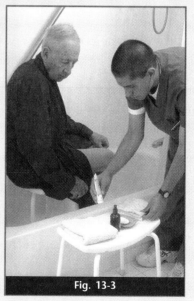

Clients who can get out of bed to take a shower or bath will need different levels of assistance and supervision. Follow the instructions in the care plan on what kind of bathing the client will do.

1. Explain what you will do.

2. Assemble supplies:
   - two bath towels
   - washcloth
   - soap or other cleanser
   - bath thermometer, if available
   - rubber bath mat
   - tub or shower chair, if appropriate
   - table for bath supplies and bell (for clients who bathe without assistance)
   - nonskid bath rug
   - deodorant, powder, lotion and other toiletries
   - clean clothes or a robe
   - shoes or nonskid slippers
   - disposable gloves

3. Clean tub or shower if necessary. Place rubber mat on tub or shower floor. Set up tub or shower chair. Place skid-resistant bath rug on the floor next to the tub or shower.

4. Provide privacy for the client.

5. Wash your hands.

6. Put on gloves.

7. Fill the tub with warm water (105° F to 110° F on the bath thermometer, or test the water on the inside of your wrist to see if it is comfortable) or adjust the shower water temperature.

8. Ask the client to undress, and assist as needed. Help client transfer to bathtub or step in the shower.

9. If the care plan allows you to leave the client to bathe alone, place the bathing supplies on a small table within the client's reach. Place a bell or

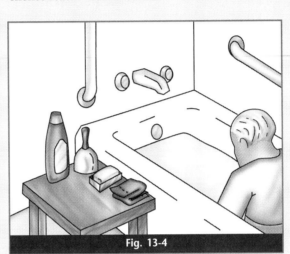

Fig. 13-4

other signal on the table (**Fig. 13-4**). Tell the client to signal when you are needed. Also tell the client not to add more hot or warm water and not to remain in the tub more than twenty minutes. Do not lock the bathroom door. Check on your client every five minutes. If the client is weak, remain in the bathroom. Otherwise, you can make the client's bed while he is in the tub.

10. For a shower, stay with the client and assist with washing hard-to-reach areas. Observe for signs of fatigue.

11. If the client needs more assistance in the bath or shower, help him wash himself. Always wash from clean areas to dirty areas, so you don't spread dirt into areas that have already been washed. Make sure all soap is rinsed off the client so his skin does not become dry or irritated.

12. Assist the client with shampooing hair, if necessary (see Procedure 5). Make sure all shampoo is rinsed out of hair.

13. When the bath or shower is finished, help the client get out of the tub. Wrap him in a towel. Have the client sit in a chair or on the toilet seat, and provide him with another towel for drying himself (**Fig. 13-5**). Offer assistance in drying hard-to-reach places.

Continued on page 162

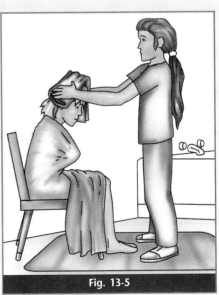

Fig. 13-5

Continued from page 161

The client may need help applying powder, deodorant, or lotion. If necessary, help the client get dressed.

14. If your client is tired after the bath or shower, help him back to the bed. Other personal care, such as mouth care, can be done later or while the client is in bed.

15. Clean the tub and place soiled laundry (towels, washcloths, dirty clothes) in the laundry hamper.

16. Wash your hands.

17. Put away supplies.

18. Document the procedure and your observations. Did you observe any redness or blanching on the skin? Was there any broken skin? How did the client tolerate bathing or showering? Has there been a change in the client's abilities since the last bath or shower?

Talk with your supervisor if the client makes a request that is not included in the care plan. For example, if the client wants a tub bath that is not included in the care plan, you must talk with your supervisor.

1. Explain what you will do.

2. Assemble supplies and place them on a table near the bed:

- basin
- bath thermometer, if available
- soap
- two washcloths
- two or three towels
- orangewood stick or nail brush, if available
- lotion, powder, deodorant
- soft cotton blanket or a large towel
- clean clothes for the client
- clean bed linens
- disposable gloves (two pairs)

3. Provide privacy for the client by closing the door, and closing shades or curtains. Be sure the room is a comfortable tempera-

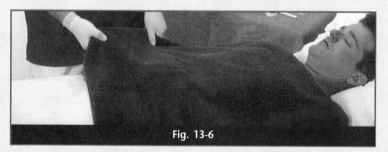
Fig. 13-6

ture and there are no drafts.

4. If the client has an adjustable bed, raise it to a comfortable working height.

5. Wash your hands.

6. Put on gloves.

7. Ask your client to remove glasses and jewelry and put them in a safe place. Offer to bring bedpan or urinal for the client to use before the bath

(see Procedure 13 and 14 in this chapter).

8. Place a soft cotton blanket or towel over your client and ask him or her to hold on to it as you remove the top sheet and blanket. Check the sheets for spills or body discharges.

9. Fill the basin with warm water and check the temperature with a bath thermometer or against the inside of your wrist. Water temperature should be between 105° F and 110° F on a thermometer. Allow the client to check the temperature to see if it is adequate. During the bath, change the water when it becomes too cool, soapy, or dirty.

10. Ask the client to move to the side of the bed near where you are standing. Assist if necessary. Place a clean towel across the client's chest (**Fig. 13-6**).

11. Fold the washcloth over your hand like a mitt and hold it in place with the thumb (**Fig. 13- 7**). Before you put soap on the cloth, wash the client's eyes and face. Start with the eye farther away from you and wipe from the inner corner, near the bridge of the nose, to the outer corner (**Fig. 13-8**). Use a different section of the washcloth for the other eye.

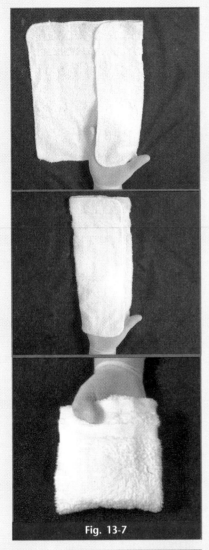

Fig. 13-7

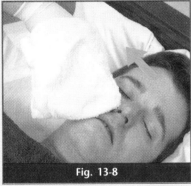

Fig. 13-8

12. Wash the face from the middle outward using firm but gentle strokes. Then wash the neck and ears. Rinse and pat dry. If the client's face is oily, ask the client if you may use soap. Some people prefer creams for cleansing their faces.

13. Remove the client's top clothing, then cover the client with the cotton bath blanket and towel again. Expose one arm. Using long strokes from the shoulder down to the elbow, wash the upper arm and axilla with a soapy washcloth (**Fig. 13-9**). Rinse and pat dry. After washing the elbow, wash, rinse, and dry from the elbow down to the wrist.

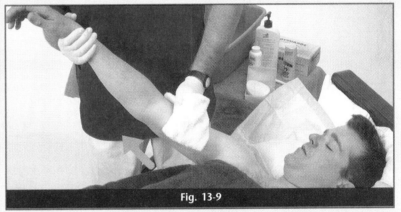

Fig. 13-9

14. To wash the hand, place it in the basin, wash the hand and clean under the nails with an orangewood stick or nail brush, if available (**Fig. 13-10**). Rinse and pat dry. Provide nail care (see

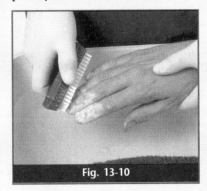

Fig. 13-10

Procedure 4) if it has been assigned to you. Do not provide nail care for diabetic clients. Repeat steps 13 and 14 for the other arm and hand. Put moisturizing lotion on the client's elbows and hands.

15. Place the towel once again across the client's chest and pull the blanket down to the waist. Lift the towel only enough to wash the chest, rinse it, and pat dry. Be sure to wash under a woman's breasts and check the skin in this area for signs of irritation and chafing. Ask the client if you may apply powder to the skin under the breasts after the area is dry.

16. Fold the cotton blanket down so that it still covers the pubic area. Wash the abdomen, rinse, and pat dry. If the client has an ostomy (AH-stoh-mee), or opening in the abdomen for getting rid of body wastes, provide skin care around the opening (Chapter 14 includes more information about ostomies). Cover with the towel. Pull the cotton blanket up to the client's chin and remove the towel.

Continued on page 164

Continued from page 163

17. Expose one leg and place a towel under it. Wash the thigh, using long, downward strokes, then rinse and pat dry. Do the same from the knee to the ankle (**Fig. 13-11**). Place another towel under the foot and transfer the basin to the towel. Place the client's foot into the basin. Wash the foot and between the toes (**Fig. 13-12**). Perform nail care if it has been assigned to you (see Procedure 4). Do not perform nail care if the client is diabetic or if nail care is not included in the care plan. Remember home care aides *never* clip a client's toenails.

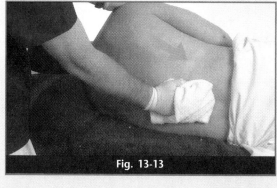
Fig. 13-13

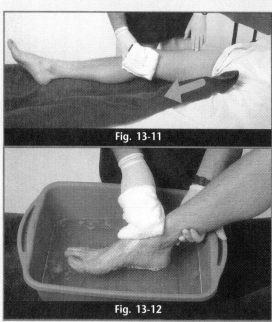
Fig. 13-11

Fig. 13-12

18. Rinse the foot and pat dry, making sure the area between the toes is dry. Apply lotion to the foot, especially at the heels. Repeat steps 17 and 18 for the other leg and foot.

19. Help the client move to the center of the bed then turn onto his side so his or her back is facing you. If the bed has rails, raise the rail on the opposite side for safety. Fold the cotton blanket away from the back. Place a towel lengthwise next to the back. Wash the back, neck, and buttocks with long, downward strokes (**Fig. 13-13**). Rinse and pat dry. Apply powder or lotion.

20. Place the towel under the buttocks and upper thighs. Help the client turn onto his or her back. Ask the client if he or she is able to complete the bath by washing the perineal area. If the client wants to and is able to do this, place a basin of clean, warm water within reach, along with a washcloth and towel. Leave the room for five minutes if the client would like privacy. If the client has a urinary catheter in place, remind him or her not to pull or disturb it.

21. If the client is unable to provide perineal care, you must do so.

Wearing gloves will prevent your hands from coming in contact with body secretions. Use clean water and a clean washcloth.

22. For a female client, always wash the perineum with soap and water from front to back, using single strokes (**Fig.13-14**). Do not wash from the back to the front, as this

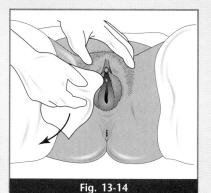
Fig. 13-14

may cause infection. First wipe the center of the perineum, then each side. Turn the washcloth to a clean side and spread the labia majora (LAY-bee-a ma-JOHR-a), the outside folds of perineal skin that protect the urinary meatus and the vaginal opening. Wipe from front to back on each side. Rinse the area in the same way. Ask the client to turn on her side, then wash and rinse the anal area. Dry the perineum thoroughly and cover the client with the cotton blanket.

23. For a male client, hold the penis by the shaft and wash in a circular motion from the top down to the base (**Fig. 13-15**).

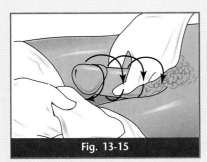

Fig. 13-15

Rinse the penis, then rinse the washcloth and wash the scrotum and **groin**. The groin is the area from the pubis to the upper thighs. Rinse and pat dry. Rinse the washcloth again, ask the client to turn on his side, then wash the anal area. Rinse and pat dry. Cover the client with the cotton blanket.

24. Place soiled washcloths and towels in the hamper or laundry basket. Dispose of the dirty bath water in the toilet. Discard gloves into a trash receptacle.

25. If time permits, a bed bath is a good time to give the client a back rub if he wants one (Chapter 12 explains how to give a back rub).

26. Provide the client with deodorant. Place a towel over the pillow and brush or comb the client's hair (Procedure 8 in this chapter). Help the client put on clean clothing and get into a comfortable position with good body alignment.

27. If the client uses a signaling device, place it within reach. Take the bath supplies away, and wash and store everything. Change bed sheets and blanket. Place used bed linens in the hamper or laundry basket.

28. Wash your hands.

29. Document the procedure and your observations. Did you observe any redness or blanching on the skin? Was there any broken skin? How did the client tolerate bathing or showering? Did the client tell you about any symptoms? Has there been a change in the client's abilities since the last bath or shower?

Procedure 4: Assisting with foot and nail care

Nail care should only be provided by the home care aide if it has specifically been assigned. Never cut a client's toenails. In some clients, poor circulation can lead to infection if skin is accidently cut while caring for nails. In a diabetic client, such an infection can lead to a severe wound or even amputation.

If you are directed to provide nail care for a client, be sure you know exactly what care you are assigned to provide.

1. Explain what you will do.

2. Assemble the following equipment:

- orangewood stick
- emery board
- small basin or bowl
- large basin
- cuticle softener or remover
- hand towel
- pumice stone
- two bath towels
- disposable gloves

If the client uses nail polish, you will need:

- nail polish
- nail polish remover
- cotton balls

3. Wash your hands.

4. Put on gloves if the client has any broken skin.

5. If necessary, remove nail polish with a cotton ball soaked with nail polish remover.

6. Fill the basin halfway full with warm water, and soak the client's nails in the water. If a tub bath or shower has just been given, soaking is not necessary. If you need to soften cuticles to push them back (step 9, below), add a cuticle softener to the water or apply to the cuticles following the directions on the container. Soak all ten fingertips for two to four minutes.

7. Fill a larger basin halfway full with warm water. Place it on a bath towel on the floor (if the client is sitting in a chair) or on a towel at the foot of the bed (if

Continued on page 166

Continued from page 165

the client is in bed). Soak the client's feet for ten minutes. Add warm water to the basin as necessary.

8. Remove the hand basin. Dry the client's hands with a towel.

9. Place the client's hands on the towel and push back the cuticles using the flat end of the orangewood stick or a towel (**Fig. 13-16**).

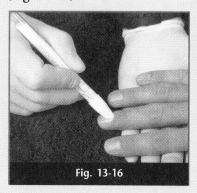

Fig. 13-16

10. If you have been assigned to clip fingernails, be sure to clip

them straight across the nail rather than curved.

11. Use the pointed end of the orangewood stick or a nail brush to remove dirt from under the nails, and wash the hands again. Apply lotion.

12. Remove feet from basin. Smooth any rough areas with the pumice stone or a washcloth (**Fig. 13-17**).

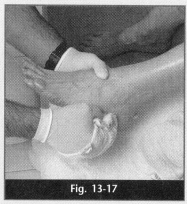

Fig. 13-17

13. Dry each foot thoroughly, especially between the toes, with bath towel. Apply lotion. *Do not*

attempt any further care of the toenails.

14. While you are giving foot care, observe the feet for sores, irritated or reddened areas (especially on the heels), any discoloration or darkening on the foot, discoloration of the toes or toenails, swelling, infection, or differences in temperature. If your client receives foot care from another person, you should still observe for these signs of problems or illness on a regular basis.

15. Discard the water and clean the basins. Dispose of the towels in the laundry hamper, and store supplies.

16. Wash your hands.

17. Document procedure and any observations. Was there any redness, blanching, or broken or discolored skin? Were there any differences in temperature?

Procedure 5: Shampooing hair

Clients who can get out of bed may have their hair shampooed in the sink, tub, or shower. For clients who cannot get out of bed, special rubber or plastic troughs exist for shampooing the hair in bed. Troughs fit under the client's head and neck and have a spout or hose that drains the water into a basin at the side of the bed (see below). Your agency should be able to provide this equipment. You may also use a plastic garbage bag formed around a rolled towel.

1. Explain what you will do.

2. Assemble the following supplies:

- shampoo
- hair conditioner
- washcloth
- pitcher, plastic cup, or hand-held shower or sink attachment
- disposable gloves
- chair (for washing hair in sink)
- large garbage bag or plastic

sheet (for washing hair in sink)

- towel (*two* towels if washing hair in bed)
- cotton blanket (for washing hair in bed)
- waterproof mat (for washing hair in bed)
- trough, or garbage bag and extra towel (for washing hair in bed)
- catch basin (for washing hair in bed)

3. Wash hands.

4. Put on gloves.

5. Position the client and wet the client's hair.

a. *For washing hair in the sink,* seat the client in a chair covered with plastic. Use a pillow under the plastic to support the client's head and neck. Have the client lean her head back toward the

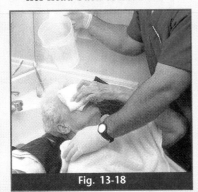
Fig. 13-18

sink. Give the client a folded washcloth to hold over her forehead or eyes. Wet hair using a plastic cup or a hand-held sink attachment (**Fig. 13-18**).

b. *For washing hair in the tub,* have the client tilt her head back. Give the client a folded washcloth to hold over her forehead or eyes. Wet hair using a plastic cup or hand-held shower attachment.

c. *For washing hair in the shower,* have the client turn so her back is toward the shower head. Ask the client to tilt her head backwards. Direct the flow of water over the hair to wet it.

d. *For washing hair in bed,* arrange the supplies within reach on a nearby table. Remove all pillows, and place

the client in a flat position. Place a waterproof sheet or mat beneath the client's head and shoulders. Cover the client with the cotton blanket, and fold back the top sheet and regular blankets. Place the trough under the client's head, then connect the trough to the catch basin (**Fig. 13-19**). Using the pitcher, pour enough water on the client's hair to make it thoroughly wet.

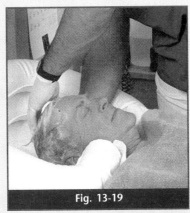
Fig. 13-19

6. Apply a small amount of shampoo to your hands and rub them together. Using both hands, massage the shampoo to a lather in the client's hair. With your fingertips, massage the scalp in a circular motion, from front to back (**Fig. 13-20**).

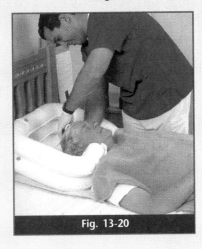
Fig. 13-20

7. Rinse the hair in the same way you wet it. Repeat the shampoo, rinse again, and use conditioner if the client wants it. Be sure to rinse the hair thoroughly to prevent the client's scalp from getting dry and itchy.

8. Wrap the client's hair in a towel. If shampooing at the sink, return the client to an upright position. If shampooing in the bath or shower, assist the client from the tub or shower as in Procedures 1 and 2. If shampooing in bed, remove the trough. Using the washcloth or a face towel, wipe water from the head and neck.

9. Remove the hair towel and comb or brush hair (see Procedure 7).

10. Dry hair with a hair dryer on the low setting. Style hair as the client prefers.

11. Wash and store equipment. Put soiled towels and washcloth in the hamper or laundry basket.

12. Wash your hands.

13. Document the procedure and your observations. How did the client tolerate having her hair washed? Was the client able to help? Have the client's abilities changed since the last time her hair was washed?

3. Describe guidelines for assisting with grooming

When assisting a client with grooming, remember to always allow the clients to do all they can for themselves. Follow the instructions in the care plan for what care to provide. Some clients may have particular ways of grooming themselves, or they may have a routine. Try to work with the client to establish a routine that includes everything in the care plan *and* satisfies the client. Check with your supervisor if you have any questions or problems.

Remember that some clients may be embarrassed or depressed because they need help with grooming tasks they have performed for themselves all their lives. Be professional, respectful, and cheerful while assisting your clients with grooming. Your attitude can go a long way toward helping your clients maintain self-respect and feel good about themselves.

Guidelines: Helping a client dress and undress

As with all care, the client's preferences should be asked and followed. Remember client-directed care is the client's right and your responsibility. Allow the client to choose clothing for the day. However, check to see if it is clean, appropriate for the weather, and in good condition. Encourage the client to

Procedure 6: Helping a client shave

Be sure the client wants you to shave him or help him shave before you begin.

1. Explain what you will do.

2. Assemble supplies:
- clean safety razor or clean electric razor
- shaving cream or gel (if using a safety razor)
- basin filled with warm water (if using a safety razor)
- bath towel
- washcloth
- mirror
- aftershave lotion
- disposable gloves

3. Wash your hands.

4. Put on gloves. Place the equipment on a table within reach of the client if he will shave himself. If the client is confined to bed, use pillows or a backrest to help the client sit up in a comfortable position. If the client wears dentures, be sure they are in place. Place the towel across the client's chest.

5. If you are using an electric razor, use a small brush to clean it. Turn on the razor and shave the face, pulling the skin tight over the mouth and cheeks if necessary to shave more smoothly (**Fig. 13-21**). Shave the chin and under the chin.

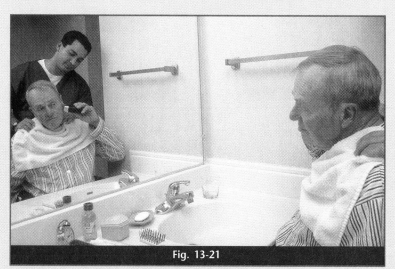
Fig. 13-21

6. If you are using a safety razor, use a blade that is sharp. A dull blade is hard on the skin. Soften the beard with a warm wet towel on the face for a few minutes before shaving. Lather the face with shaving cream or

gel and warm water. Warm water and lather make shaving more comfortable. Shaving in the direction of hair growth is also more comfortable and will result in a more even shave (**Fig. 13-22**). Use short strokes on the chin and longer strokes on the cheeks. Rinse the blade frequently in the basin.

7. When you have finished, rinse the client's face with a warm, wet washcloth or let him use the washcloth himself. If the client wants aftershave, moisten

Procedure 7: Combing or brushing hair

1. Explain what you will do.

2. Assemble equipment:
   ▶ comb, brush, or hair pick
   ▶ bath towel
   ▶ mirror
   ▶ hair lotion or oil if needed
   ▶ detangler, leave-in conditioner, or rubbing alcohol and cotton ball if the hair is tangled
   ▶ accessories such as barrettes, bobby pins, small combs, or coated rubber bands, depending on the client's style preference
   ▶ disposable gloves

3. If the client is confined to bed, raise the head of the bed, use a backrest, or use pillows to raise the client's head and shoulders. Place the towel under the client's head. If the client is ambulatory, provide a comfortable chair. Place the towel around the client's shoulders.

4. Wash your hands.

5. Put on gloves according to your agency's policies and procedures, and especially if the client has broken skin on the scalp or face.

6. Brush two-inch sections of hair at a time. Brush from roots to ends.

7. If the hair is tangled, work on the tangles first. Put a small amount of detangler or leave-in conditioner on the tangle, or dab a small amount of alcohol on the tangles. Hold the lock of hair just above the tangle so you don't pull at the scalp, and gently comb or brush through the tangle (**Fig. 13-23**).

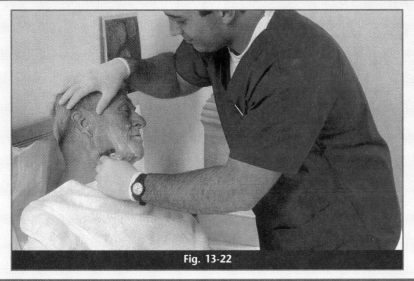

Fig. 13-23

8. Clients who have dry, brittle hair may require a special treatment with oil or hair lotion. Clients whose hair is tightly curled may use a comb with large teeth or a pick.

9. Style hair in the way the client prefers (**Fig. 13-24**).

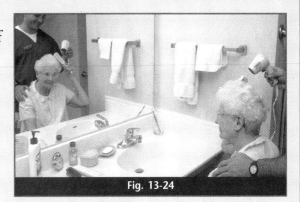

Fig. 13-24

10. Remove the towel and shake excess hair in the wastebasket. Place the soiled towel in the hamper. Store supplies. Remove your gloves.

11. Wash your hands.

12. Document the procedure and any observations.

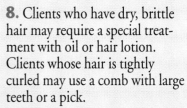

your palms with aftershave lotion and pat it onto the client's face.

8. Clean the equipment and store it. Dispose of the used razor blade or disposable razor. Put the towel and washcloth in the hamper or laundry basket. Remove and discard gloves.

9. Wash your hands.

10. Document the procedure and any observations.

Fig. 13-22

dress in regular clothes rather than nightclothes. Wearing regular daytime clothing encourages more activity and out-of-bed time. Elastic-waist pants or skirts are easy to pull on over legs and hips. Be sure the elastic waistband of underpants, slip, panty-hose, pants, or skirt fits comfortably at the waist. Clothing that is a size larger than the client would normally wear is easier to put on. Use the following guidelines when assisting a client with dressing or undressing:

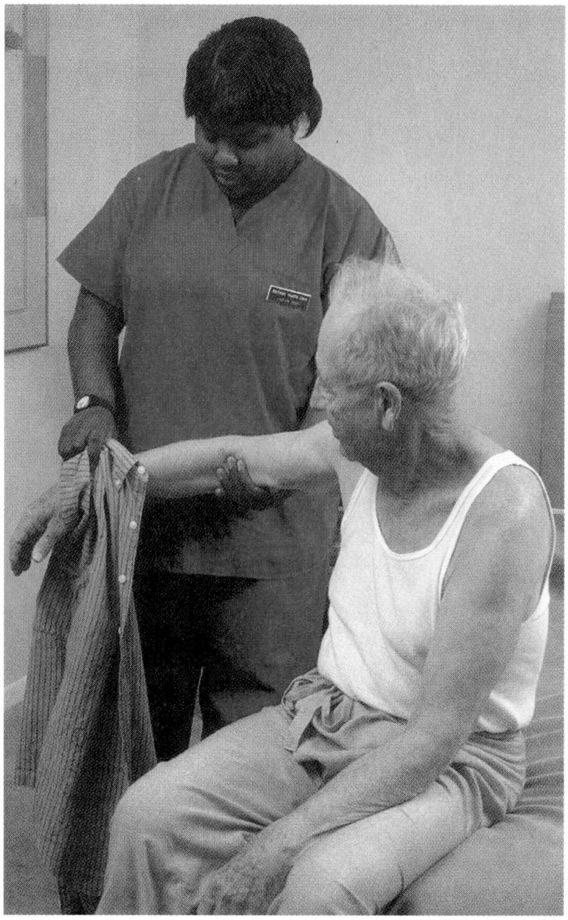

▶ The client should do as much to dress or undress himself as possible. It may take longer when the client dresses himself, but it helps maintain independence and regain self-care skills. Ask where your assistance is needed.

Fig. 13-25. When dressing assist with the involved (weaker) side first.

▶ Provide privacy. If the client has just had a bath, cover him with the cotton bath blanket and put on undergarments first. Never expose more than you need to.

▶ When putting on socks or stockings, roll or fold them down so they can be slipped over the toes and foot, then unrolled up into place on the leg. Make certain toes, heels, and seams of socks or stockings are in the right place.

▶ For a female client, make sure bra cups fit over the breasts. Front-fastening bras are easier for clients to manage by themselves. Bras that fasten in back can be put around the waist and fastened first, then rotated around and moved up, putting arms through the straps last. This can be done in reverse for undressing.

▶ For clients who have weakness or paralysis on one side, place the weak arm or leg through the garment first, then the strong arm. When undressing, do the opposite (**Fig. 13-25**).

▶ Several types of adaptive aids for dressing, such as long-handled hooks and pulls, are available to help clients maintain independence in dressing themselves (**Fig. 13-26**). An occupational therapist may be involved in teaching clients to perform ADLs using adaptive equipment.

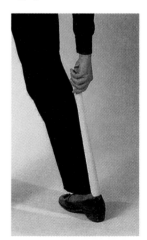

Fig. 13-26.

❏ 4. Identify guidelines for good oral care

Oral care, or care of the mouth, teeth, and gums, is performed at least twice each day to cleanse the mouth of food particles and secretions. Oral care should be done after breakfast and after the last meal or snack of the day. Oral care includes brushing teeth and gums, **flossing** teeth, and caring for dentures. **Dental floss** is a special kind of string used to clean between teeth.

Procedure 8: Assisting with mouth care

1. Explain what you will do.

2. Assemble supplies:
- soft-bristled toothbrush
- toothpaste or powder
- glass of water
- two towels
- moisturizer for lips
- basin and a drinking straw (if the client is in bed)
- disposable gloves

3. Provide privacy if the client desires it.

4. If your client is in bed, have him sit up, propped up by pillows. Place a towel under your client's head and one across the chest.

5. Wash your hands.

6. Put on gloves.

7. Remove any dental bridgework (Procedure 11 in this chapter explains how to remove dentures) or ask your client to do so.

8. Put toothpaste on the toothbrush.

9. Gently brush the teeth, or help the client brush teeth using short strokes and brushing back and forth on all surfaces. Brush the tongue gently as well.

10. Give the client water to rinse the mouth and place the basin

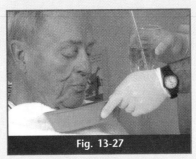

Fig. 13-27

under the client's chin for him to spit the water into (**Fig. 13-27**).

11. Replace any dental bridgework (Procedure 12 in this chapter explains how to reinsert dentures). Apply moisturizer to the lips.

12. Put the soiled towel in the laundry hamper. Dispose of the water in the basin by pouring it into the toilet. Clean the basin and put away supplies. Remove your gloves and discard them.

13. Wash your hands.

14. Document the procedure and any observations. Did you observe any mouth ulcers or other broken skin? What was the condition of the mucous membrane? Did the client's breath smell unusual?

Procedure 9: Performing mouth care for the unconscious client

Although clients who are unconscious are not eating, breathing through the mouth causes saliva to dry in the mouth. Good mouth care needs to be performed more frequently to keep the mouth clean and moist. Swabs with a mixture of lemon juice and glycerine are traditionally used to soothe the gums, but these may further dry the gums if used too often. Mouthwash may be used in place of glycerine if appropriate.

1. Always explain to the client what you will do before beginning any procedure. Even clients who are unconscious may be able to hear you. Always speak to them as you would to any client.

2. Assemble supplies:
- cotton swabs or **Toothettes**, a brand name for sticks with a small sponge at the end
- lemon glycerine swabs
- padded tongue blade (**Fig. 13-28**)

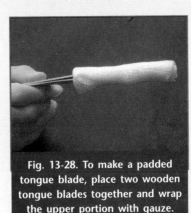

Fig. 13-28. To make a padded tongue blade, place two wooden tongue blades together and wrap the upper portion with gauze. Tape the gauze in place.

- mouthwash or a solution of hydrogen peroxide and water supplied by your agency
- basin
- lip moisturizer
- disposable gloves

3. Wash your hands.

4. Put on gloves.

5. Turn your client's head to the side and place a towel under his cheek and chin. Place a small kidney-shaped basin or other low-rimmed pan or basin next to the cheek and chin so that excess fluid flows into the basin.

6. Dip the plain cotton swab or Toothette in the mouthwash.

Continued on page 172

Continued from page 171

Do not dip a lemon glycerine swab in mouthwash.

7. Separate the upper and lower teeth with the padded tongue blade. Using the swab, cleanse all surfaces in the mouth cavity, including the teeth and underneath the tongue. Remove debris with the swab or toothette (**Fig. 13-29**). Repeat this step until the mouth is clean.

8. Swab again, this time with the lemon glycerine swab.

9. Remove the towel and basin.

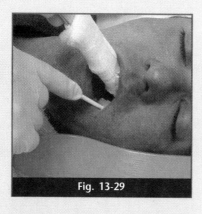
Fig. 13-29

Pat lips or face dry if needed. Apply lip moisturizer.

10. Place the towel in the laundry hamper. Clean the basin and put away supplies. Remove your gloves and discard them.

11. Wash your hands.

12. Document the procedure and your observations. Did you observe any mouth ulcers or other broken skin? What was the condition of the mucous membrane? Did the client's breath smell unusual?

Procedure 10: Flossing teeth

Flossing the teeth removes plaque and tartar buildup around the gum line and between the teeth. Teeth may be flossed immediately after or before they are brushed, as the client prefers.

1. Explain what you will do.

2. Assemble supplies:
- about 18 inches of dental floss
- glass of water
- basin
- face towel
- disposable gloves

3. Position the client as you would for brushing teeth.

4. Wash your hands.

5. Put on gloves.

6. Wrap the ends of the floss securely around each of your index fingers (**Fig. 13-30**).

7. Starting with the back teeth, place the floss between teeth and move it down the surface of the tooth using a gentle sawing

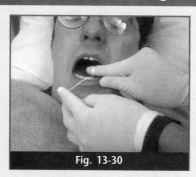
Fig. 13-30

motion (**Fig. 13-31**). Continue to the gum line. At the gum line, curve the floss into a letter C, slip it gently into the space between the gum and tooth, then go back up, scraping that side of the tooth (**Fig. 13-32**). Repeat this on the side of the other tooth.

8. After every two or three teeth, unwind floss from your fingers and move it so you are using a clean area. Floss all teeth.

9. Occasionally offer water so that the client can rinse debris from the mouth into the basin.

10. Offer the client a face towel when done flossing all teeth.

11. Discard floss. Pour water from the basin into the toilet. Clean and store the basin. Put the soiled face towel in the laundry hamper. Remove your gloves and discard them.

12. Wash your hands.

13. Document procedure and observations.

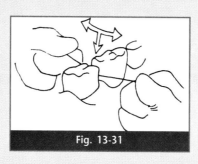
Fig. 13-31

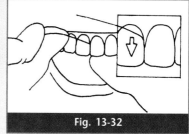
Fig. 13-32

Remember to ask the client how you can assist with denture care. Each person has his own preference about when and how denture care should be done.

1. Explain what you will do.

2. Assemble supplies:

- denture cup for storage
- denture cleaner or toothpaste
- denture brush or soft toothbrush
- two face towels
- basin or sink
- gauze squares
- mouthwash or a cotton swab or Toothette
- disposable gloves

3. Line the sink or a basin with a face towel and fill with water. The towel and water will prevent the dentures from breaking if they slip from your hands and fall into the sink.

4. Provide privacy if the client desires it.

5. Wash your hands.

6. Put on gloves.

7. Ask the client to remove the dentures and place them in the denture cup. If the client is unable to remove them, do it yourself. Remove the lower denture first. The lower denture is easier to remove because it floats on the gum line of the lower jaw. Grasp the lower denture with a gauze square (for a good grip) and remove it. Place it in a denture cup filled with water.

8. The upper denture is sealed by suction. Firmly grasp the upper denture with a gauze square and give a slight downward pull to break the suction. Turn it at an angle to take it out of the mouth.

9. Take the denture cup to the sink or basin. Apply denture cleanser to a denture brush or soft toothbrush, and brush the dentures under warm, running tap water to remove all material (**Fig. 13-33**). Do not use hot water, or dentures may warp. Rinse out the denture cup and place dentures in it.

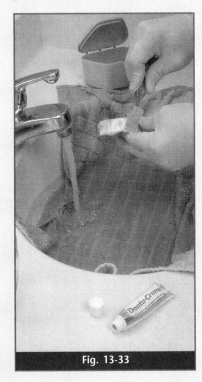
Fig. 13-33

10. Your client may prefer to clean the dentures with a soaking solution. Read the directions on the bottle and prepare the solution. Soak the dentures for the amount of time indicated (**Fig. 13-34**). Rinse and place in denture cup.

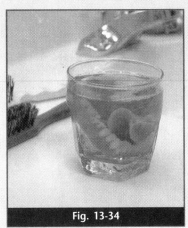
Fig. 13-34

11. Store dentures in water or solution to prevent them from warping. To avoid accidently throwing dentures away, always store them in a labeled denture cup when the client is not wearing them.

12. Offer the client mouthwash, a cotton swab, or a Toothette to cleanse the mouth.

13. Discard gauze pads and swabs. Put towels in laundry hamper. Clean out sink or basin. Rinse and store toothbrush and other supplies. Remove your gloves.

14. Wash your hands.

15. Document procedure and any observations.

Procedure 12: Reinserting dentures

Ask if the client needs your assistance in inserting dentures.

1. Explain what you will do.

2. Assemble supplies:
- denture cup with dentures
- denture cream or adhesive
- face towel
- disposable gloves

3. Provide privacy if the client desires it.

4. Position client as you would for brushing teeth (help him to as upright a position as possible).

5. Wash your hands.

6. Put on gloves.

7. Apply denture cream or adhesive to the dentures if needed.

8. Ask client to open mouth. Insert the upper denture into the mouth by turning it at an angle. Straighten it and press it onto the upper gum line firmly and evenly (**Fig. 13-35**).

9. Insert the lower denture onto the gum line of the lower jaw and press firmly.

10. Offer the client the face towel.

11. Rinse and store the denture cup. Remove the gloves and discard them.

12. Wash your hands.

13. Document the procedure and any observations.

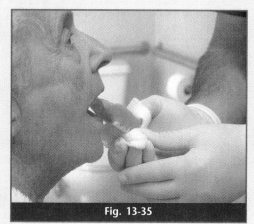

Fig. 13-35

When you perform or assist with oral care, you have the opportunity and responsibility to observe the mouth. Observe and report any of the following signs:

- irritation
- infection
- raised areas
- coated tongue
- **ulcers**, such as **canker sores** or small, painful, white sores
- flaky, white spots
- dry and cracked or chapped lips
- loose or decayed teeth
- swollen, bleeding, or whitish gums
- breath that smells bad or fruity

❏ 5. Explain care guidelines for hearing aids and prosthetic devices

Caring for a hearing aid. Many different types of hearing aids exist (**Fig. 13-36**). Follow manufacturer's directions for cleaning the hearing aid. In

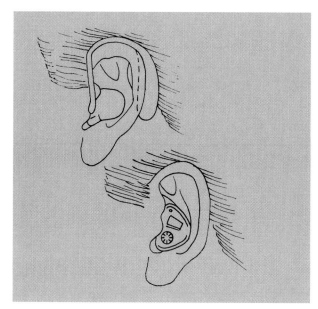

Fig. 13-36. Several types of hearing aids are available, depending on a person's needs.

general, use a little soap and water on a cloth, cotton swab, or pipe cleaner to keep the earpiece free of wax and dirt. Do not submerge the hearing aid or allow the section that houses the battery to get wet. Handle the hearing aid carefully. Do not drop it. Keep the hearing aid in a safe place when it is not being worn. Remind clients it is a good idea to have an extra battery on hand.

Caring for a prosthesis (pros-THEE-sis). A prosthesis is a device that replaces a body part that is missing or deformed because of an accident, injury, illness, or birth defect. You may work with clients who have prosthetic feet, legs, hands, arms, or eyes. Because prostheses are specially fitted, expensive pieces of equipment (an artificial leg may cost from $10,000 to $20,000), you should only care for prostheses as assigned in the client care plan. Make sure you know exactly how you are to care for the equipment before you begin. If you have any questions, call your supervisor.

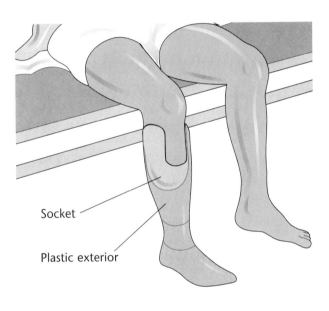

Socket

Plastic exterior

Fig. 13-37. Prostheses are specially fitted, expensive pieces of equipment.

Caring for an artificial eye. As with any procedure, wash your hands, provide privacy, and put on gloves before beginning to care for an artificial eye. Artificial eyes are held in by suction, so they will come out quickly when pressure is applied below the lower eyelid. Wash eye with solution and rinse in warm water. Moisten the artificial eye and place it far under upper eyelid. Pull down on lower eyelid and the artificial eye should slide into place.

❑ *6. Explain guidelines for assisting with toileting*

Clients who are unable to get out of bed to go to the bathroom may be given a **bedpan** (a) or a **urinal** (b) (**Fig. 13-38**). A **fracture pan** (c), a bedpan that is flatter than the regular bedpan, is used for clients who cannot assist with raising their hips onto a regular bedpan. Women will use a bedpan for urination and bowel movements. Men will generally use a urinal for urination and a bedpan for a bowel movement.

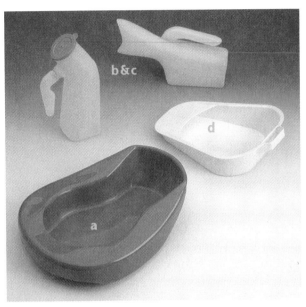

Fig. 13-38. a) A bedpan is used for persons who are unable to get out of bed to go to the bathroom; **b&c)** Male or female clients may use a urinal; **d)** A fracture pan is a flat version of the bedpan, used for persons who are unable to assist with raising their hips onto a bedpan.

Some clients are able to get out of bed, but may still need help walking to the bathroom and using the toilet. Others are able to get out of bed, but cannot walk to the bathroom and so use a portable commode. A portable commode is a chair with a toilet seat and a removable container underneath (see Procedure 15). In homes where the bathroom is on a different floor, portable commodes are very useful. When clients need assistance to get to the bathroom or use the toilet or commode, offer to help frequently. This can avoid accidents and embarrassment. Toilets can be fitted with raised seats to

1. Explain what you will do.

2. Assemble equipment:
   - bedpan
   - bedpan cover (newspaper or washable cloth)
   - protective plastic or latex sheet
   - talcum powder or corn-starch
   - cotton bath blanket
   - toilet paper
   - disposable or regular wash-cloths
   - disposable gloves

3. Provide privacy by closing doors and shades and using a covering blanket.

4. Wash your hands.

5. Put gloves on.

6. Warm outside of the bedpan with warm water in the bathroom and cover it when you bring it to the client. Dust the top of the bedpan with talcum powder to prevent it from sticking to the client's skin. Do not use talcum powder if the client has open sores on the buttocks or genitals. If a stool or urine sample is not needed, place a few sheets of toilet paper in the bedpan to make cleanup easier.

7. Cover the client with the cotton bath blanket and ask him to hold it while you pull down the top covers underneath it.

8. Place a protective sheet under the client. To do this, have the client roll toward you. If the client is unable to roll toward you unassisted, you must roll the client

(Procedure 9 in Chapter 12). Be sure the client cannot roll off the bed. Move to the empty side of the bed and place the protective sheet on the area where the client will lie on his back. The side of the protective sheet nearest the client should be fanfolded (folded several times into pleats) (**Fig. 13-39**). Ask the client to roll onto his back, or roll him as you did before. Unfold the rest of the protective sheet so it completely covers the area under and around the client's hips (**Fig. 13-40**).

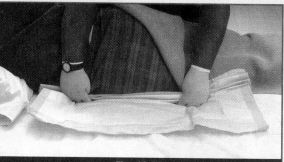
Fig. 13-39

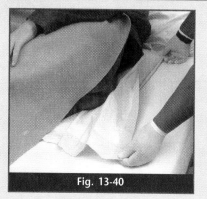
Fig. 13-40

9. Ask the client to remove undergarments, or help him do so.

10. With the client lying on his back, adjust the bed or use a backrest or pillows to prop up the upper body. Place the bedpan near his hips with the open end facing the foot of the bed (**Fig. 13-41**).

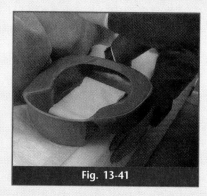
Fig. 13-41

11. Ask the client to help by raising his hips. Slide the bedpan under his hips. If the client cannot do this himself, place your arm under the small of his back and tell him to push with his heels and hands on your signal as you raise his hips (**Fig. 13-42**). If a client cannot help you in any way, keep the bed flat and roll the client onto the far side. Slip the bedpan under the hips and roll the client back onto

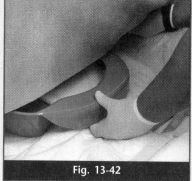
Fig. 13-42

the bedpan. Then prop the client into a semi-sitting position using pillows.

12. Check the bedpan to be certain it is in the correct position. Make sure the bath blanket is still covering the client. Provide the client with toilet paper, dispos-

able washcloths, and a bell or other way to call you. Tell the client you will return when called. Make sure the client is comfortable before you leave.

13. If the client is unable to clean the anal area and the rest of the perineum, you must do this. With gloves on, help the client to roll onto his side. Use the toilet paper to clean the perineal area first. For female clients, wipe from the front to the back. Use one disposable washcloth to cleanse the front part of the perineum and another to cleanse the anal area.

14. Wrap the toilet paper and disposable washcloths in a plastic bag and discard them. Dry the perineal area with a towel. Place the towel in a hamper. Remove your gloves and discard them. Immediately replace gloves with a clean pair.

15. Offer a wet washcloth and soap and water to the client to wash hands. Cover the client and remove the cotton bath blanket. Help the client put on undergarment.

16. Cover the bedpan and take it to the bathroom. Empty the bedpan carefully into the toilet and flush. If you notice anything unusual about the stool or urine (for example, the presence of blood), do not discard it. Remove and discard your gloves, wash your hands, and notify your supervisor. He or she may ask you to save a specimen (Chapter 14 describes how to collect stool specimens). Put on new gloves.

17. Turn the faucet on with a paper towel. Rinse the bedpan with cold water first and empty it into the toilet. Then clean the bedpan with hot, soapy water and store.

18. Remove and discard gloves.

19. Wash your hands.

20. Document the time of the elimination, the contents, and any observations.

make it easier for clients to get up and down (**Fig. 13-43**). Hand rails can also be installed next to the toilet. Observe and report if these assistive devices are needed but not present in a home.

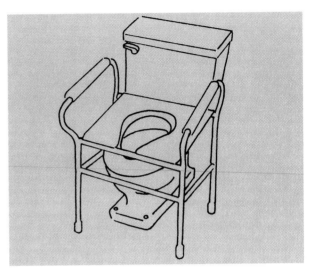

Fig. 13-43. A raised toilet seat makes it easier for a client to get up and down.

Your client may ask for the bedpan, or you may need to ask if he needs it at regular times listed on the assignment sheet. Remember that clients may be embarrassed about needing assistance with bodily functions. Always be professional when providing assistance. Provide as much privacy as possible.

❑ 7. List guidelines for care of the male and female perineal areas

Good perineal care is essential to prevent infection, skin irritation, and odor. Clients who are incontinent need regular and thorough perineal care. Never let you or your clients' embarrassment keep you from providing good perineal care. You can protect privacy without neglecting perineal care.

Remember to always wear gloves when providing or assisting with perineal care. Specific instructions for perineal care are found earlier in this chapter in the procedure for assisting with a bed bath (steps 21, 22, and 23 of Procedure 3 in this chapter).

Your client may ask for the urinal, or the assignment sheet may direct you to ask if he needs it at regular times.

1. Explain what you will do.

2. Assemble equipment:

- urinal
- protective plastic or latex sheet
- cotton bath blanket
- soap
- washcloth
- basin
- towel
- disposable gloves

3. Wash your hands.

4. Provide privacy by closing doors and shades and using a covering blanket.

5. Put on disposable gloves.

6. Place a protective pad under the client's buttocks and hips, as in Procedure 13.

7. Hand the urinal to the client. If the client is not able to help himself, place the urinal between his legs and position the penis inside the urinal. Replace covers.

8. Give the client a bell or another way to call you. Leave the room and close the door.

9. When the client signals that he is finished, remove the urinal or have him hand it to you. Follow the correct procedure if a specimen has been ordered (see Chapter 14). Discard urine in the toilet. Use a paper towel to turn on the faucet. Rinse the urinal with cold water and store it away.

10. Remove your gloves and discard them. Wash your hands.

11. Give the client a washcloth, soap, and water to wash his hands.

12. After taking the washcloth from the client and placing it aside (to be washed separately from other laundry), wash your hands again.

13. Document the time, the amount of urine (if monitoring intake and output), and any other observations.

❏ 8. Describe how to dispose of body wastes

Remember that wastes such as urine and feces can carry infection. Always dispose of wastes in the toilet, being careful not to spill or splash. Wear gloves when handling bedpans, urinals, or basins that contain wastes, including dirty bath water. Wash these containers thoroughly. Remove your gloves and wash your hands. Put on a new pair of gloves if you are not through with client care.

Washcloths used to wash perineal areas must be washed in hot water. Handle such laundry carefully, with gloves. Washing it separately from other family laundry is safest. Disposable washcloths may or may not be flushable. Read the package to be sure. If they are not flushable, dispose of them in a waste container lined with a plastic bag. Remove and replace the plastic bag frequently to prevent odors.

If a client has expressed a need to use the toilet or a portable commode, she may need your help.

1. Explain what you will do.

2. Assemble supplies, or be sure supplies are available in the bathroom:

- toilet paper
- disposable washcloths
- soap, washcloth, and basin (if using portable commode)
- disposable gloves

3. Wash your hands.

4. Put on gloves.

5. Help client out of bed and to the bathroom or portable commode.

6. If needed, help client remove clothing and sit on toilet seat.

7. Provide privacy. Leave the room or area. Close the door, but do not lock it. Provide a bell or another way for the client to call you. Don't go too far away in case you are needed soon.

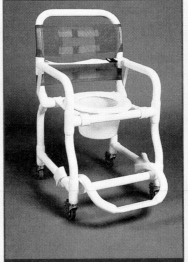

Fig. 13-44. A portable commode can be used for clients who can get out of bed but may not be able to move to the bathroom easily.

8. When the client calls you, return. If assistance is needed to clean the perineal area, provide it. Remember to wipe female clients from front to back. Use disposable washcloths if necessary. Dispose of these in the toilet, or in the wastebasket if they are not flushable. If your gloves become soiled, discard them and put on fresh gloves.

9. Help the client up and be sure she washes her hands before returning to bed. Use the sink or a basin, soap, and a washcloth.

10. When using a portable commode, remove waste container and empty it into the toilet unless a specimen is needed or the client's urine is being measured for intake/output monitoring (Chapter 14 explains how to measure output). Clean the container as you would a bedpan, rinsing first with cold water and then washing with hot water and cleanser.

11. Remove your gloves and discard them.

12. Wash your hands.

13. Document the procedure and any observations.

Chapter 14

Performing Basic Health Care Skills

❑ **1. List and explain the importance of each of the four vital signs that must be monitored**

As a home care aide, you will be responsible for monitoring, documenting, and reporting the **vital signs** of your clients. Vital signs

---

Learning Objectives

In this chapter you will learn to:

are important indicators of how well the vital organs of the body, such as the heart and lungs, are functioning. Measuring a client's vital signs consists of the following:

1. taking the body temperature
2. counting the pulse
3. counting the rate of respirations
4. measuring the blood pressure

You need to be able to detect changes in the vital signs that may indicate a client's condition is worsening. Always notify your supervisor if the client is running a fever (temperature is above average for the client or outside the normal range listed below), has a respiratory or pulse rate that is too rapid or too slow, or has an elevated or abnormally low blood pressure. Table 14-1 shows normals ranges for vital signs.

Table 14-1.
Normal Ranges for Vital Signs

Vital Sign Normal Range Temperature:

	Fahrenheit	Celsius
Oral	97.6°–99.6°	36.5°–37.5°
Rectal	98.6°–100.6°	37.0°–38.1°
Axillary	96.6°–98.6°	36.0°–37.0°

Pulse: 60–80 beats per minute

Respirations: 12–20 respirations per minute

Blood Pressure: Systolic 100–140,
Diastolic 70–90

Vital sign: Temperature

Body temperature is normally very close to 98.6°F (Fahrenheit) or 37°C (Celsius). Body temperature reflects a balance between the heat created by our bodies and the heat lost to the environment. Increases in body temperature may indicate an infection or disease.

There are four sites for taking body temperature:

1. the mouth (oral)
2. the rectum (rectal)
3. the armpit (axillary)
4. the ear (tympanic)

The different sites require different thermometers, so the site you use will depend on what kind of thermometer is available. Temperatures are most often taken orally. Use a different site if the client is unconscious, using oxygen, confused or disoriented, paralyzed from stroke, has facial trauma, or is younger than six years old. Taking a rectal temperature on an uncooperative client, such as a small child, can be dangerous. Axillary temperature is considered the least accurate.

Glass bulb or **mercury thermometers** may be for either oral or rectal use, and can also be used to take axillary temperatures. Glass rectal thermometers are thicker than oral thermometers, have a rounded, stubby bulb, and are less fragile (**Fig. 14-1**). The glass bulb thermometer is inexpensive, but it may take longer to use, be more difficult to read, or be dangerous if broken. If you break a glass thermometer, never touch the mercury or the broken glass. Clean up the pieces using a broom and dustpan, and discard.

The point of a glass thermometer, known as the bulb end, contains mercury that will move along the length of the thin hollow tube to register the client's temperature. Numbers on the thermometer let you read the temperature after it registers. Most thermometers show the temperature in degrees Fahrenheit (F), with each long line representing one degree and each short line representing two-tenths of a degree. Some thermometers show the temperature in degrees Celsius (C), with the long lines representing one degree and the short lines representing one-tenth of a degree. The small arrow points to the normal temperature: 98.6° F and 37° C. See **Fig. 14-1** to practice reading a thermometer.

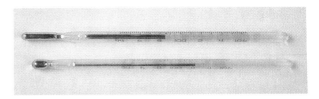

Fig. 14-1. Glass bulb thermometer registering a normal temperature, and glass bulb rectal thermometer registering a high temperature.

Battery-powered, digital, or electronic thermometers are becoming more affordable and more common in the home (**Fig. 14-2**). These thermometers display the results digitally and register the temperature more quickly than glass bulb thermometers. Digital thermometers usually take two to sixty seconds to register the temperature. The thermometer will beep or flash when the temperature has registered. Digital thermometers may be used to take oral, rectal, or axillary temperatures. You must follow manufacturer's guide for proper use of these thermometers.

The **tympanic thermometer**, or ear thermometer, is the quickest way to take a temperature (**Fig. 14-2**). However, these thermometers are expensive and not

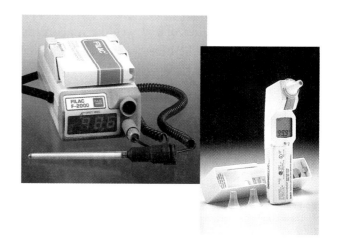

Fig. 14-2. Digital and tympanic thermometers register a temperature quickly and are easy to read.

Procedure 1: Taking body temperature orally

A glass thermometer can be used to take oral temperature:

1. Explain what you will do. You need the client's cooperation to take an oral temperature.

2. Assemble equipment: glass thermometer and disposable plastic thermometer covers.

3. Wash your hands.

4. Make sure the thermometer is clean. If not, or if you're not sure, rinse it in tepid (lukewarm) water and dry it. Check that the mercury has been shaken down below 96° F or 35° C. To shake the thermometer down, hold it at the side opposite the bulb with the thumb and two fingers. With a snapping motion of the wrist, shake the thermometer. Be sure you are standing away from furniture and walls so you don't accidently hit something and break the thermometer. Recheck the mercury level.

5. Make sure that the client has not smoked, eaten, drunk hot or cold fluids, or exercised for at least 10 minutes prior to taking

the temperature.

6. In some cases you will use disposable plastic covers over the glass thermometer. If plastic covers are available, slide the thermometer into the plastic cover.

7. Place the thermometer at least halfway to the back of the mouth, slightly to one side, under the tongue. It should lie next to the frenulum (FREN-yoo-lum), the connecting fold of tissue under the tongue (**Fig. 14-3**).

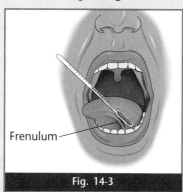

Frenulum

Fig. 14-3

8. Instruct the client not to bite down or talk. Client should keep the mouth closed and breathe through the nose.

9. Remove the thermometer

after three or four minutes.

10. Read the temperature in a place with good lighting, and hold the thermometer at eye level so that the lines are on top. Roll the thermometer between your thumb and forefinger until you see the silver stripe of mercury (**Fig. 14-4**).

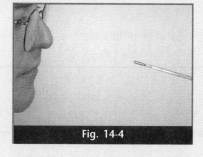

Fig. 14-4

11. Read and document the number that corresponds to the point where the line of mercury ends. Document the temperature, date, time, and method used (oral).

12. Rinse and dry the thermometer and store it away from a heat source.

13. Wash your hands.

as common in the home. They also require more practice to consistently take accurate temperatures.

Remember that there is a range of normal temperatures. Some people's temperatures normally run low while others in completely good health will run slightly higher temperatures. Normal temperature readings also vary according to the method used to take the temperature. Table 14-1 shows the normal range of temperatures.

To use a digital thermometer to take an oral temperature, follow the procedure for using a glass thermometer, with the following exceptions:

▶ You do not have to shake down the thermometer.

▶ Always use disposable plastic covers over the oral probe.

▶ Replace batteries if the thermometer is not registering the temperature properly.

▶ Wait for the final, correct temperature to register before documenting.

▶ For rechargeable thermometers, return the probe to the charger once you have noted the temperature.

You may need to take a rectal temperature, using either a glass or digital thermometer, when a tympanic thermometer is unavailable and you are caring for unconscious clients, clients who suffer from seizures, combative clients, clients with poorly-fitted dentures or missing teeth, anyone having difficulty breathing through the nose, and infants or young children. Always explain what you will do before beginning any procedure. You need the client's cooperation to take a rectal temperature. Advise the client to hold still, and reassure him or her that the procedure will only take a few minutes.

If you are using a digital thermometer to take a rectal temperature, the procedure is similar to using a glass thermometer, with the following exceptions:

▶ There is no need to shake down the digital thermometer.

▶ Plastic disposable sheaths are always used to cover the probe of a digital thermometer.

▶ Insert the thermometer only about one half inch into the rectum.

▶ Hold the probe in place until you obtain a digital reading. It usually takes less than a minute to get the results.

▶ For rechargeable thermometers, return the probe to the charger once you have noted the temperature.

Procedure 2: Taking body temperature rectally

A glass thermometer can be used to take temperature rectally:

1. Explain what you will do.
2. Assemble equipment:
   ▶ glass thermometer
   ▶ disposable plastic cover
   ▶ lubricant
   ▶ wipes or tissues
   ▶ disposable gloves
3. Provide privacy for the client.
4. Wash your hands.
5. Put on gloves.
6. Shake down the thermometer and make sure it is clean and in good condition.
7. Cover the thermometer with a disposable plastic cover

if available.

8. Using water-soluble lubricant on a tissue or wipe, lubricate one inch of the bulb end of the thermometer.
9. An adult or older child can lie on his side, with his back to you and knees slightly bent. An infant can be placed on his back or stomach for measuring the rectal temperature.
10. Separate the buttocks and gently insert the thermometer about one inch into the rectum. If you meet resistance, do not force the thermometer in. Hold the thermometer in place to avoid tissue damage in the rectum.

11. After three or four minutes, remove the thermometer by gently pulling it straight out.
12. Discard the plastic sheath if you used one. Otherwise, wipe the thermometer with a tissue from the flat end toward the bulb.
13. Read the thermometer at eye level as you would for an oral temperature. Document the temperature, date, time, and method used (rectal).
14. Rinse and dry the thermometer and store it away from a heat source.
15. Remove and discard gloves.
16. Wash your hands.

With a little practice, tympanic thermometers can be used to take a fast and accurate temperature reading. Many of your older clients may not be familiar with tympanic thermometers. As always, explain what you will do before beginning any procedure. Tell the client that accurate temperatures can now be obtained by placing a thermometer in the ear canal. Reassure the client that the procedure is entirely painless, and that the short tip of the thermometer will only go into the ear one-quarter to one-half inch. Because thermometer models vary, follow the manufacturer's instructions for the thermometer you will use.

Axillary temperatures are much less reliable than temperatures taken at any of the other sites. For this reason the axillary site should only be used as the last resort if no other site is possible.

Procedure 3: Taking a tympanic temperature

1. Explain what you will do.

2. Assemble equipment: tympanic thermometer and disposable probe cover.

3. Wash your hands.

4. Place a disposable probe cover over the cone-shaped end of the thermometer.

5. Position the client's head so that the ear is in front of you. You must seal the opening to the ear canal with the probe to get an accurate temperature reading. To do this, straighten the ear canal by pulling up and back on the pinna (PIN-na), or outside edge of the ear, for an adult, or by gently pulling straight back on the pinna for infants and children (**Fig. 14-5**).

6. Insert the covered probe into the ear canal and press the button. Remove the thermometer after one second.

7. Read and document the results.

8. Discard the disposable probe cover. Return the thermometer to the battery charger if the thermometer is a rechargeable model.

9. Wash your hands.

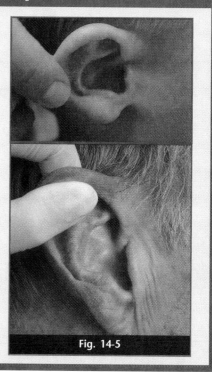

Fig. 14-5

Procedure 4: Taking an axillary body temperature

1. Explain what you will do.

2. Assemble equipment: glass or digital thermometer.

3. Wash your hands.

4. Adjust or remove enough of the client's clothing to allow skin contact with the end of the glass or digital thermometer. Make sure that the axilla is dry before placing the thermometer under the arm.

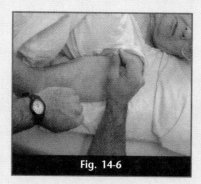

Fig. 14-6

5. Hold the thermometer in place, with the arm close against the side, for eight to ten minutes (**Fig. 14-6**).

6. Read and document the temperature and method.

7. Clean and store the thermometer as you would for an oral or rectal temperature.

8. Wash your hands.

Vital sign: Pulse

The pulse is essentially the number of heart beats per minute. The beat that you feel at certain pulse points in the body represents the wave of blood moving as a result of the heart pumping. The most common site for monitoring the pulse is on the inside of the wrist, where the radial artery runs just beneath the skin (**Fig. 14-7**). Other pulse points are in the elbow, the groin, the neck, the feet, and behind the knees.

For adults, the normal pulse rate is 60–80 beats per minute. Small children have more rapid pulses, in the range of 100–120 beats per minute. A newborn baby's pulse may be as high as 120–140 beats per minute. Many things can affect the pulse rate, including exercise, fear, anger, anxiety, heat, medications, and pain. An unusually high or low rate does not necessarily indicate disease. However, sometimes the pulse rate can be a signal that serious illness exists. For example, a rapid pulse may result from fever, infection, or heart failure. A slow or weak pulse may indicate dehydration, infection, or shock.

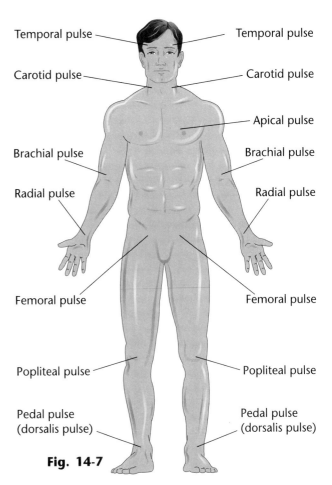

Temporal pulse — Temporal pulse
Carotid pulse — Carotid pulse
Apical pulse
Brachial pulse — Brachial pulse
Radial pulse — Radial pulse
Femoral pulse — Femoral pulse
Popliteal pulse — Popliteal pulse
Pedal pulse (dorsalis pulse) — Pedal pulse (dorsalis pulse)

Fig. 14-7

Procedure 5: Counting radial (wrist) pulse

1. Explain what you will do.

2. Assemble equipment: watch with a second hand.

3. Wash your hands.

4. Have your client sit or lie comfortably.

5. Find the radial pulse by pressing the tips of your first two fingers on the inside of the wrist, between the tendons and the wrist bone (**Fig. 14-8**).

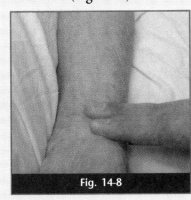

Fig. 14-8

6. When you have found the pulse, look at your watch. Count the beats for thirty seconds. For example, wait for the second hand to reach the 12 and count the beats until the second hand reaches the 6 (**Fig. 14-9**).

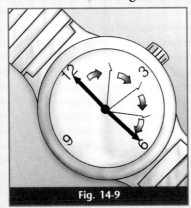

Fig. 14-9

7. Multiply the number of beats by two to get the actual pulse rate.

8. If you detect an irregular rhythm or feel that the volume of beats is abnormal, feel the pulse for a full minute.

9. Count the client's respirations while your fingers are still on the client's wrist (see Procedure 6).

10. Document the pulse rate, date, time, and method (radial). Notify your supervisor if the pulse is less than 60 beats per minute, over 100 beats per minute, or if the rhythm is irregular.

11. Wash your hands.

Procedure 6: Counting apical pulse

1. Explain what you will do.

2. Assemble equipment: stethoscope and watch with second hand.

3. Wash your hands.

4. Fit the earpieces of the stethoscope snugly in your ears. Place the flat metal diaphragm on the left side of the chest, just below the nipple (**Fig. 14-10**). Listen for the heartbeat.

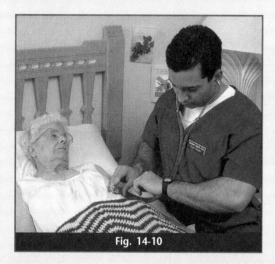

Fig. 14-10

5. Use the second hand of your watch as you would for a radial pulse. Count the heartbeats for one minute. Each "lub-dub" that you hear is counted as one beat. A normal heartbeat is rhythmical. Leave the stethoscope in place to count respirations (see Procedure 7).

6. Document the pulse rate, date, time, and method used (apical). Note any irregularities in the rhythm.

7. Store stethoscope.

8. Wash your hands.

The apical (AY-pi-kul) pulse is heard by listening directly over the heart with a stethoscope. This is often the easiest method for measuring the pulse in infants and small children because their pulse points are harder to find. A **stethoscope** is an instrument designed to listen to sounds within the body,

such as the heart beating or air moving through the lungs.

Vital sign: Respirations

Respiration is the process of breathing air into the lungs, or **inspiration**, and exhaling air out of the lungs, or **expiration**. Each respiration consists of an inspiration and an expiration. The chest rises during inspiration and falls during expiration.

The normal respiration rate for adults ranges from 12–20 breaths per minute. Infants and children have a faster respiratory rate; infants can breathe normally at a rate of 30–40 respirations per minute. Because people may breathe more quickly if they know they are being observed, count respirations immediately after taking the pulse, while your fingers are still on the client's wrist or the stethoscope is still over the heart. Do not make it obvious that you are observing the client's breathing.

Note: If you find it difficult to remember the pulse rate after taking the respiratory rate, use a paper and pencil and jot down the pulse rate before counting respirations. Then document the pulse and respiration rates on the visit notes when you are finished.

Vital sign: Blood Pressure

Blood pressure is one of the most important vital signs that home care aides will measure. Blood pressure, measured in millimeters of mercury (mmHg), is an indicator of how well the heart is functioning. There are two components of blood pressure, the systolic (sis-TOL-ik) and diastolic (DYE-a-stol-ik).

The systolic phase occurs when the heart is at work, contracting and pushing the blood from the left ventricle of the heart. The pressure reading you obtain reflects the pressure that is being exerted on the walls of arteries as the blood is pumped through the body. The normal range for systolic blood pressure is 100–140 mmHg.

The second measurement reflects the diastolic phase, which occurs when the heart relaxes. The diastolic measurement is always lower than the systolic measurement and represents the pressure in the arter-

Procedure 7: Counting respirations

1. For this procedure, you do not need to explain what you will do. Many people will breathe more quickly if they know they are being watched.

2. Immediately after measuring the pulse rate, count the breaths taken in thirty seconds. Multiply by two to get the rate per minute. If the rate is very rapid or if you are having difficulty counting, place your hand over the chest and count by watching your hand rise with the chest (**Fig. 14-11**).

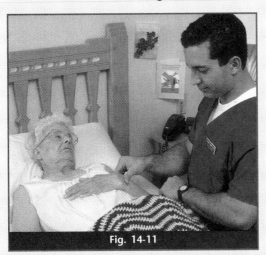
Fig. 14-11

3. Observe for the pattern and character of the client's breathing. Normal breathing is smooth and quiet. If you see signs of difficult breathing, shallow breathing, or noisy breathing, such as wheezing, report it to your supervisor.

4. Document the respiratory rate and the pattern or character of breathing.

5. Wash your hands.

ies when the heart is at rest. The normal range for adults is 60-90 mmHg.

Blood Pressure Abnormalities. People with high blood pressure, or hypertension (high-per-TEN-shun), have elevated systolic and/or diastolic blood pressures. Many factors can cause increased blood pressure, including aging, exercise, physical or emotional stress, pain, medications, and the volume of

blood in the circulation. For example, loss of blood will lead to abnormally low blood pressure, or hypotension (high-poh-TEN-shun), which can be life threatening if not corrected.

Blood Pressure Equipment. The tools you will use to measure blood pressure are a stethoscope and a blood pressure cuff, or sphygmomanometer (sfig-moh-ma-NOM-e-ter) (**Fig. 14-12**). Inside the cuff is an inflatable balloon that expands when air is pumped into the cuff. Two pieces of tubing are connected to the cuff. One leads to a rubber bulb that pumps air into the cuff. A pressure control button allows you to control the release of air from the cuff after it is inflated. The other piece of tubing is connected to a pressure gauge with numbers. The gauge is either a mercury column or a round dial.

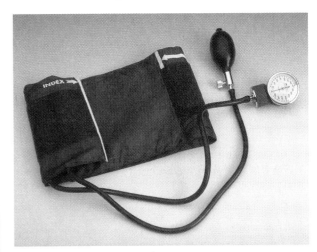
Fig. 14-12. The sphygmomanometer, or blood pressure cuff, is used to measure blood pressure.

There may be an electronic sphygmomanometer in some homes. The systolic and diastolic pressure readings and pulse are displayed digitally. Some units have automatic inflation and deflation. You do not need a stethoscope with an electronic sphygmomanometer. Ask your supervisor for instructions on the proper use of the equipment.

How Blood Pressure is Measured. Inflating the blood pressure cuff placed around the upper arm puts pressure over the brachial (BRAY-kee-al) artery and stops the blood flow. With the stethoscope placed over the brachial artery, on the inside of the elbow, you will first listen for the rush of blood filling the artery

1. Explain what you will do.

2. Assemble equipment: sphygmomanometer and stethoscope.

3. Wash your hands.

4. Have client sit or lie comfortably.

5. Select the left or the right arm. Never measure the blood pressure on an arm that has an intravenous line, dialysis shunt, or other medical equipment. Avoid a side that has a cast, recent trauma, or breast surgery (mastectomy).

6. Ask the client to roll up his or her sleeve. Do not measure the blood pressure over clothing.

7. Wrap the blood pressure cuff around the upper arm, about 1-1/2 inches above the elbow. Fasten so that the tubing is positioned over the inner portion of the arm. Line up the arrow on the cuff with the brachial artery.

8. Find the brachial pulse at the inner part of the elbow. Place the stethoscope diaphragm flat over the pulse (**Fig. 14-13**).

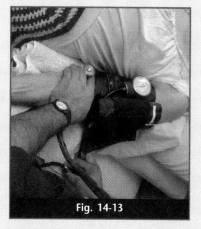

Fig. 14-13

9. Close the pressure valve on the bulb by turning the metal knob to the right (clockwise).

10. Grasping the bulb, pump air into the cuff while watching the mercury move in the column or the needle rise on the dial. Inflate the cuff until the gauge reads 30 mmHg over the client's normal systolic pressure or a palpated (PAL-payt-ed) blood pressure. If you do not know what the client's normal blood pressure is, you must obtain a palpated blood pressure first:

a. To palpate means to examine or feel with your hands or fingers. To take a palpated blood pressure, find the brachial pulse with your fingers. Close the blood pressure cuff and inflate it until you no longer feel the pulse. Note the number on the gauge. Continue to inflate the cuff an additional 30 mmHg.

b. Slowly turn the pressure control knob to the left (counterclockwise) until you first feel the pulse again. Note the number (this is the palpated systolic pressure).

c. The palpated systolic pressure can be used as a substitute for the client's normal blood pressure in step 10, above. Wait at least thirty seconds after taking a palpated blood pressure before taking the client's actual blood pressure.

11. Too much pressure causes discomfort in the arm, so keep your thumb and forefinger on the pressure control knob. Slowly and evenly turn the pressure control knob to the left (counterclockwise) to release air, watching the column of mercury or the pressure dial as the cuff deflates.

12. Listen for the first sound of the blood entering the artery and the pulse returning. Read the gauge at eye level. This is the systolic pressure.

13. Continue to deflate the cuff and note where on the gauge the last sound is heard. This is the diastolic pressure.

14. Fully deflate the cuff and remove it from the client's arm.

15. Document the blood pressure results, noting which arm was used. Write the numbers like a fraction, with the systolic reading on top and the diastolic reading on the bottom (for example: 120/80). Note which arm was used, writing "RA" for right arm, and "LA" for left arm (**Fig. 14-14**).

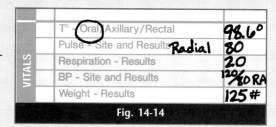

VITALS		
T° - Oral/Axillary/Rectal		98.6°
Pulse - Site and Results	Radial	80
Respiration - Results		20
BP - Site and Results		120/80 RA
Weight - Results		125 #

Fig. 14-14

16. Store sphygmomanometer.

17. Wash your hands.

Procedure 9: Measuring the weight of a client

1. Explain what you will do.

2. Assemble equipment: bathroom scale.

3. Wash your hands.

4. Set the scale on a hard floor surface, in a place the client can get to easily.

5. Be sure the scale reads zero with no one on it. If not, adjust the knob.

6. Help your client to the scale as needed.

7. Have the client step on the scale. Be sure she is not holding, touching, or leaning against anything, as this interferes with weighing. Be ready to help the client if he or she becomes unsteady while standing on the scale. Do not force someone to let go. If you are unable to obtain an accurate weight,

notify your supervisor.

8. When dial has stopped moving, read the weight.

9. Have client step off the scale and help him or her back to a comfortable position.

10. Document the weight.

11. Store the scale if you have moved it.

12. Wash your hands.

as you deflate the pressure in the cuff. This pressure reading is the systolic blood pressure. From this point you will hear the regular pulsating beats as you continue to deflate the cuff. The second reading to note is when the sounds stop completely. This reading is the diastolic blood pressure.

Other measurements of client status

You may be asked to check clients' weights and heights as part of your care. Height is checked less frequently than weight. Weight changes can be indicators of illness and can also affect the medication doses a client needs. For these reasons, you may need to weigh your clients daily or weekly. Clients confined to bed can be weighed using a chair scale. Your agency will provide this equipment if it is needed. Ambulatory clients can be weighed on a bathroom scale. Keep the following in mind when weighing a client:

▶ Always explain what you will do before beginning any procedure. You will need your client's cooperation to measure weight properly.

▶ Provide for privacy, as some people are sensitive about their weight.

▶ Always weigh at the same time of day, with client wearing the same amount of clothing. Have the client void, or empty her bladder, before she is weighed.

Procedure 10: Measuring the height of a client

You will need to know how to measure a client's height in bed if the client is unable to get out of bed.

1. Explain what you will do.

2. Assemble equipment: tape measure and pencil.

3. Wash your hands.

4. Have the client lie in bed, flat on his back, with his arms and legs at his sides. Be sure the bed sheet is smooth underneath the client.

5. Make a small pencil mark on the sheet at the top of the head.

6. Make another mark at the client's heel.

7. Help the client turn to the side.

8. With the tape measure, measure the distance between the two marks (**Fig. 14-15**).

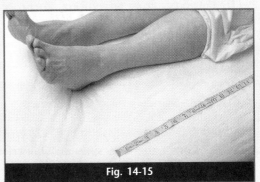

Fig. 14-15

Continued on page 190

Continued from page 189

9. Document the height in the chart.

10. Store equipment.

11. Wash your hands.

For clients who can get out of bed, you will measure height while they stand against the wall.

1. Explain what you will do.

2. Assemble equipment: tape measure and pencil.

3. Have the client stand with his back to the wall, with his arms at his sides and without shoes. A hard floor will work better than carpet.

4. Make a small pencil mark on the wall even with the top of the client's head.

5. Ask client to step away. Measure the distance between the pencil mark and the floor.

6. Document the height.

7. Store the equipment.

8. Wash your hands.

Part 2
Specimen Collection

❑ 2. List three types of specimens you may be asked to collect from a client

Sometimes you may be asked to collect a **specimen** from a client. A specimen is a sample. You may be asked to collect different types of specimens:

1. Sputum (SPYOO-tum) is the fluid and matter that a client may cough up. The specimen allows the doctor, nurse, or lab to observe what the client's body is producing. This may help diagnose illness or evaluate the effects of medication.

Procedure 11:
Collecting a sputum specimen

1. Explain what you will do.

2. Assemble equipment:
- specimen container, with cover, labeled with client's name, address, date and time
- tissues
- plastic bag
- disposable gloves
- HEPA or N-95 mask

3. Wash your hands.

4. Put on mask and gloves. If the client has known or suspected tuberculosis or another infectious disease, you should wear a HEPA, or high efficiency particulate air, respirator when collecting a sputum specimen. Coughing is one way TB germs can enter the air. Procedure 6 in Chapter 5 describes how to put on a HEPA or N-95 mask.

5. Ask the client to cough deeply, so that sputum from the lungs comes up. To prevent the spread of infectious material, give the client tissues to cover his or her mouth while coughing. Ask the client to spit the sputum into the specimen container.

6. When you have obtained a good sample (about two tablespoons of sputum), cover the container tightly. Wipe any sputum off the outside of the container with tissues, and discard the tissues. Put the specimen container in the plastic bag and seal.

7. Remove gloves and mask.

8. Wash your hands.

9. Document the procedure.

Procedure 12: Collecting a stool specimen

Ask the client to let you know when he or she can have a bowel movement. Be ready to collect the specimen.

1. Explain what you will do.

2. Assemble equipment:
   - bedpan, portable commode, or toilet attachment (hat)
   - container with lid and label bearing client's name, address and date
   - tongue depressor
   - handwashing supplies
   - disposable gloves

3. Wash your hands.

4. Put on gloves.

5. Provide privacy.

6. When the client is ready to move bowels, ask him not to urinate at the same time and not to put toilet paper in with the sample. Provide a plastic bag to discard toilet paper separately.

7. Fit hat to toilet, or provide client with bedpan. Leave the room and ask the client to call you when he is finished with the bowel movement.

8. After the bowel movement, assist as necessary with perineal care. Help the client wash his hands. Make the client comfortable. Remove gloves.

9. Wash your hands again.

10. Put on clean gloves.

11. Using the tongue depressor, take about two tablespoons of stool and put it in the container. Without touching the inside of the container, cover it tightly.

12. Wrap the tongue depressor in toilet paper and throw it away. Empty the bedpan or container into the toilet. Clean and store the equipment.

13. Store the specimen properly. It must be bagged and labeled.

14. Remove gloves.

15. Wash your hands.

16. Document the procedure.

2. Stool (feces) specimens are another type of sample collected. If the client uses a bedpan or portable commode for elimination, you will take the stool specimen from there. If the client uses the toilet, you will need a special container (often called a **hat**) that fits into the toilet bowl, to collect the stool (**Fig. 14-16**).

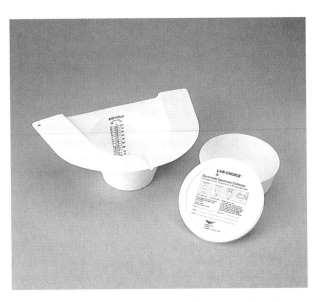

Fig. 14-16. A "hat" is a container that is placed under the toilet seat to collect specimens for clients who use the toilet rather than a bedpan or portable commode.

3. **Urine** specimens may be either clean catch (midstream) or 24-hour. The purpose of a 24-hour urine specimen is to collect all the urine voided by a client in a 24-hour period to test for certain chemicals and hormones. Usually the collection begins at 7am and runs until 7am the next day. When beginning a 24-hour urine specimen collection, the client must void and discard the first urine so that the collection begins with an empty bladder. All urine must be collected and stored properly. If any is accidentally thrown away or improperly stored, the collection will have to be done over again another day.

Note: Different states have different rules about what home care aides are allowed to do. Be sure you understand your state's guidelines before performing any procedures. Check with your supervisor if you are uncertain.

Procedure 13: Collecting a clean catch (mid-stream) urine specimen

Some clients will be able to collect their own specimens. Others will need your help. Be sure to explain exactly how the specimen must be collected.

1. Explain what you will do.

2. Assemble equipment:
   ▶ clean catch specimen kit or a sterile container, cleansing solution, and gauze
   ▶ washcloth
   ▶ towel
   ▶ bedpan or urinal if client cannot go to the bathroom
   ▶ disposable gloves

3. Provide privacy.

4. Wash your hands.

5. Explain the procedure carefully if the client will collect his or her own specimen. To assist with collecting the specimen, follow the rest of this procedure.

6. Put on gloves.

7. Open the clean catch specimen kit if you have one. Be careful never to touch the inside of the container or the inside of the lid.

8. Using the towelettes in the kit or the gauze and cleansing solution, clean the area around the urethra. For female clients, separate the labia and wipe from front to back along one side. Discard the towelette or gauze. With a new towelette or gauze, wipe from front to back along the other labia. Using a new towelette or gauze, wipe down the middle. For male clients, clean the head of the penis using circular motions with the towelettes or gauze. Clean thoroughly, changing towelettes or gauze and throwing them away after use. If the man is uncircumcised, pull back the foreskin of the penis before cleaning and hold it back during urination. Make sure it is pulled back down after collecting the specimen.

9. Ask the client to urinate into the bedpan, urinal, or toilet, and to stop before urination is complete.

10. Place the container under the urine stream and have the client start urinating again. Fill the container at least half full.

11. Cover the urine container with its lid. Wipe off the outside of the container with a paper towel.

12. If using a bedpan or urinal, discard extra urine, rinse and clean equipment, and store.

13. Remove gloves and wash your hands. Help client wash his or her hands at the sink or using the washcloth and towel.

14. Wash your hands again.

15. Complete the label for the container with the client's name, address, the date, and time.

16. Document the procedure.

❑ 3. Describe the importance of maintaining fluid balance

To maintain health, your body must take in a certain amount of fluid each day in the form of liquids you eat or drink and fluids found in semi-liquid foods like gelatin, soup, ice cream, pudding, and yogurt. Generally, a healthy person needs to take in about 64–96 ounces (oz.) of fluid each day. The fluid a person consumes is called **input**, or **intake**. If a person's input is not in a healthy range, he or she can become **dehydrated**. Dehydration is a serious medical condition that requires immediate attention.

All this fluid taken in each day cannot remain in the body, but must be eliminated as **output**. Output includes urine, feces, and vomitus. It also includes perspiration and moisture in the air we exhale. If a person's input exceeds their output, the fluid is building up in body tissues. This fluid retention can cause medical problems and discomfort.

Fluid balance is maintaining equal input and output, or taking in and eliminating equal amounts of fluid. Most people regulate fluid balance automatically, without paying particular attention to their input and output. But some clients must have their input and output, or I&O, monitored and documented. To monitor input and output, you will need to measure and document all fluids the client takes by mouth, as well as all urine and vomitus the client produces.

Procedure 14: Collecting a 24-hour urine specimen

Since you will probably not be present during all 24 hours of the test, it is important to explain the collection fully to the client and family members.

1. Explain what you will do.

2. Assemble equipment:

- container for urine: gallon bottle or a container from the lab
- bedpan or urinal for clients confined to bed
- special attachment for toilet bowl if client can get to the bathroom
- bucket of ice if the urine must be kept cold (a clearly marked container can also be put in the refrigerator)
- funnel if the container opening is small
- handwashing supplies
- disposable gloves

3. When beginning the collection, have the client completely empty the bladder. Discard the urine and note the exact time of this voiding. The collection will run until the same time tomorrow.

4. Label the container with client's name, address, dates and times the collection period began and ended (**Fig. 14-17**).

Client:	**Josie Montoya**	
Address:	**8529 Indian School**	
	Albuquerque, NM 87112	
	Date	Time
Begin Collection:	**7/6/98**	**7:20am**
End Collection:	**7/7/98**	**7:20am**

Fig. 14-17

5. Put on gloves each time the client voids.

6. Pour urine from bedpan, urinal, or toilet attachment into the container, using the funnel as needed.

7. Offer the client handwashing supplies after each voiding.

8. Be sure the client or a family member understands that all urine is to be saved, even when you are gone. Show them how to pour the urine into the container and remind them to store the container in the bucket of ice or in the refrigerator if ordered.

9. Clean equipment after each voiding.

10. Remove gloves.

11. Wash your hands.

12. Document the time of the last void before the 24-hour collection period began, and the last void of the 24-hour collection period.

Table 14-2. Conversion Table: Ounces (oz.) to Cubic Centimeters (cc)

(oz.) = (cc)	(oz.) = (cc)
1 oz. = 30 cc	5 oz. = 150 cc
2 oz. = 60 cc	6 oz. = 180 cc
3 oz. = 90 cc	7 oz. = 210 cc
4 oz. = 120 cc	8 oz. = 240 cc

Table 14-3. Conversion Table: Cups to Ounces (oz.) to Cubic Centimeters (cc)

cups	=	(oz.)	=	(cc)
¼ cup	=	2 oz.	=	60 cc
½ cup	=	4 oz.	=	120 cc
1 cup	=	8 oz.	=	240 cc

Monitoring fluid balance begins with measuring input.

1. Explain what you will do.

2. Assemble supplies:
- ▶ pencil and paper
- ▶ measuring cup

3. Wash your hands.

4. Using a measuring cup, measure the amount of fluid a client is served. Note the amount on paper, not in the visit notes.

5. When client has finished a meal or snack, measure any left-over fluids. Note this amount on paper.

6. Subtract the leftover amount from the amount served. If you have measured in ounces, convert to cubic centimeters (cc) by multiplying by 30. See Tables 14-2 and 14-3 for conversions and examples.

7. Document the amount of fluid consumed (in cc) in the visit notes, as well as the time and what fluid was taken (**Fig. 14-18**).

Measuring output is the other half of monitoring fluid balance.

1. Explain what you will do.

2. Assemble supplies:

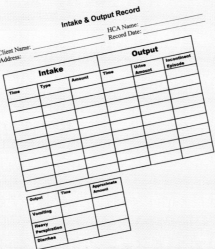

Fig. 14-18. Many employers provide a form for documenting input and output, or an Input and Output (I&O) sheet.

- ▶ measuring container
- ▶ bedpan, urinal, or toilet attachment
- ▶ plastic bag for disposal of toilet paper
- ▶ handwashing supplies
- ▶ disposable gloves

3. Wash your hands.

4. Provide privacy.

5. Put on gloves.

6. Ask the client to put used toilet paper in the bag, not in the bedpan or toilet. Ask client not to move bowels at the same time as urinating, if possible.

7. Make client comfortable, assisting as necessary or providing privacy by leaving the room if your assistance is not needed.

8. Offer the client hand-washing supplies. Assist the client as necessary with cleaning himself.

9. Pour urine into measuring container. Note the amount on paper, converting to cc if necessary.

10. Discard urine. Wash and store equipment. Flush toilet paper down the toilet and discard plastic bag.

11. Remove gloves.

12. Wash your hands.

13. Document the time, amount, and color of urine. For example: 3:45pm 200 cc urine

Note: To measure vomitus, pour from basin into measuring container, then discard in the toilet. If client vomits on the bed or floor, estimate the amount. Document emesis (EM-e-sis, or vomiting) and amount in the visit notes and/or I&O sheet (**Fig. 14-18**).

To measure these amounts, use separate measuring containers for input and output, and be careful never to mix them up. Measuring cups can be used. If a client frequently drinks out of one type of cup or glass, measure the amount that cup holds. You can even use masking tape on the outside of the cup to mark different quantities and make it easier to keep track of input.

To document input (also called intake) and output, some agencies use a special form, called an input and output, or I&O, sheet. Use this form if your employer provides it. Otherwise, make your own I&O sheet on regular paper.

Example #1: You serve Mrs. Wyant a glass of milk. You know the glass holds 180 cc. She finishes most but not all of the milk. You measure the leftover milk, and it measures ¼ cup.

First, convert ¼ cup to cc (¼ cup = 60 cc).

Now, subtract the amount leftover from the amount you served: 180 cc - 60 cc = 120 cc.

Document 120 cc milk on your input sheet.

Example #2: Mr Bernicke tells you he ate a container of yogurt in the morning. You find the container and read the label: it contained 6 oz. of yogurt. You measure what is left in the bottom, about 20 cc.

First, convert all amounts to cc: 6 oz. = 180 cc.

Then, subtract the amount leftover from the amount served: 180 cc - 20 cc = 160 cc.

So Mr. Bernicke ate about 160 cc of yogurt. Document this on the input sheet.

Practice: Miss Cahill drinks tea in the morning. Her mug holds 10 oz., and 3 oz. are left in the mug. What was her input? (answer: 210 cc)

(10 oz. = 300 cc) (3 oz. = 90 cc) (300 cc - 90 cc = 210 cc)

❑ 4. Describe the guidelines for catheter care

A urinary catheter (KATH-et-er) is a tube used to drain urine from the bladder. With an **indwelling catheter,** the tube is inserted through the urethra into the bladder, and it drains the urine into a bag. A section of the catheter is for inflating a five cubic centimeter bag, which keeps the catheter from falling out of the urethra. *Home care aides never insert, remove, or irrigate catheters.* However, you may be asked to provide daily care for the catheter, cleaning the area around the urethral opening and emptying the drainage bag.

An **external,** or **condom catheter,** has an attachment on the end that fits onto the penis. The attachment is fastened with a velcro strap or self-adhesive strip. The external catheter is changed daily. Your supervisor will teach you how to change an external catheter if that task is assigned to you. As always, provide *only* the care you are assigned to provide. In some states home care aides are allowed to change an external catheter, but in some states the nurse must perform this procedure (**Fig. 14-19**).

You may be asked to collect a urine specimen from a client who uses a catheter. You should be aware of what to report to your supervisors about clients with catheters.

Keep the following guidelines in mind when working with clients who have catheters:

▶ The drainage bag must always be kept lower than the hips. Gravity allows the urine to drain and prevents bacteria from moving back up into the bladder.

▶ Use a catheter holder strap or securely tape the tubing to the client's leg to prevent the catheter

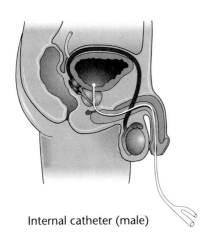
Internal catheter (male)

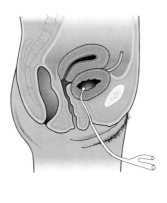
Internal catheter (female)

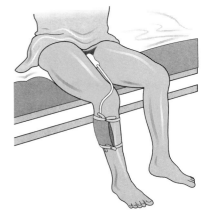
External or condom catheter (male)

Fig. 14-19. a) An internal catheter for a male; b) an internal catheter for a female; c) an external, or condom, catheter.

from being accidently pulled out of the bladder (**Fig. 14-20**).

▶ Tubing should be kept as straight as possible and should not be kinked. Kinks, twists, or pressure on the tubing (such as from the client sitting or lying on the tubing) can prevent urine from draining. A rubber band and a safety pin attached to the bottom sheet for a bed-bound client can help keep the catheter from kinking (**Fig. 14-20**).

▶ The genital area must be kept clean to prevent infection. Because the catheter goes all the way into the bladder, germs can enter the bladder more easily when a catheter is in place. Daily care of the genital area is especially important for clients with catheters.

Report any of the following to your supervisor:

▶ blood in the urine or any other unusual appearance

▶ catheter bag does not fill after several hours

▶ catheter bag fills suddenly

▶ catheter is not in place

▶ urine leaks from the catheter

▶ client reports pain

If you are asked to collect a urine specimen from a client who is wearing a catheter, you will disconnect the tubing from the drainage bag and allow the specimen to drip directly into the specimen container. If the client's input and output is being monitored, be sure to measure the amount of urine collected. Collecting a specimen this way may take some time. Do *not* collect a urine sample from the drainage bag unless ordered to do so.

Emesis, or vomiting, must be documented. It may be a sign of illness or of a reaction to medication. Some clients, such as cancer patients undergoing chemotherapy, may vomit frequently as a result of treatment. Vomiting is unpleasant for the client. Learn to handle it calmly and provide comfort to the client.

Keep these guidelines in mind when a client vomits:

▶ Treat vomitus as you treat urine and other potentially infectious wastes. Follow standard precautions and always wear gloves when handling it. Vomitus should be flushed down the toilet and spills should be cleaned thoroughly with a disinfecting solution of bleach and water.

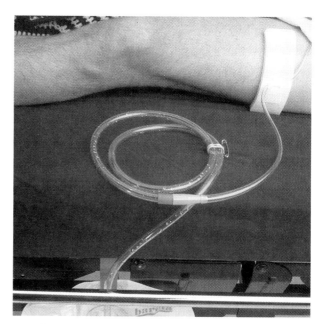

Fig. 14-20. Use a catheter holder strap or securely tape the tubing to the client's leg to prevent the catheter from being accidently pulled out of the bladder.

▶ Provide comfort to a client who has vomited. Stay calm, and offer a basin if you think he or she may vomit more. Remove soiled sheets or clothing promptly. Provide a wet washcloth to wipe face, mouth or hands. Offer a drink of water or toothbrushing to clean the mouth.

▶ Provide plenty of fluids to the client who has vomited. Water, diluted juices, or sports drinks may help prevent dehydration. Discontinue solid foods when vomiting occurs. Check with your supervisor for what you can serve. Clear liquids or a bland diet may be recommended.

> ### Part 3
> ### Special Procedures

❑ **5. Explain the benefits of warm and cold applications**

Applying heat or cold to injured areas can have several beneficial effects. Heat tends to relieve pain and muscular tension, reduce swelling, elevate the temperature in the tissues, and increase blood flow. Increased blood flow brings more oxygen and nutrients to the tissues for healing.

Procedure 16: Daily cleaning of a catheter site

Many clients can clean the catheter site themselves. If you need to provide this care for a client, follow the steps below.

1. Explain what you will do.

2. Assemble supplies:

▶ basin of warm water, soap, and washcloth or antiseptic wipes

▶ gauze pads

▶ plastic bag for waste

▶ disposable gloves

3. Provide privacy if the client desires it.

4. Wash your hands.

5. Put on gloves.

6. Position the client on his or her back and undress as necessary to expose catheter.

7. Using the washcloth dipped in soap and water, or the antiseptic wipes, clean the genital area around the catheter. Rinse the washcloth frequently, or use

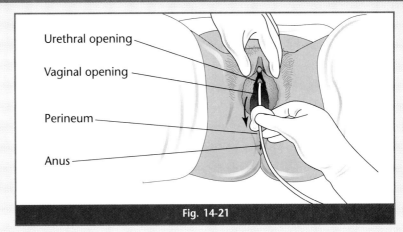

Urethral opening

Vaginal opening

Perineum

Anus

Fig. 14-21

each wipe once and discard in the plastic bag.

8. Using the wipes or gauze pads dipped in water, clean the catheter tubing. Wipe once and discard the wipe or gauze. Begin at the urethral opening and wipe down the tubing away from the body (**Fig. 14-21**).

9. Dispose of water in the toilet.

10. Remove gloves.

11. Wash your hands.

12. Help the client dress. Arrange covers. Check that catheter tubing is free from kinks and twists and that it is securely taped to the leg. Tubing can also be secured to the sheet with a pin and a rubber band if the client is bed bound.

13. Wash your hands again.

14. Document procedure and any observations.

Procedure 17: Emptying the catheter drainage bag

1. Explain what you will do.

2. Assemble equipment:

▶ alcohol wipes

▶ measuring container

▶ paper towels

▶ disposable gloves

3. Wash your hands.

4. Put on gloves.

5. Place paper towel on the floor under the drainage bag. Place measuring container on the paper towel.

6. Open the drain or spout on the bag so that urine flows out of the bag into the measuring con-

tainer (**Fig. 14-22**).

7. When urine has drained, close spout. Using alcohol wipe, clean the drain spout. Replace the drain in its holder on the bag.

8. Mentally note the amount and the appearance of the urine. Empty into toilet.

9. Clean and store measuring container.

10. Remove gloves.

11. Wash your hands.

12. Document procedure and amount of urine.

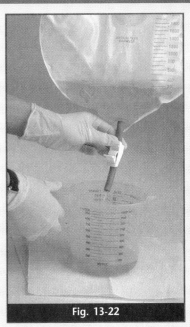

Fig. 13-22

Because you may not know when a client is going to vomit, you may not have time to explain what you will do and assemble supplies ahead of time. Talk to the client soothingly as you help him clean up, and tell him what you are doing to help him.

1. Put on gloves when client has vomited.

2. Provide a basin and remove it when vomiting has stopped.

3. Remove soiled linens or clothes, set aside for laundering, and replace with fresh linens or clothes.

4. If client's I&O is being monitored, measure and note amount of vomitus.

5. Flush vomit down the toilet and wash and store basin.

6. Remove gloves.

7. Wash your hands.

8. Put on fresh gloves.

9. Provide comfort to client: wipe face and mouth, position comfortably, offer a drink of water or toothbrushing (**Fig. 14-23**).

10. Launder soiled linens and clothes promptly in hot water.

11. Remove gloves.

12. Wash your hands again.

13. Document time, amount, color, and consistency of vomitus. Look for blood in vomitus

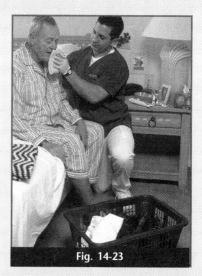

Fig. 14-23

or blood-tinged vomitus.

14. Report to your supervisor immediately and get instructions for diet.

Cold applications can help stop bleeding, reduce swelling and pain, and bring down high fevers. Cold is usually applied using ice bags or cold compresses immediately following an injury to stop bleeding and reduce swelling.

In the past, home care aides were allowed to prepare and apply different types of heat and cold applications. Now, most states allow only warm water bottles, heating pads, warm compresses or soaks, ice packs, and cold compresses. If your agency and state allow you to use other methods, your supervisor will train you. *Never perform a procedure you are not trained or allowed to do. Only perform procedures that are assigned to you in the care plan or otherwise directed by your supervisor.*

Be alert for excessive redness, pain, blisters, or numbness at the site of a heat or cold application. If you observe these signs, the application may be causing tissue damage. Persons at greater risk of complications during heat and cold applications include the elderly, fair-skinned persons, and persons with circulatory problems, central nervous system damage, or receiving strong pain medication.

Electric heating pads can also be used as heat applications. As always, follow the instructions in the care plan. Do *not* use a heating pad unless it has been ordered in the care plan or by your supervisor. Remember the following safety precautions:

- Be sure to check the skin frequently for redness or pain. Because electric heating pads do not cool down, having it just a little too hot can be very dangerous for the client.

- Make sure any electric heating pad you use is in good shape. Do not use it if the cord is frayed or if wires are exposed.

- Do not use a pin to fasten the pad. The pin could contact a wire inside the pad and cause a shock.

- Do not allow the client to lie on top of an electric heating pad.

- Do not allow the client to use an electric heating pad near a source of water.

There are two types of wound dressings: sterile or nonsterile (dry). Home care aides generally work only with nonsterile, or dry dressings.

1. Explain what you will do.

2. Assemble supplies:
   ▶ a package of four-inch-square gauze dressings
   ▶ adhesive tape
   ▶ a waste bag
   ▶ disposable gloves
   ▶ scissors
   ▶ two pairs of disposable gloves

3. Wash your hands.

4. Open the waste bag. Cut pieces of tape long enough to secure the dressing and hang the tape on the edge of a table within reach. Open the four-inch gauze square package without touching the gauze. Place the opened package on a flat surface.

5. Put on gloves.

6. Remove the soiled dressing by gently peeling the tape toward the wound. Lift the dressing off the wound (**Fig. 14-24**). Do not drag it over the wound. Observe the dressing for odor, amount, and color of drainage. Place the used dressing in the waste bag. Remove your gloves and place them in the waste bag.

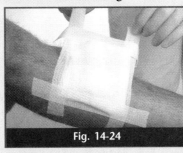
Fig. 14-24

7. Put on clean gloves. Touch-ing only the outer edges of the new four-inch gauze square, remove it from the package and apply it to the wound. Tape the gauze in place, being sure to secure it firmly (**Fig. 14-25**). The care plan will list any specific instructions for changing the dry dressing.

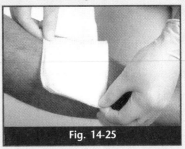
Fig. 14-25

8. Remove gloves and discard in waste bag. Discard the waste bag.

9. Wash your hands.

10. Document the procedure and your observations.

An **embolism** (EM-boh-lizm) is a blood clot. Blood clots can be very serious. Some clients need a special elastic hose to prevent swelling and blood clots and to promote circulation in the feet and legs. These stockings are called anti-embolic hose, or ted hose.

1. Explain what you will do.

2. Assemble supplies: anti-embolic hose and powder.

3. Wash your hands.

4. With client lying down, remove his or her socks, shoes, or slippers, and expose one leg.

5. Roll stocking down to the toe. Place the stocking over the client's toe and heel, being sure

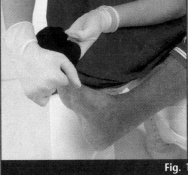
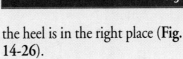
Fig. 14-26

the heel is in the right place (**Fig. 14-26**).

6. Unroll the stocking up the leg. Check that the stocking is smooth and even over the leg. If you have trouble putting the stocking on, try applying pow-der to the client's leg before unrolling the stocking.

7. Repeat for the other leg.

8. Wash your hands.

9. Document the procedure.

Procedure 21: Preparing and applying warm compresses

1. Explain what you will do.
2. Assemble equipment:
   ▶ washcloth
   ▶ plastic wrap
   ▶ towel
   ▶ basin
   ▶ bath thermometer
3. Wash your hands.
4. Fill basin one-half to two-thirds full with hot water. Check temperature with thermometer (should be between 105°F and 115° F), or against the inside of your wrist.
5. Soak the washcloth in the water and wring it out. Immediately apply it to the area needing a hot compress. Note the time. Quickly cover the washcloth with plastic wrap and the towel to keep it warm (**Fig. 14-27**).

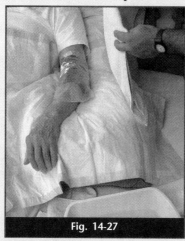
Fig. 14-27

6. Check the area every five minutes. Remove the compress if the area is red or numb or if the client complains of pain or discomfort. Change the compress if cooling occurs. Remove the compress after twenty minutes.
7. Commercial warm compresses are also available (**Fig. 14-28**). If these are provided, follow the package directions and your supervisor's instructions.

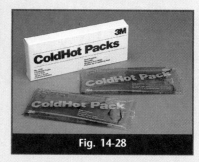
Fig. 14-28

8. Discard water in the toilet. Clean and store basin and other supplies. Put laundry in hamper. Discard plastic wrap.
9. Wash your hands.
10. Document the time, length, and site of procedure, and any observations.

Procedure 22: Administering warm soaks

1. Explain what you will do.
2. Assemble equipment:
   ▶ basin or bathtub, depending on the area to be soaked
   ▶ bath thermometer
   ▶ bath blanket
   ▶ towel
3. Wash your hands.
4. Fill the basin or tub half full of warm water (105°–110°F).
5. Immerse the body part in the basin, or help the client into the tub. Pad the edge of the basin with a towel if needed (**Fig. 14-29**). Use a bath blanket to cover the rest of the client if needed for extra warmth.

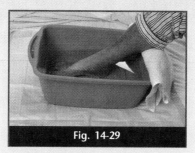
Fig. 14-29

6. Check water temperature every five minutes and add hot water as needed to maintain the temperature. To prevent burns, tell the client not to add hot water him- or herself. Observe the area for redness and discontinue the soak if the client complains of pain or discomfort.
7. Soak for fifteen to twenty minutes, or as ordered in the care plan.
8. Remove basin or help the client out of the tub. Use the towel to dry client.
9. Drain the tub or discard water. Clean and store basin and other supplies. Put laundry in hamper.
10. Wash your hands.
11. Document the time, length, and site of procedure. Report the client's response and any of your observations about the skin.

Another type of heat application is a **sitz bath**, or a warm soak of the perineal area. Sitz baths clean perineal wounds and reduce inflammation and pain. Circulation in the perineal area is increased, and voiding may be stimulated by a sitz bath. Clients with perineal swelling (such as hemorrhoids), or perineal wounds (such as those that occur after childbirth), may be ordered to take sitz baths. Because the sitz bath causes increased blood flow to the pelvic area, blood flow to other parts of the body is decreased. Clients may feel weak, faint, or dizzy after taking a sitz bath.

❑ 6. Define the terms ostomy, colostomy, and ileostomy

An ostomy (OS-toh-mee) is the surgical removal of a portion of the intestines. In a client with an ostomy, the end of the intestine is brought out of the body through an artificial opening in the abdomen. This opening is called a stoma (STOH-ma). Stool, or feces, are eliminated through the ostomy rather than through the anus. People with cancer or bowel disease, and victims of trauma may require ostomies.

Procedure 23: Using a hot water bottle

1. Explain what you will do.
2. Assemble equipment:
   ▶ hot water bottle
   ▶ cloth cover or towel
   ▶ bath thermometer
3. Wash your hands.
4. Fill the bottle half full with warm water (105° F–115° F, or 98° F–110° F for infants and small children or older adults).

5. Press out excess air and seal the bottle.
6. Dry the bottle and check for leaks. Cover with a cloth cover or towel.
7. Apply the bottle to the area ordered. Check skin every five minutes for redness or pain. If redness or pain are present, add cold water to the bottle to reduce the temperature.

8. Remove the bottle after 20 minutes or as ordered in the care plan.
9. Empty the hot water bottle. Wash and store supplies.
10. Wash your hands.
11. Document the time, length, and site of procedure. Document the client's response and any of your observations about the skin.

Procedure 24: Assisting with a sitz bath

A disposable sitz bath fits on the toilet seat and is attached to a rubber bag containing warm water.
1. Explain what you will do.
2. Assemble equipment:
   ▶ disposable sitz bath
   ▶ bath thermometer
   ▶ towels
   ▶ disposable gloves
3. Wash your hands.
4. Fill the sitz bath two-thirds full with hot water. Place the disposable sitz bath on the toilet seat. If the sitz bath is prescribed

for cleaning the perineal area, the temperature should be 100° F–104° F. For a sitz bath given for pain and to stimulate circulation, the water temperature should be 105°F–110° F. Check the water temperature using the bath thermometer.
5. Provide privacy. Help the client undress and be seated on the sitz bath. A valve on the tubing connected to the bag allows the client or you to replenish the water in the sitz bath with hot water.

6. Leave the room, but check on the client every five minutes to make sure he or she is not dizzy or weak. Stay with a client who seems unsteady.
7. Assist the client out of the sitz bath in 20 minutes. Provide towels and help with dressing if needed.
8. Clean and store supplies.
9. Wash your hands.
10. Document the procedure, including the time started and ended, the client's response, and the water temperature.

Procedure 25: Applying ice packs

1. Explain what you will do.

2. Assemble equipment: ice pack or sealable plastic bag and crushed ice, towel to cover pack or bag.

3. Wash your hands.

4. Fill plastic bag one-half to two-thirds full with crushed ice. Remove excess air. Cover bag or ice pack with towel.

5. Apply bag to the area as ordered (**Fig. 14-30**). Note the time. Use another towel to cover bag if it is too cold.

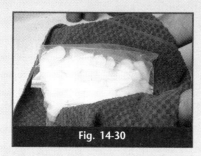

Fig. 14-30

6. Check the area after ten minutes for blisters, pale, white, or gray skin. Stop treatment if client complains of numbness or pain.

7. Remove ice after 20 minutes or as ordered in the care plan.

8. Return ice bag or pack to freezer.

9. Wash your hands.

10. Document the time, length, and site of procedure. Report the client's response and any of your observations about the skin.

Procedure 26: Applying cold compresses

1. Explain what you will do.

2. Assemble equipment:
- basin filled with water and ice
- two washcloths
- plastic or rubber sheet
- towels

3. Wash your hands.

4. Position client on plastic sheet. Rinse washcloth in basin and wring out. Cover the area to be treated with a cloth sheet or towel and apply cold washcloth to the area as directed (**Fig. 14-**31). Change washcloths often to keep area cold.

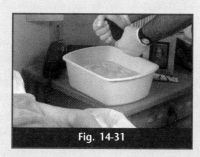

Fig. 14-31

5. Check the area after five minutes for blisters, pale, white, or gray skin. Stop treatment if client complains of numbness or pain.

6. Remove compresses after 20 minutes or as ordered in the care plan. Give client towels as needed to dry the area.

7. Clean and store basin.

8. Wash your hands.

9. Document the time, length, and site of procedure. Report the client's response and any observations about the skin.

The terms colostomy (koh-LOS-toh-mee) and ileostomy (il-ee-OS-toh-mee) indicate what section of the intestine was removed and the type of stool that will be eliminated. In a colostomy, stool will generally be semi-solid. With an ileostomy, stool may be liquid and irritating to the client's skin.

Clients who have had an ostomy wear a disposable bag that fits over the stoma to collect the feces. The bag is attached to the skin by adhesive. The bag may also be secured by a belt. These materials are frequently referred to as an **ostomy appliance**.

Many people manage the ostomy appliance by themselves. Your employer should provide further training before you are expected to provide this care. If

1. Explain what you will do.

2. Assemble equipment:
- bedpan
- disposable bed protector
- bath blanket
- clean ostomy bag and belt/appliance
- toilet paper
- basin of warm water
- soap or cleanser
- washcloth
- skin cream as ordered
- two towels
- plastic trash bag or old newspaper
- disposable gloves

3. Provide privacy.

4. Wash your hands.

5. Place the protective sheet under the client. Cover the client with a bath blanket, and have the client hold the bath blanket while you pull down the top sheet and blankets. Expose ostomy site. Offer the client a towel to keep clothing dry.

6. Put on gloves.

7. Remove the ostomy bag carefully. If it will be washed and reused, place it in the bedpan. If it will be discarded, wrap it in newspaper or the plastic trash bag. Note the color, odor, consistency, and amount of stool in the bag.

8. Wipe the area around the stoma with toilet paper. Discard paper in bedpan.

9. Using a washcloth and warm soapy water, wash the area around the stoma. Pat dry with another towel. Apply cream as ordered (**Fig. 14-32**).

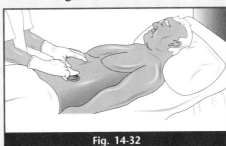

Fig. 14-32

10. Place the clean ostomy appliance on the client, following your supervisor's instructions. Make sure the bottom of the bag is clamped.

11. Remove the plastic protector sheet and discard.

12. Remove gloves. Make the client comfortable. Put on fresh gloves and change linens if necessary. Cover the client and remove bath blanket and towel.

13. Put on a new pair of gloves. Take bedpan and other supplies to bathroom. Empty bag into toilet and flush, along with used toilet paper. Wash out bag and use a deodorant in the bag as directed.

14. Wash out the bedpan and store. Clean basin and store.

15. Remove gloves.

16. Wash your hands.

17. Document procedure and any observations.

Note: Call your supervisor if stoma appears very red or blue, or if swelling or bleeding is present.

you are providing ostomy care, make certain the client receives good skin care and hygiene. The ostomy bag should be emptied and cleaned or replaced whenever a stool is eliminated. Always wear gloves and wash hands carefully when providing ostomy care. Teach thorough handwashing techniques to clients with ostomies.

Many clients with ostomies feel they have lost control of a basic bodily function. They may be embarrassed or angry about the ostomy. Be sensitive and supportive when working with these clients. Always provide privacy for ostomy care.

Chapter 15

Promoting Independence: Rehabilitation and Restorative Care

Part 1
What is Restorative Care?

❑ **1. List four goals of restorative home care programs**

Restorative care or **rehabilitation** involves helping clients move from illness, disability, and dependence, toward health, ability, and independence. Goals of a restorative or rehabilitative program can include the following:

❭ To help a client regain abilities or recover from illness

❭ To develop and promote a client's independence

Learning Objectives

In this chapter you will learn to:

▶ To allow a client to feel in control of his or her life

▶ To help a client accept or adapt to limitations of a disability

Rehabilitation will be a goal of care for many of your clients, particularly those who have suffered a stroke, accident, trauma, or other disabling condition. Because you will spend many hours in the home with these clients, you can play a critical role in helping clients recover and regain their independence. Rehabilitation is one of the great joys of working as a caregiver. You should enjoy seeing clients progress toward independence or recovery, and take pride in the contributions you make to their improving health.

❑ 2. Explain the home care rehabilitation model

Just as with any client, when you work with clients who need restorative care you will be working as part of a team of caregivers. Some different members of the team and their roles may include those in **Figure 15-1:**

❑ *3. Describe guidelines for assisting with restorative care*

When assisting with rehabilitation or restorative care, there are attitudes you can adopt that will be critical to your clients' progress:

▶ **Patience.** Progress may be slow, and it will seem slower to you and your client if you are impatient. Your clients must do as much for themselves as they can, regardless of how long it takes or how poorly they are able to do it. This means that although you could do it faster or better, you must encourage them to perform as much self-care as possible. The more patient you are, the easier you will make it for them to regain abilities and confidence.

▶ **Positive attitude.** Your attitude can set the tone in the home. Family members as well as clients will take cues from you as to how they should behave. If you are encouraging and positive, you will help create an atmosphere that supports and motivates the client in rehabilitation.

In addition, your expectations and reactions can contribute to rehabilitation efforts. Keep the fol-

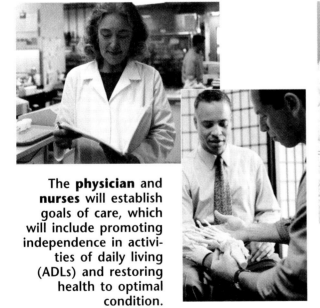

You, the **home care aide**, will be in the home, carrying out the instructions of the other care team members, assisting in achieving the client goals, and observing and reporting the client's progress.

The **physician** and **nurses** will establish goals of care, which will include promoting independence in activities of daily living (ADLs) and restoring health to optimal condition.

The **physical therapist, occupational therapist**, or **speech therapist** will work with the client to help restore or adapt specific abilities. **Social workers** or other **counselors** may see the client to help promote attitudes of self-sufficiency and acceptance.

Fig. 15-1.
The home care rehabilitation model

lowing tips in mind to help you have a positive effect on the client's rehabilitation.

▶ **Focus on small tasks and small accomplishments.** For example, dressing themselves may seem like an overwhelming task to some clients. It may take weeks or even months until they are able to dress without assistance. If you break the task down into smaller steps, clients will be able to develop a sense of accomplishment sooner. For example, today or this week the goal might be putting on a shirt without buttoning it. Next week the goal could be buttoning the shirt, if that seems manageable. When the client is able to put the shirt on without assistance, congratulate him or her on this accomplishment. Take everything one step at a time.

▶ **Recognize that setbacks occur.** Progress occurs at different rates, and sometimes a client can do something one day that he or she cannot do the next. Downplay these setbacks so clients don't become discouraged. Reassure clients that setbacks are normal. However, do document in your notes any decline in a client's abilities that occurs.

▶ **Be sensitive to the client's needs.** Some clients may need more encouragement than others. Some may feel embarrassed by certain kinds of encouragement. For example, some clients may welcome a

hug or a pat on the back to show you are proud of their efforts. Others may feel uncomfortable if you touch them or make too much of what they have done. Get to know your clients and understand what motivates them. Adapt your encouragement to fit an individual's personality.

Part 2
Range of Motion Exercises

❑ 4. Describe how to assist with range of motion exercises

Exercise helps people regain strength and mobility and prevent disabilities from developing. People who are bedridden for long periods of time are particularly prone to developing disabilities such as contractures (kon-TRAK-churs). A contracture is the permanent and often very painful stiffening of a joint and muscle, caused by immobility and resulting in loss of ability. Range of motion (ROM) exercises, or ROME, refer to exercises that put a particular joint through its full arc of motion. The purpose of range of motion exercises is to decrease or prevent contractures, improve strength, and increase circulation.

Passive range of motion (PROM) exercises are used when clients do not have the ability to execute the movements on their own. If you are assisting with PROM exercises, you will support the client's joints and move them through the range of motion. Active range of motion (AROM) exercises are performed by a client himself, using his own muscle power. Your role in AROM exercises is to encourage the client. Active assisted range of motion (AAROM) exercises are performed by the client with some assistance and support from you.

You should be oriented to each client's exercise program by the nurse or physical therapist before providing care. Depending on what the care plan specifies, you will repeat each exercise two to five times, once or twice a day, working on both sides of the body. Exercise the upper extremities before the lower

1. Explain what you are going to do.

2. Provide privacy if the client desires it.

3. Wash hands.

4. Put on gloves according to your agency's policies and procedures, or if the client has open sores.

5. Position the client supine on the bed.

6. **Shoulder.** Place one hand above the elbow and the other hand around the wrist. Move the arm upward so that the upper arm is aligned with the side of the head (*forward flexion*). Move the arm downward to the side (*extension*) (**Fig. 15-2**).

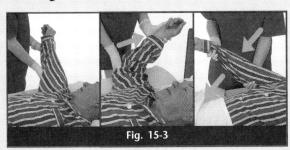

Fig. 15-2

Bring the arm sideways away from the body to above the head (*abduction*) and back down (*adduction*) (**Fig. 15-3**).

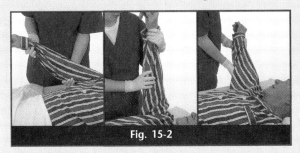

Fig. 15-3

Bend the elbow and position it at the same level as the shoulder. Move the forearm down toward the body (*internal rotation*). Now move the forearm toward the head (*external rotation*) (**Fig. 15-4**).

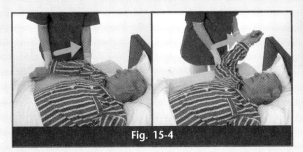

Fig. 15-4

7. **Elbow.** Hold the client's wrist with one hand, the elbow with the other hand. Bend the elbow so that the hand touches the shoulder on that same side (*flexion*). Straighten the arm (*extension*) (**Fig. 15-5**).

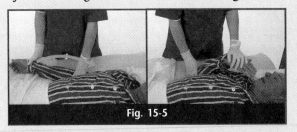

Fig. 15-5

Exercise the forearm by moving it so the palm is facing downward (*pronation*) and then the palm is facing upward (*supination*) (**Fig. 15-6**).

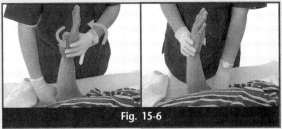

Fig. 15-6

8. **Wrist.** Hold the wrist with one hand and use the fingers of the other hand to help the joint through the motions. Bend the hand down (*flexion*); bend the hand backwards (*extension*) (**Fig. 15-7**).

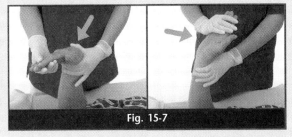

Fig. 15-7

Turn the hand in the direction of the thumb (*radial flexion*); turn the hand in the direction of the little finger (*ulnar flexion*) (**Fig. 15-8**).

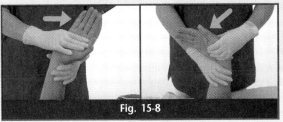

Fig. 15-8

Continued on page 208

Continued from page 207

9. Thumb. Move the thumb away from the index finger (*abduction*). Move the thumb back next to the index finger (*adduction*) (**Fig. 15-9**).

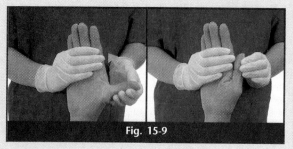

Fig. 15-9

Touch each fingertip with the thumb (*opposition*) (**Fig. 15-10**).

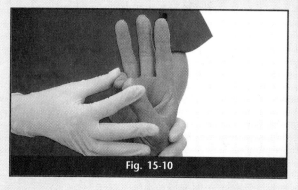

Fig. 15-10

Bend thumb into the palm (*flexion*) and out to the side (*extension*) (**Fig. 15-11**).

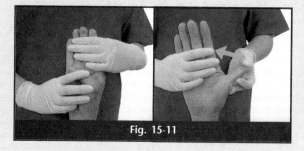

Fig. 15-11

10. Fingers. Make the hand into a fist (*flexion*). Straighten out the fist (*extension*) (**Fig. 15- 12**).

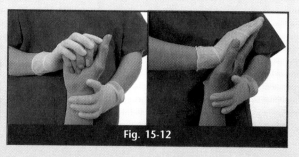

Fig. 15-12

Spread the fingers and the thumb far apart from each other (*abduction*). Bring the fingers next to each other (*adduction*) (**Fig. 15-13**).

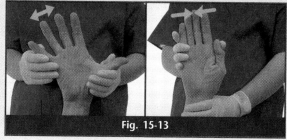

Fig. 15-13

11. Hip. Support the leg by placing one hand under the knee and one under the ankle. Straighten the leg and raise it gently upward. Move the leg away from the other leg (*abduction*). Move the leg toward the other leg (*adduction*) (**Fig. 15-14**).

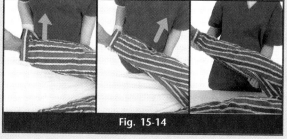

Fig. 15-14

Gently turn the leg inward (*internal rotation*), then turn the leg outward (*external rotation*) (**Fig. 15-15**).

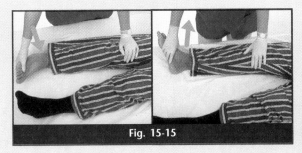

Fig. 15-15

12. Knees. Bend the leg at the knee (*flexion*). Straighten the leg (*extension*) (**Fig. 15-16**).

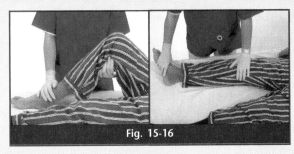

Fig. 15-16

13. Ankles. Bend the foot up toward the leg (*dorsiflexion*). Turn the foot down away from the leg (*plantar flexion*) (**Fig. 15-17**).

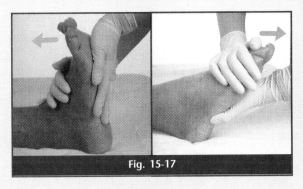

Fig. 15-17

Turn the inside of the foot inward toward the body (*supination*) and the sole of the foot so that it

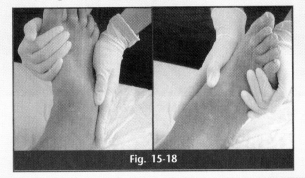

Fig. 15-18

faces away from the body (*pronation*) (**Fig. 15-18**).

14. Toes. Curl and straighten the toes (*flexion* and *extension*) (**Fig. 15-19**).

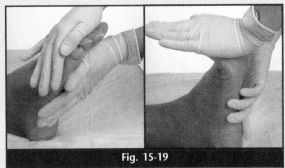

Fig. 15-19

Spread the toes apart (*abduction*) (**Fig. 15-20**).

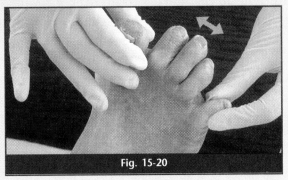

Fig. 15-20

15. Return the client to a comfortable resting position and cover as appropriate.

16. Wash your hands.

17. Document the procedure. Note any decrease in range of motion or any pain experienced by the client. Notify the supervisor or the physical therapist if you find increased stiffness or physical resistance. Resistance may be a sign that a contracture is developing.

Note any decrease in range of motion or any pain experienced by the client. Notify the supervisor or the physical therapist if you find increased stiffness or physical resistance. Resistance may be a sign that a contracture is developing.

extremities. Move the extremity as far as the joint's normal arc in a smooth manner. Slight discomfort or stiffness may occur initially but should improve as you continue the exercises. Stop the motion if the client complains of pain. Give support above and below the joint and move the affected extremity through the prescribed range of motion. Exercise one side and then the other.

❏ 5. Explain the guidelines for assisting a client with maintaining proper body alignment

Clients in restorative care, particularly those confined to bed, need to maintain good body alignment to promote recovery and prevent injury to muscles and joints. Chapter 12 includes specific instructions for positioning clients. The following guidelines are intended to help you ensure that clients maintain good alignment and allow clients to make more rapid progress when they can get out of bed.

▸ **Observe principles of alignment.** Remember that proper alignment is based on straight lines. The spine should lie in a straight line. Pillows or rolled or folded blankets may be needed to support the small of the back and raise the knees or head in the supine position, or to support the head and one leg in the lateral position (**Fig. 15-21**).

▸ **Keep body parts in natural positions.** In a natural hand position, the fingers are slightly curled. Use a rolled washcloth, gauze bandage, or a rubber ball inside the palm to support the fingers in this position. Use footboards to keep covers from resting on feet in the supine position.

▸ **Prevent external rotation of hips.** When legs and hips are allowed to turn outward during prolonged bedrest, hip contractures can result. A trochanter (troh-KAN-ter) roll is a rolled blanket or towel that is tucked alongside the hip and thigh to prevent the leg from turning outward.

▸ **Change positions frequently.** Clients confined to bed should change positions frequently, at least every two hours, to prevent muscle stiffness and pressure ulcers. You can help your clients by teaching the caregivers at home the importance of position changes and how to perform them safely.

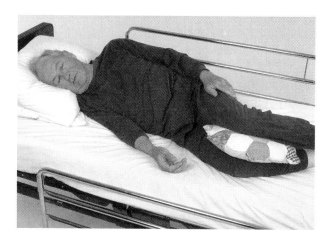

Fig. 15-21. Pillows or rolled or folded blankets may be needed to support the small of the back and raise the knees or head in the supine position, or to support the head and one leg in the lateral position.

Part 3
Skin Care

Immobility reduces the amount of oxygen-carrying blood that circulates to the skin. Clients who have restricted mobility have increased risk of skin deterioration at **pressure points**. Pressure points are areas of the body that bear much of the body weight. Pressure points are mainly located at **bony prominences**, areas of the body where the bone lies close to the skin. These areas include elbows, shoulder blades, tailbone, hip bones, ankles, heels, and the knob at the back of the neck, and the back of the head (see **Fig. 9-5** in Chapter 9 for an illustration of pressure sore danger zones).

Other areas of skin deterioration are the ears, the area under the breasts, and the scrotum. The pressure on these areas reduces circulation, decreasing the amount of oxygen the cells receive. Warmth and moisture also contribute to skin breakdown. Once the surface of the skin erodes, micro-organisms can invade and cause infection. When infection occurs, the healing process slows down.

❏ 6. List five important observations to make about changes in a client's skin

When the skin begins to break down, it becomes pale, white or a reddened color. The client may also complain of tingling or burning in the area. This white or reddened area does not go away, even when the client's position is changed. If pressure is allowed to continue, the area will further deteriorate, first breaking the skin surface, then eroding the next layer. The resulting wound is called a **pressure sore**, **bed sore**, or decubitus ulcer (dee-KYOO-bi-tus) (**Fig. 15-22**). Once a pressure sore forms, it can get bigger, deeper, and infected. Because pressure sores are difficult to heal, prevention is very important.

Report any of the following changes or abnormalities in the client's skin to your supervisor:

▶ pale, white or reddened areas, or blistered or bruised areas on the skin

▶ complaints of tingling, warmth, or burning of the skin

▶ dry or flaking skin

▶ itching or scratching

▶ rash or any skin discoloration

▶ swelling

▶ blisters

▶ fluid or blood draining from skin

▶ broken skin

▶ wounds or ulcers on the skin

▶ changes in an existing wound or ulcer (size, depth, drainage, color, odor)

▶ redness or broken skin between toes or around toenails

❑ 7. List five guidelines for providing basic skin care and preventing pressure sores

The following are guidelines for basic skin care. It is important that family caregivers also understand and follow these guidelines.

▶ Provide regular care for skin to keep it clean and dry. When complete baths are not given or taken every day, check the client's skin and provide skin care daily.

▶ Reposition immobile clients frequently (every two hours).

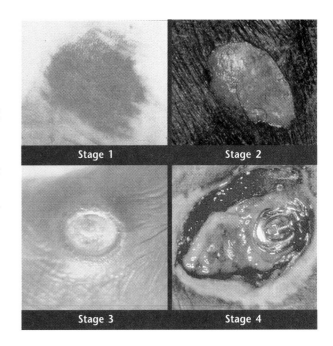

Fig 15-22. Pressure sores are categorized by Stage 1 through Stage 4.

▶ Provide frequent and thorough skin care and change clothing and linens as often as needed for incontinent clients.

▶ Avoid scratching or irritating the skin in any way. Report to your supervisor if a client wears shoes or slippers that cause blisters or sores.

▶ Massage the skin frequently, using light, circular strokes to increase circulation. Use little or no pressure on bony areas. If you observe a pale, white or reddened area that does not go away, do not massage the area or put any pressure on it. Massage the healthy skin and tissue surrounding the area.

For clients who are confined to bed or who spend a great deal of time in bed or in a certain position, remember the following:

▶ Keep the bottom sheet tight and free from wrinkles and the bed free from crumbs.

▶ Avoid pulling the client across sheets during transfers or repositioning. Dragging the client's skin across the surface of the sheet causes **shearing**, or pressure, when the surfaces rub against each other. Shearing can lead to skin breakdown, as explained in Chapter 12.

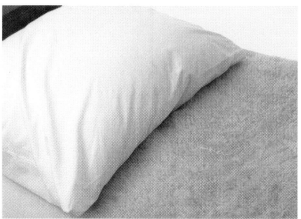

Fig. 15-23. To absorb moisture or perspiration that may accumulate and to protect the skin from irritating bed linens, place a sheepskin or chamois skin under the back and buttocks.

▶ Place a sheepskin or chamois skin under the back and buttocks to absorb moisture or perspiration that may accumulate and to protect the skin from irritating bed linens (**Fig. 15-23**).

▶ Relieve pressure under bony prominences. Place foam rubber or sheepskin pads under them. Heel and elbow protectors made of foam and sheepskin are available. These devices are shaped to conform to the heel and elbow and are held in place with straps (**Fig. 15-24**).

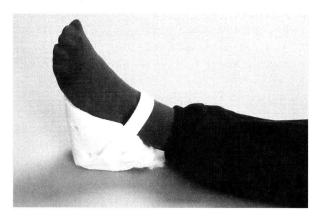

Fig. 15-24. Heel and elbow protectors made of foam and sheepskin are available. These devices are shaped to conform to the heel and elbow and are held in place with straps.

▶ A bed or chair can be made softer with flotation pads or an egg crate mattress. **Flotation pads** are made of a gel-like substance encased in heavy plastic (**Fig. 15-25**). The pad is put into a pillowcase or sheet for skin protection. The **egg crate mattress** is made of foam and looks like an egg carton. The peaks distribute the client's weight more evenly. An

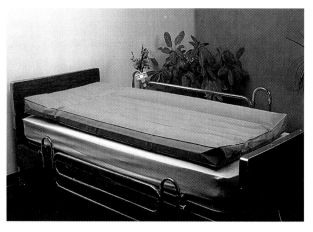

Fig. 15-25. Flotation pads are made of a gel-like substance encased in heavy plastic.

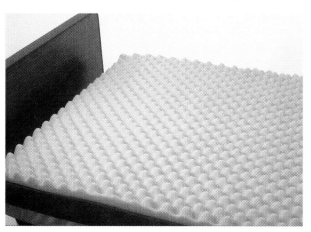

Fig. 15-26. The egg crate mattress is made of foam and looks like an egg carton. The peaks distribute the client's weight more evenly. An egg crate mattress is placed on top of a regular mattress.

egg crate mattress is placed on top of a regular mattress (**Fig. 15-26**).

▶ Use a bed cradle to keep top sheets from rubbing the client's skin. A **bed cradle** is made of metal or you can make a homemade variety with a cardboard box (see Chapter 12). Top sheets are tucked in at the bottom of the bed and mitered at the corners, then brought up over the cradle.

❑ 8. Describe the guidelines for caring for clients who have fractures or casts

Fractures are broken bones caused by accidents or by osteoporosis (os-tee-oh-poh-ROH-sis), the condition that produces porous and brittle bones that easily crack or break. Osteoporosis occurs more frequently in elderly people, particularly women, as a result of a loss of calcium from the bones. Signs and symptoms of a fracture are pain, swelling, bruising, changes in skin color at the site of the fracture, and limited movement.

When bones are fractured, the sections of broken bone must be placed in alignment so the body can heal itself. The body has the capacity to grow new bone tissue and fuse the sections of fractured bone together. The bone must be immobilized to allow this healing to occur. Immobilization is often accomplished by the use of a **cast**.

Some casts will allow the client to bear weight, and some will not. A client who has had a cast applied must wait until the cast is completely dry before bearing weight on it. A wet cast is grey, dull, cool, and smells musty. A dry cast is white, shiny, and odorless. Plaster of paris casts take 24 to 48 hours to dry. Fiberglass casts dry within an hour of application, come in different colors, and are lighter in weight (**Fig. 15-27**). As a cast dries, it gives off heat. This heat must be allowed to escape or it will burn the skin, so never cover a cast with any material until it has completely dried.

Guidelines for caring for a client who has a cast

Follow instructions in the care plan. Keep the following in mind:

▷ If caring for a client who has a wet cast, do not

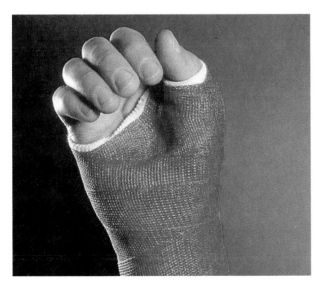

Fig. 15-27. A plaster cast is white and shiny. A fiberglass cast comes in many colors.

cover the cast until it is dry. Assist the client in changing positions to allow the cast to dry evenly. Do not place the cast on a hard surface; place it on pillows. A hard surface alters the shape of the cast. Use the palms of the hands to lift the cast; fingers will dent it and dents will cause pressure on the client's skin.

▷ Elevate the extremity that is in a cast to allow swelling in the injured tissue around the break to subside (**Fig. 15-28**).

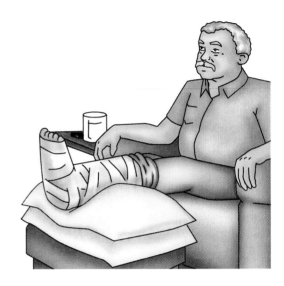

Fig. 15-28. To help swelling go down, elevate the extremity that is in a cast. Place the cast on pillows to prevent flattening or changing the shape of the cast (especially if it is still drying).

▷ Observe the affected extremity for swelling, skin discoloration, odor, and loss of sensation or feeling cold. Compare to the extremity that does not have a cast. Report any one of these to a supervisor.

▷ Protect the client's skin from the rough edges of the cast. The stockinette that lines the inside of the cast can be pulled up and over the edges and secured with tape. Inform your supervisor if cast edges are irritating the client's skin.

▷ Keep the cast dry at all times. Wet casts lose their shape.

▷ Do not insert or allow the client to insert anything inside the cast, even when skin itches. Pointed or blunt objects may injure the skin, which is already dry and fragile. Skin can become infected under the cast.

❑ 9. List the guidelines for caring for a client who has a hip fracture

The weakening of bones caused by osteoporosis makes elderly clients especially susceptible to hip fractures. A sudden fall can result in a fractured hip that takes months to heal. Hip fractures can also occur because of weakened bones that fracture and then cause a fall. A hip fracture is a serious condition. The elderly heal slowly and are at risk for secondary illnesses and disabilities.

Most fractured hips require surgery. A cast or traction may also be used to immobilize the hip. A client in traction will require special care that will be detailed in his or her care plan. Home care aides should *never* disconnect the traction assembly. Good skin care and repositioning according to the care plan are the foundations of care for all clients who are immobilized. Skin will rapidly deteriorate over pressure points.

The home care aide assignment sheet and your supervisor will explain the type of care to be provided, depending on the client's stage of recuperation. The assignment sheet may specify the use of trochanter rolls and sandbags to prevent external rotation, or rolling outward, of the injured hip. It may also specify that the hip be kept in **abduction**, a position away from the midpoint of the body, with the use of pillows or abductor splints. You should only provide this care when it is prescribed by the care plan and you have been trained by a nurse.

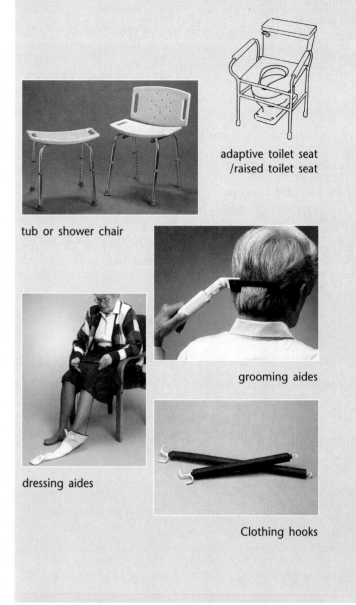

adaptive toilet seat /raised toilet seat

tub or shower chair

grooming aides

dressing aides

Clothing hooks

Part 4
Assistive Devices

❑ 10. List five ways to adapt the environment for people with physical limitations

Many devices are available to assist people who are recovering from or adapting to a physical condition. Always be on the lookout for hazards that could cause weak or confused clients to trip or otherwise injure themselves. The items shown in **Fig. 15-29** can be useful as your clients relearn old skills or adapt to new limitations.

Part 5
Bowel and Bladder Retraining

❑ 11. Identify three reasons clients lose bowel or bladder control

When people cannot control the muscles of the bowels or bladder, they are said to be incontinent (in-KON-ti-nent). Incontinence can occur in clients who are confined to bed, ill, elderly, paralyzed, or who have circulatory or nervous system diseases or injuries. Diarrhea can also cause temporary incontinence.

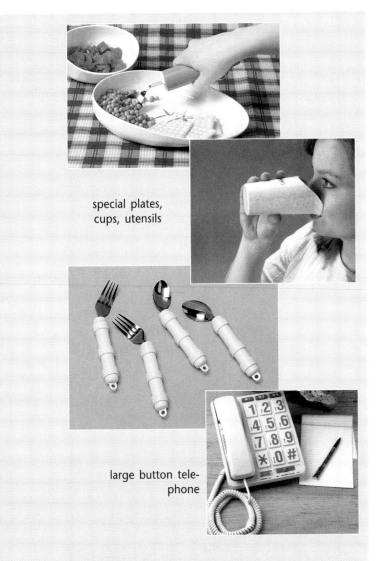

special plates, cups, utensils

large button telephone

Fig. 15-29. Many adaptive items are available to help make it easier for clients to adapt to physical changes.

Clients who are incontinent need reassurance and understanding. Offer them a bedpan or take them to the bathroom more frequently and keep them clean, dry, and free from odor. They will need good skin care as well. Urine and feces are very irritating to the skin, and should be washed off completely by bathing and good perineal care.

Clients who are confined to bed should have a plastic, latex, or disposable sheet placed under them to protect the bed. Place a **draw sheet** over the protective sheet to absorb moisture and protect the client's skin from the rubber or plastic. A draw sheet can be made by doubling a regular flat sheet. Disposable incontinence pads or briefs for adults

are available to keep body wastes away from the skin (**Fig. 15-30**). Always check the care plan assignment, as certain types of mattress and bed therapies require no bed pads or require that a particular type is used.

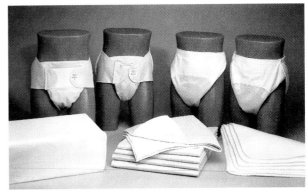

Fig. 15-30.

❑ 12. Explain the guidelines for assisting with bowel or bladder retraining

Clients who have had a disruption in their bowel and bladder routines from illness, injury, or inactivity may need assistance in re-establishing a regular routine and normal function. The physician may order suppositories, laxatives, stool softeners, or enemas to assist the client.

You can help the client in the following ways:

▶ Always be professional and matter-of-fact when handling incontinence or working to re-establish routines. It is hard enough for clients to handle incontinence without having to worry about your reactions. Offer a trip to the commode or a bedpan before beginning long procedures or bathing.

▶ Keep a record of the client's bowel and bladder habits. When you can see a pattern of voiding or elimination, you can predict when the client will need a bedpan or a trip to the bathroom.

▶ Encourage the client to drink a sufficient amount of fluids each day. About thirty minutes after fluids are taken, offer to take your client to the bathroom. If a client cannot get out of bed, offer the bedpan or urinal.

▶ Encourage the client to eat foods that are high in fiber, as appropriate or assigned. Chapter 22 provides more information on diet and nutrition.

- If a client has difficulty urinating once he or she is on the commode or toilet, try running water from the tap or having the client lean forward slightly to put pressure on the bladder.

- Offer positive reinforcement for successes or even attempts to control bladder and bowels.

- Never show frustration or anger toward clients who are incontinent. The problem is out of their control and your negative reactions will only make things worse.

Part 6
Other Restorative Measures

❑ 13. Describe the benefits of deep breathing exercises

Deep breathing exercises help expand the lungs, clearing them of mucus and preventing infections (such as pneumonia). Clients who are paralyzed or who have had abdominal surgery are often instructed to do deep breathing exercises to expand the lungs regularly.

If you are instructed to assist a client with breathing exercises, your supervisor or another member of the health care team will train you to assist with this procedure. The care plan may include using a deep breathing device called an **incentive spirometer**, or even a balloon for deep breathing exercises (**Fig. 15-31**). Do not assist with these exercises if you have not been trained. Ask your supervisor for instruction. The following procedure is intended as general instruction only.

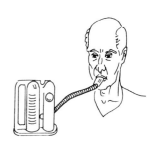

Fig. 15-31. Incentive spirometers are used for deep breathing exercises.

Procedure 2: Assisting with deep breathing exercises

1. Explain what you will do.

2. Assemble equipment:
- disposable gloves
- tissues
- waste container
- small basin
- mouth care supplies

3. Provide privacy if the client desires it.

4. Wash your hands.

5. Put on a mask, eye shield, and gown as indicated by standard precautions. Be sure to put on a HEPA (high efficiency particulate air) or N-95 mask if the client has known or suspected tuberculosis. Deep breathing exercises may stimulate the client to cough and produce mucus.

6. Put on gloves.

7. With client sitting up, if possible, have him or her breathe in as deeply as possible through the nose. You should see the chest and then the abdomen expand and fill with air.

8. Have the client exhale through the mouth until all air is expelled.

9. Repeat this exercise five to ten times, as specified in the care plan.

10. If the client coughs or brings up mucus from the lungs during the exercise, offer the client tissues or the basin to catch the mucus.

11. Dispose of the used tissues and clean the basin.

12. Remove gloves, eye shield, mask, and gown.

13. Wash your hands.

14. Put on fresh gloves.

15. Provide mouth care as desired, and help the client return to a comfortable position.

16. Remove gloves.

17. Wash your hands again.

18. Document the procedure and any reactions you observe, including pain, prolonged coughing, and color or amount of mucus.

Chapter 16

Observations about Medications and Technology in Home Care

> **Part 1**
> **The Home Care Aide's Role**

❑ 1. Identify four guidelines for promoting safe and proper use of medications

People who need home care often need medications. Elderly clients who have problems with several body systems, such as coronary artery disease, high blood pressure, and diabetes, may take numerous drugs, all with different actions. Although home care aides do not usually handle or administer medications, you need to have a clear understanding of the kinds of medicine your clients may be taking and what to do if a client experiences side effects or refuses to take medication.

The following are four guidelines for promoting the safe and proper use of medications:

1. **Never handle or administer medications unless specifically trained and assigned to do so.** Unless you have been trained and assigned to handle medications, you should *never* touch the inside of a medicine bottle or the pills or other medicines themselves. *Never* put any medication in a client's mouth. If you handle or administer medication, you can be held liable for any consequences of your action. You are not trained to administer medications.

2. **Observe clients' self-administration of medication.** Although you cannot handle or administer the medication, you can remind clients to take their medications. You can also bring medication containers to clients, and provide water or food as needed to take with the medication. Always observe, report, and document as appropriate.

3. **Know the difference between prescription drugs and over-the-counter or nonprescription drugs.** Antibiotics (such as penicillin), heart

drugs (such as nitroglycerin), and potent pain medication (such as codeine) are examples of prescription drugs. Aspirin or cold medications, such as antihistamine or decongestant preparations, are over-the-counter drugs (**Fig. 16-1**).

4. Be aware of all medications a client is taking, both prescription and nonprescription. There are many possible side effects and interactions among medications. Be on the watch for symptoms such as itching, palpitations, anxiety, stomach-ache, diarrhea, confusion, vomiting, rash, hives, or headache. Any of these symptoms could indicate a side effect or interaction. Report any of these symptoms to your supervisor. Remember to report and document only the facts and your observations. Your supervisor will evaluate whether the symptom is caused by medications.

❑ 2. Identify the five "rights" of medications

Knowing and remembering the five "rights" of medications will help prevent mistakes with medications.

1. The Right Client. Always check the label on the medication container to make sure the client's name is on it.

2. The Right Medication. Check the expiration date and the name of the medication before giving the container to the client. Make sure the medication name on the container matches the name listed in the care plan.

3. The Right Time. Make sure the instructions on the

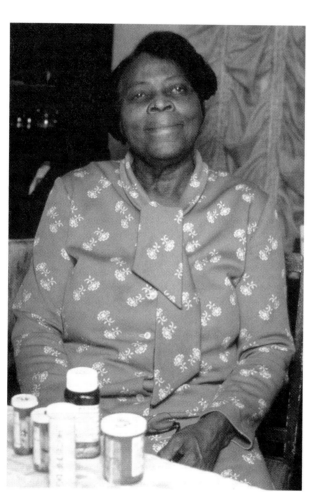

Fig. 16-1. Always know what medications the client is taking. Be aware of the difference between prescription and over-the-counter medications.

container label for what time or how often to take the medication match the instructions in the care plan.

4. The Right Route. Check the medication label for instructions on how the medication is to be taken. Make sure the instructions on the label match those in the care plan.

5. The Right Amount. Make sure the instructions on the container label for how much medication to take match the instructions in the care plan.

If the medication container label and the care plan do not agree on any of the five "rights," call your supervisor for instructions. Similarly, if there is not enough information, or if you have noticed another problem with the medication (for example, the client's name is not on the container), call your supervisor. Explain to the client that you need to check on his or her medication, and that you will get clarification as soon as possible.

❑ 3. Explain how to assist a client with self-administered medications

Some elderly people have a hard time remembering to take all their medications. In addition, there may be various instructions to remember, such as taking pills with food or on an empty stomach, or drinking plenty of fluids. Pay close attention to the medication schedule, which is usually set by the nurse in charge. Become familiar with all the physicians instructions on how and when to take specific medications. If

Reading the label on a prescription medication container

A prescription medication container will contain the following information.

If specified in your assignment sheet, you may be instructed to help the client with self-medication by doing any of the following:

▶ Remind the client when it is time for medication.

▶ Bring the bottle or container of medication to the client.

▶ Provide food or water to take with the medication, as directed.

▶ Observe the client taking the medication.

▶ Document that the client took the medication, the time, and any other medications or food taken at the same time (Fig. 16-3).

▶ Report any possible reactions to your supervisor.

Hartman Pharmacy

8529-A Indian School Rd NE
Albuquerque, NM 87112

DEA No. AW-968958   505-291-1274

No. 52989986   Dr. Michaels

John D. Client 505 Main St.
Take one tablet by mouth four times a day until all are gone

Erythromycin 250 mg
8/26/98

Discard after 8/99

Fig. 16-2

cations, document all medication that is taken and report drugs, prescription or nonprescription, that the client takes that are not part of the treatment plan. Even a pill as innocent as aspirin should be noted. Aspirin inhibits platelets and can cause prolonged bleeding. If a client is already on a certain kind of drug called an anticoagulant, taking aspirin for a simple headache may cause unwanted effects. Another example is a common over-the-counter decongestant/antihistamine cold pill, which can make high blood pressure worse. It is extremely important that you report to your supervisor and document any reactions the client may have to medications.

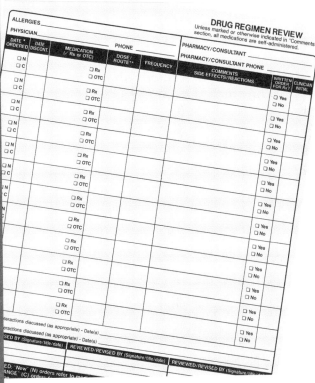

Fig. 16-3. The care plan or your assignment sheet may direct you to document that a client took medication. Many home care agencies use medication forms to help the client or aide document the client's self-medication.

the specified time for a dose passes, remind the client to take the medicine. Report to your supervisor if the client does not take a medication that has been ordered.

Sometimes clients have reactions to certain medications, or one medication taken will interact with another, causing problems. To avoid these compli-

Avoiding certain foods or substances can be important when taking certain medications. For example, drugs that have sedative or calming effects should never be mixed with alcohol. Clients who are on certain antidepressant medications and antibiotics are instructed to avoid certain foods. If the client fails to comply with these restrictions, notify your supervisor immediately. The physician and the pharmacist will usually inform the client and the family members of any side effects that can occur with the drugs prescribed. Make sure you are aware of what side effects to watch for. Common side effects include dizziness, drowsiness, headache, nausea and vomiting, or confusion. More serious side effects occur when there is an allergic reaction to the medication or a hypersensitivity reaction. Allergic reactions with symptoms like hives, fever, rash, or difficulty breathing, can be life threatening, and may require emergency intervention.

Part 2
Observing, Reporting, and Safety

❏ 4. Identify observations about medications that should be reported right away

If a client shows signs of a reaction to a medication, or complains of side effects, report these right away. Again, your supervisor can assess whether the symptom is caused by the medication. Your responsibility is to report your observations. Signs include the following:

- dizziness, fainting
- nausea, vomiting
- rash, hives, itching
- difficulty breathing, swelling of throat or eyes
- drowsiness
- headache, blurred vision
- abdominal pain
- diarrhea
- any other unusual sign

In addition, report any of the following problems immediately:

- Client refuses to take medication as directed.
- Client takes the wrong dose (amount) of medication.
- Client takes medication at the wrong time.
- Client takes the wrong medication.
- A medication container is missing or empty.

❏ 5. Describe what to do in an emergency involving medications

If a client has a severe allergic reaction to a medication, takes the wrong dose of a medication, or takes medications together that cause complications, emergency medical treatment is necessary. Treat an overdose of medication, whether it was accidental or intentional, as a poisoning. Call the local poison control number immediately and follow their instructions. Poison control will send paramedics or an ambulance if needed.

For severe drug reactions or interactions, call 911 or 0 for emergency help. Stay with the client. Do not give any liquids, food, or other medications unless instructed to do so by emergency personnel. Notify your supervisor as soon as possible.

❏ 6. Identify methods of medication storage

You may be required to assist with the proper storage of medications. Keep the following in mind:

- The client's medications should be kept in one place, separate from medicine used by other members of the household.
- If there are young children or a disoriented elderly person in the home, recommend to the family that medications be stored in a locked cabinet.
- All medications should be kept in child-proof containers if children are in the home. To avoid an accidental overdose, keep medications out of reach of children.
- If medicine requires refrigeration, make sure the bottle is on an upper shelf in the back, out of a child's reach (**Fig. 16-4**).
- All medications should be stored away from heat and light, as appropriate.
- The client or a family member should discard medications that have expired, are not labeled, or are discolored. Make sure these medications are not discarded in the trash, where children or animals may have access. Consult your supervisor for specific disposal instructions or if the client or family will not dispose of expired medications. *Do not* dispose of them yourself.

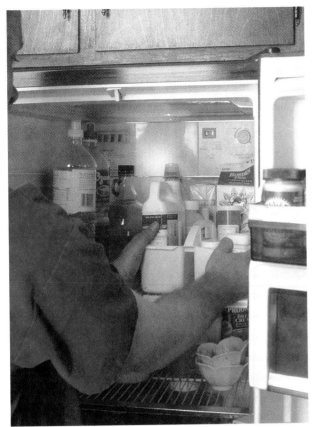

Fig. 16-4. Keep medications out of the reach of children.

❏ 7. Identify signs of drug misuse and abuse and know how to report these

Drug misuse and abuse may be accidental or deliberate. It can include refusing to take medications, taking the wrong dose or taking it at the wrong time, mixing the medication with alcohol, taking drugs that have not been prescribed for the client, and taking illegal drugs. Misuse and abuse of drugs is extremely dangerous and can even be fatal.

What should you do if your client refuses to take certain medications? You can encourage the client to take the medication and explain that recovery often depends on taking the right medication. If the client still refuses, you must notify your supervisor. Do not push the client to take the medication, but try to find out what is making him or her reluctant to take it. Getting the client to open up and express uncertainties or dislikes may enable you to communicate needed information to members of the health care team. A physician or nurse can then either persuade the client to

take the medication or change or adjust the treatment regimen.

Two common reasons people avoid taking prescribed medication are because they can't afford them and because they have difficulty obtaining them. Sometimes the client is confused about which drugs to take, at what hour, and in what quantities. You can be quite helpful in clarifying the schedule. If the client wants to know why he needs to be taking certain medications, ask the nurse or physician to provide an explanation. People who have conditions such as Alzheimer's disease, that affect mental function, will greatly benefit from your friendly reminders. Other reasons people do not take medicine are the dislike of side effects and difficulty swallowing the pills. These problems can be overcome once you have informed your supervisor.

Be alert to the signs of misuse or abuse and report them to your supervisor immediately. These signs include the following:

- depression
- anorexia
- change in sleep patterns
- withdrawn behavior or moodiness
- secrecy
- verbal abusiveness
- poor relationships with family members

The drugs that pose the highest risk for causing drug dependency are pain medications and tranquilizers.

> **Part 3**
> **Safe Use of Oxygen**

❏ 8. Demonstrate an understanding of oxygen delivery equipment

Some clients with breathing difficulties may receive oxygen in a form more concentrated than what we breathe in the air. Oxygen is prescribed by a physician. The rules that apply to you regarding med-

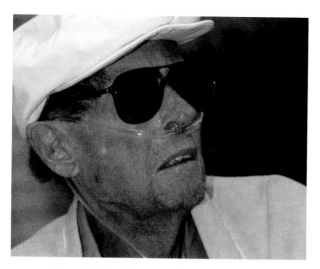

Fig. 16-5. Client with nasal cannula

ications also apply for oxygen. You should *never* handle or administer oxygen for a client. Oxygen will be delivered to the home in tanks or produced by an oxygen concentrator, which changes air in the room into air with a higher oxygen concentration. The agency that supplies the oxygen will also service the equipment and train the client and family members in its use.

Oxygen passes from the tank or concentrator, through a tube, and eventually to the client's nose or mouth. Because oxygen is very drying, it is generally passed through a humidifier and mixed with moisture before it is given to the client. Oxygen can be administered to a client in several ways, depending on the client's condition.

Some clients receive oxygen through a nasal cannula (KAN-ye-la). A nasal cannula is a piece of plastic tubing that fits around the face and is secured by a strap that goes over the ears and around the back of the head (**Fig. 16-5**). The face piece has two short prongs made of tubing. These prongs fit inside the nose, and oxygen from the tank or concentrator is delivered through them. The cannula is fitted by a respiratory therapist, and the length of the prongs (usually no more than half an inch) is adjusted for the client's comfort. The client can talk and eat while wearing the cannula.

Clients who do not need to receive concentrated oxygen all the time may use a face mask when they need oxygen. The face mask fits over the client's nose and mouth. It is secured by a strap that goes over the ears and around the back of the head. It is difficult for a client to talk when wearing an oxygen face mask. The mask must be removed for the client to eat or drink anything.

No matter how it is administered, oxygen can be irritating to the nose and mouth. The strap of a nasal cannula or face mask can also cause irritation around the ears. Wash and dry skin carefully, and provide frequent mouth care. Offer the client plenty of fluids. Report and document any irritation you observe.

Oxygen is a highly combustible (kom-BUS-ti-bel) gas. It can very easily explode or catch fire. Working around oxygen requires special safety precautions.

Guidelines for working safely around oxygen equipment:

▶ Remove all fire hazards from the room or area. Fire hazards include electric shavers, hair dryers, or other electrical appliances. Notify your supervisor if a fire hazard is present and the client does not want it removed.

▶ Post "No Smoking" and "Oxygen in Use" signs, and never allow smoking in the room or area where oxygen is used or stored.

▶ Never allow candles or other open flames around oxygen.

▶ Learn how to turn oxygen off in case of fire. *Never* adjust oxygen level.

▶ Report if the nasal cannula or face mask is causing skin irritation.

Part 4
Clients Using Special Equipment

❑ **9. Explain guidelines for the care of a client with an IV**

IV stands for intravenous (in-tra-VEE-nus), or into a vein. A client with an IV is receiving medication, nutrition, or fluids through a vein (**Fig. 16-8**). When

Having an IV in place makes some basic care procedures more difficult. Always be careful not to pull or catch on IV tubing when performing or assisting with routine care of clients with IVs.

1. Explain what you will do.

2. Assemble equipment: clean clothes.

3. Provide privacy if the client desires it.

4. Wash your hands.

5. If the bed is adjustable, lower it as far as possible.

6. Help the client sit up at the edge of the bed, if possible. Procedures 1 and 2 in Chapter 12 explain how to do this.

7. Have the client remove the arm without the IV from clothing. Assist as necessary.

8. Help the client gather the clothing on the arm with the IV. Carefully lift the clothing over the IV site and move it up the tubing toward the IV bag (**Fig. 16-6**).

9. Lift the IV bag off its pole and, keeping it higher than the IV site, carefully slide the clothing over the bag. Place the IV bag back on the pole.

10. Set the used clothing aside to be placed with the soiled laundry when the client is finished changing clothes.

11. Gather the sleeve of the clean clothing.

12. Lift the IV bag off its pole and, keeping it higher than the IV site, carefully slide the clothing over the bag (**Fig. 16-7**). Place the IV bag back on the pole.

13. Carefully move the clean clothing down the IV tubing, over the IV site, and onto the client's arm.

14. Have the client put his other arm in the clothing. Assist as necessary.

15. Check that the IV is dripping properly. Make sure none of the tubing is dislodged and the IV site dressing is in place.

16. Assist the client with changing the rest of his clothing, as necessary.

17. Place soiled clothes in the laundry basket.

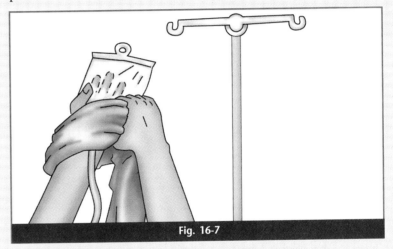
Fig. 16-7

18. Adjust bed if necessary.

19. Wash your hands.

20. Document the procedure and any observations.

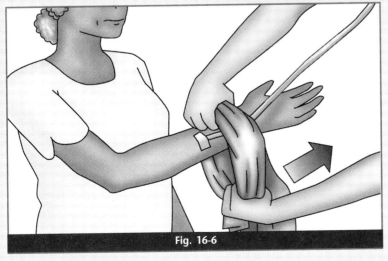
Fig. 16-6

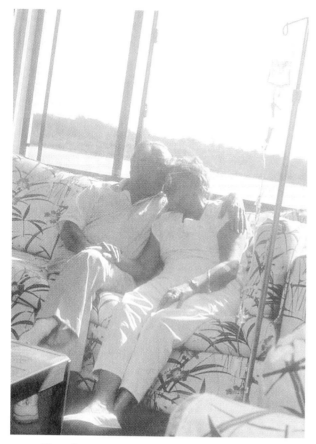

Fig. 16-8. Client receiving intravenous medication.

a physician prescribes an IV, a registered nurse inserts a needle into a vein, allowing direct access to the bloodstream. Medication, nutrition, or fluids either drip from a bag suspended on a pole or are pumped by a portable pump through a tube and into the vein. Some clients with chronic conditions may have a permanent opening that has been surgically created in a vein to allow easy access for IV fluids.

Home care aides *never* insert or remove IV lines. You will not be responsible for care of the site. Your only responsibility for IV care is to report and document any observations of changes or problems with the IV. Signs to report include the following:

▶ The needle falls out or is removed.

▶ The dressing around the IV site is loose or not intact.

▶ Blood is visible in the tubing or around the site of the IV.

▶ The site is swollen or discolored.

▶ The client complains of pain.

▶ The bag is broken, or the level of fluid does not seem to decrease.

▶ The IV fluid is not dripping.

▶ The IV fluid is nearly gone.

▶ The pump beeps, indicating a problem, and the client or caregiver cannot fix it.

▶ The pump is dropped.

As always, document your observations, your call, instructions received, and care provided.

❑ *10. Define hyperalimentation*

Hyperalimentation (high-per-al-i-men-TAY-shun) is the process of delivering nutrients directly into the blood stream through a special catheter inserted in a vein. Hyperalimentation may be ordered when a client is severely malnourished or unable to eat.

Hyperalimentation feedings are prescribed by a doctor, and prepared and supplied by a special pharmacy. Feedings are usually delivered on a regular schedule. Bottles may need refrigeration. You will *not* be responsible for administering feedings or caring for the catheter or the site of insertion. Any duties you are expected to perform will be explained to you by your supervisor. Report any discomfort associated with the catheter or the site, or any signs of irritation or infection you notice at the site.

SECTION V
Special Clients, Special Needs

Chapter 17

Assisting Clients with Disabilities

Part 1
Understanding Clients with Disabilities

A **disability** is the absence or impairment of a physical or mental function. Disability may result from a disease, a complication of pregnancy, or an injury sustained in an accident or in childbirth. For example, blindness is a disability because it is the permanent absence of sight. Vision loss can have a number of causes, including disease or injury.

Depending on the type and the extent of the disability, a person may not be able to perform certain activities, including activities of daily living (ADLs). Work and social activities may be limited as well. People with disabilities may be more vulnerable to illness. By strictly following the client care plan and your assignments, and carefully observing and reporting, you can help your clients with disabilities avoid illness.

Families of people with disabilities, especially the parents of children with severe problems, may find it difficult to cope with the stress a disability can cause. They may feel resentment, disappointment, guilt or shame, and anger or frustration. Caring for someone with a disability can be a tremendous responsibility that stretches a family's time, energy, patience, and financial resources to the limit. As a home care aide, you can give family members a much needed break.

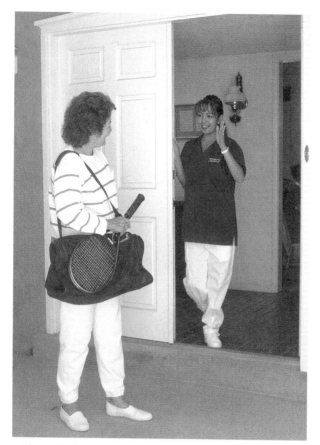

Fig. 17-1. The time a home care aide spends with a client with disabilities may be the only break a family caregiver receives.

Clients and their families may need additional support, including counseling, as they attempt to deal with the disability and adapt to it. Tell your supervisor or another member of the care team if you think a client or family member needs additional support to cope with a disability.

Many clients with disabilities develop strong emotional attachments to their caregivers. Clients may also become angry with a caregiver, either because the client resents being dependent or because the client is afraid of the caregiver's efforts to encourage independence. Be patient with clients who have disabilities. If a client's emotions are more than you can handle, speak to your supervisor.

❑ 1. Identify common causes of disabilities

There are hundreds of diseases and disorders that may cause disability. Among them are diabetes, stroke (CVA), muscular dystrophy (DIS-troh-fee, or MD), con-

gestive heart failure, AIDS, chronic obstructive pulmonary disease (COPD), Parkinson's disease, rheumatoid (ROOM-a-toyd) arthritis, osteoarthritis (ah-stee-oh-ar-THRYE-tis), and multiple sclerosis (skler-OH-sis, or MS).

Disabilities are also frequently caused by accidents. Head or spinal cord injuries can cause severe disabilities, including paralysis and brain damage. Accidents can also cause vision loss, hearing loss, or a number of other disabilities.

A person may also be born with a disability due to a complication of pregnancy or childbirth, or because of his or her inherited genetic pattern. Cerebral palsy, which can cause mild to severe physical disability, can result from premature birth. Malnutrition or drug or alcohol abuse during pregnancy can cause lasting disability in babies. Down syndrome is a genetic abnormality that causes physical and mental disability.

❑ 2. Describe daily challenges a person with a disability may face

Which activities are challenging for a person with a disability depends on the nature of the disability. A person who is mentally retarded will face different challenges than a person who is confined to a wheelchair. However, any of the following activities may pose a challenge for a person with a disability:

▶ getting out of bed

▶ preparing or eating meals

▶ washing, dressing, or grooming him- or herself

▶ getting to the bathroom

▶ communicating with family, friends, or caregivers

▶ meeting basic human needs for acceptance, belonging, and community

▶ getting from one place to another

▶ finding a job or functioning in a job

▶ making ends meet financially

Understand that even the most basic ADLs can be challenges for a client with a disability. You can make a big contribution by helping a client with a disability to meet these challenges successfully each day.

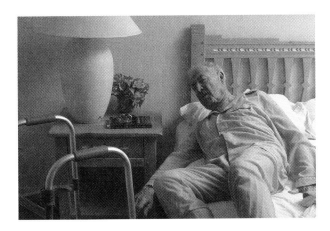

Fig. 17-2. Even getting out of bed in the morning may pose a challenge for a person with a disability.

❑ 3. Define terms related to disabilities and explain why they are important

Over the last decade the terms used to describe people with disabilities have changed. For example, it used to be common to call a person in a wheelchair a "cripple." Now most people find that term offensive. As a member of a professional health care team working with people with disabilities, you must be sensitive to the terms used to describe your clients.

Many people with disabilities want to be viewed and described as people first, rather than identified by their disability. Thus, someone may prefer to be called "a person who is deaf" rather than "a deaf person." Someone else may prefer the term "hearing-challenged," while others may prefer the commonly used term "hearing-impaired."

Some people find even the term "disabled" offensive, implying that they are less competent than others. These people may prefer to be called "differently abled." It is true that sometimes people with a loss of one function, such as sight, may have other functions, such as hearing, that are very well-developed. Thus, they are indeed differently abled.

Avoid using terms that may be offensive to your clients. Find out how they or their families prefer to refer to the disability, and use those terms. Be sensitive in discussing any disability, and remem-

ber that you should only discuss your clients with the care team and, if appropriate, the family.

❑ 4. Identify social and emotional needs of persons with disabilities

Most people with disabilities have the same social and emotional needs we all have. However, some disabilities may make it more difficult to meet those needs. As with all your clients, understand and help meet these needs when appropriate. As discussed in Chapter 8, basic social and emotional needs include:

▶ independence

▶ dignity

▶ social interaction

▶ a sense of worth

Help your clients with disabilities learn to do all they can for themselves. Give them opportunities to show you what they can do. Don't take over a task just because you can do it faster or better; it may be more important for the client to do it for him- or herself. The need for feelings of independence, dignity, social interaction, and self-worth are all boosted when the client is able to perform a task for him- or herself. On the other hand, do not push a client beyond his or her abilities. Humiliation and failure do not help fulfill social or emotional needs! Treat all clients with respect. Think about how you would want to be treated if you were in their position.

❑ 5. Explain how a disability may affect sexuality and intimacy

Depending on a person's disability, sexual desires, needs, and abilities can all be affected. Clients may be especially sensitive about how an illness or injury has affected their sexuality. As a caregiver, you must remember that sexual desire may not have been lessened by a disability, although ability to meet sexual needs may have been limited. Many people confined to wheelchairs can have sexual and intimate relationships, though adjustments may have to be made. Don't assume you know what impact a physical disability has had on sexuality. Be sensitive to privacy needs.

❑ 6. Identify skills you have already learned that can be applied to clients with disabilities

Many of the basic skills you have learned or will learn in other sections of this book apply to working with clients with disabilities:

- communication (Chapter 4)
- safety and body mechanics (Chapter 6)
- safe and comfortable transfers, ambulation, and body positioning (Chapter 12)
- assisting with ADLs (Chapter 13)
- taking vital signs and specimens (Chapter 14)
- housekeeping and meal preparation (Chapter 21 and Chapter 23)

Of course there are some adjustments you will make in caring for each client, but generally you should find that working with a client who is disabled is no different that working with any of your clients. Treat each person as an individual and with respect, and you will be on your way to providing excellent care for all types of clients.

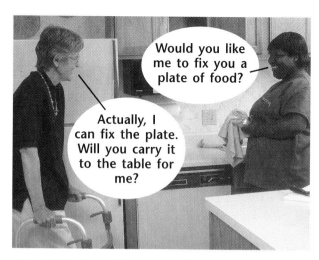

Fig. 17-3. By asking your client about personal preferences, you may find ways of performing tasks, within the care plan and assignment, that please the client and promote her self-care. In addition, you show the client that she still has some control over her life.

Part 2
The Home Care Aide's Role in Caring for Clients with Disabilities

---

The goals of home care for clients who are disabled include maintaining or improving health and comfort while promoting self care and independence. If these goals are met, clients are better able to maintain their dignity and self-esteem. In addition to health services and personal care, home care aides also help stabilize the household and promote a safe, secure environment.

❑ 7. List five goals to work toward when assisting clients who have disabilities

1. **Promote self-care and independence.** It is important to consult with your client about how much assistance he or she thinks will be needed to perform certain personal care tasks. Inform your client about the goals of the care plan and involve him or her in discussions regarding the goals of care and how assigned tasks should be performed. Ask your client about personal preferences (**Fig. 17-3**). Self care and independence cannot be accomplished without the client's cooperation.

2. **Assure the client's safety.** Be aware of the types of accidents that commonly occur in the home. Most of these accidents can be avoided if you think ahead. Remember that each client is an individual with special needs. Think critically about each client's abilities and disabilities. Safety concerns will vary depending on the disability. For example, storing personal care items on high shelves can cause safety problems for a client who uses a wheelchair. Clutter on the floor could cause falls for clients with impaired vision or mobility. Look over the home each day for things that might be unsafe. Being able to consider each client and foresee potential problems is very important. Use good body mechanics when you are working, and encourage your clients to do the same to avoid physical strain on any part of the body (see Chapter 6).

3. **Promote the client's health and comfort.** Help your clients achieve good health by maintaining nutrition

and hydration and by assisting with personal care. The care plan and your assignment sheet will include instructions for this type of care. To provide further comfort, you should watch and listen to the client. If you think about how you might feel in similar situations, you may be able to anticipate your client's needs. You may see, for example, that an extra pillow under the client's arm would help keep his shoulder from drooping and would make him more comfortable. Some clients with disabilities may be unable to communicate their wishes to you.

4. Maintain the client's dignity and self-worth. Never discuss a client with anyone other than a member of the health care team or, if appropriate, the client's immediate family (see Chapter 3 for more on client confidentiality). Treat a client who is disabled with the same respect you would give any client. Recognize that a person with a disability may have many feelings about his or her situation. Be sensitive to these feelings and find ways to make your clients feel good about themselves. Remember to allow and encourage the client to direct how and when care is provided. Even when someone is physically unable to perform a task, he or she should be allowed the opportunity to decide how and when the task is done.

5. Maintain the stability of the client's household. Disability can disrupt the stability of a family and home, causing insecurity, anxiety, and disorder. As a home care aide, you are in the home longer than any member of the health care team. You will help maintain the stability of the household by being punctual and dependable, respecting the schedules and routines of the family, and working cheerfully, calmly and efficiently. In addition, you act as a role model for the family, showing acceptance of and encouragement for the client.

❏ 8. Identify five qualities of excellent service needed by clients with disabilities

When asked what qualities they need and value most in home care workers, people with disabilities list the following:

1. Punctuality: Being on time for all scheduled visits makes a big difference to a client who needs your assistance.

2. Reliability: Clients with disabilities may depend on your help to meet basic needs, so being reliable is essential.

3. Responsiveness to needs: A client's needs may change, and you should be willing (with the approval of your supervisor) to adapt your service to be most helpful.

4. Continuity: Constantly changing caregivers may be disruptive or inconvenient for people with disabilities.

5. Positive attitude: Your cheerful and encouraging attitude is important to clients with disabilities.

❏ 9. Explain how to adapt personal care procedures to meet the needs of clients with different disabilities

The guidelines below are intended to help you understand what special needs clients with various disabilities may have. When working with clients who are disabled, you will need to adapt your care to the individual client's needs. The care team will work together to discover and address any other needs a client may have. Because you are probably with the client more than anyone else on the care team, it is very important for you to report your observations to your supervisor.

Developmental Disabilities

Developmental disabilities refer to disabilities that are present at birth or emerge during childhood. These disabilities prevent a child from developing mentally or physically at a "normal" rate or in an established pattern. The role of the home care aide in helping clients with developmental disabilities is often to offer respite for the family caregivers. Home care aides help teach the client self care and assist with ADLs. They also provide a role model for families in dealing with the disability.

Mental Retardation. Mental retardation causes below average intellectual abilities. There are different levels or degrees of mental retardation. Children with this disability are usually slow to develop, and may be slow to sit up, crawl, or walk. They may also have difficulty in chewing, swallowing, eating by themselves, and talking. Some may display extreme behavior that is either withdrawn or hyperactive. In addition to their special needs, children who are mentally retarded also have the same emotional and physical needs that other children have (**Fig. 17-4**).

Care of a person with mental retardation. The care of a child or adult who is mentally retarded and living at home may involve health specialists, such as a psychologist, a social worker, and a physician. It may also involve special education facilities, day care centers, and community resources. A case manager coordinates health care services.

For clients who are mentally retarded, the main goal of care and treatment is the same as it is for all persons with disabilities: to help the person have as normal a life as possible. For a person with mental retardation, this means recognizing his or her individuality, basic human rights, and physical and emotional needs, as well as chronological age, mental ages, and special needs. This goal is often referred to as **normalization**. Other goals of care for clients who are mentally retarded include maintenance and improvement of physical health, development of new skills, performance of ADLs, communication, and social interaction.

To achieve the goals of care for clients who are mentally retarded, home care aides may help train the client to perform ADLs by dividing a task into smaller units. Although independence is promoted, home care aides may also assist clients with activities and motor functions that are difficult to perform. Children and adults with mental retardation should also be encouraged to use positive behavior that will permit social interaction with people of their own age group.

Down's Syndrome. People who are born with Down's syndrome experience varying degrees of mental retardation, along with physical symptoms. A person with Down's syndrome typically has a small skull, a flattened nose, short fingers, and a wider space between the first two fingers of each hand and the first two toes of each foot. As with other types of mental retardation, a person with Down's syndrome can become fairly independent.

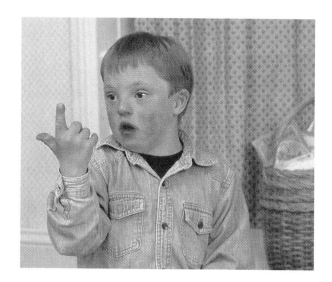

Fig. 17-4. Children who are mentally retarded have the same emotional and physical needs as other children.

Care of a person with Down's syndrome. A home care aide provides the same type of care and instruction for a Down's syndrome client as for any other person with mental retardation. Home care aides may assist with a range of tasks, from teaching and performing ADLs to encouraging positive behavior.

Cerebral Palsy. People with cerebral palsy have suffered brain damage either while in the uterus or during birth. They may have both physical and mental disabilities. Damage to the brain retards or stops the development of the child or causes the child to develop in a disorganized and abnormal way. Muscle coordination and nerves are affected. People with cerebral palsy may lack control of the head, have difficulty using the arms and hands, have poor balance or posture, be either stiff and spastic or limp and flaccid, and may have speech impairment. Intelligence may also be affected.

Care of a person with cerebral palsy. When caring for a person with cerebral palsy, remember the following:

- Allow the client to move slowly. People with cerebral palsy take longer to adjust their body position and may repeat movements several times.

- Maintain the client's body in as normal alignment as possible.

- Remember to talk to the client, even if he or she is incapable of speaking. Give those who can talk opportunities to speak by being patient and listening.

- Use touch as a form of nonverbal communication.

- Avoid activities that require excessive effort and are likely to produce fatigue and frustration.

- Be gentle when handling parts of the body that may be painful (**Fig. 17-5**).

- Support the client's efforts to be independent and socialize.

- Spend time with the client even though he or she may appear to be unaware that you are there.

Spina Bifida (spy-na BIF-e-da). Spina bifida literally means "split spine." When part of the backbone is not well enough developed at birth, the spinal cord may bulge out of the person's back. Depending on how severe the condition is, where on the spinal column the spinal cord sticks out, and what treatment a baby receives, spina bifida can cause a range of disabilities. Some babies born with spina bifida

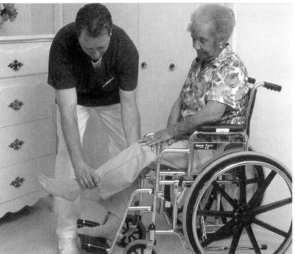

Fig. 17-5. Help a client with cerebral palsy stay in normal body alignment, but be gentle when moving body parts that might be painful.

will be able to walk and will experience no lasting disabilities. Others may be in a wheelchair and/or may have little or no bladder or bowel control. In some cases, complications of spina bifida may cause brain damage.

Care of the person with spina bifida. The type and severity of disabilities caused by spina bifida varies. A home care aide may provide assistance with range of motion exercises, assist the client with ADLs, and perform light housecleaning duties if the client is an adult. If assigned to a family with an infant or child who has spina bifida, a home care aide may perform tasks that help the parents

manage and stabilize the home. As in any assignment, home care aides should provide a positive role model for the family and the client in learning to deal with the client's disabilities.

Physical Disabilities

Physical disabilities that are not developmentally related are the result of disease or accident. Clients with these types of disabilities are faced with learning to adjust not only physically, but also mentally, to a gradual or sudden loss of ability.

Muscular Dystrophy (MD) and Amyotrophic (a-me-o-TRO-fic) **Lateral Sclerosis (ALS).** MD refers to a number of progressive diseases that cause a variety of physical disabilities due to muscle weakness. Most forms of MD are present at birth or become apparent during childhood. Many forms of MD are very slow to progress. Often people with MD can live to middle or even late adulthood.

ALS, often called Lou Gehrig's disease, is a progressive disease that causes muscle atrophy (weakening or wasting) and eventually leads to death. A person may be diagnosed with ALS at any age. The average time a person lives with ALS is between three and five years, though some people can live longer. Physical disabilities caused by ALS may begin with muscle weakness in the limbs or throat. Because ALS is progressive, disabilities usually get worse. Eventually, people with ALS usually have to breathe and be fed with the assistance of ventilators and tubes.

Care of a person with MD or ALS. The care provided by a home care aide depends on the severity of the client's disability. For someone in the early stages of one of these diseases, the home care aide may assist with ADLs or range of motion exercises. For a client in the more advanced stages of ALS or MD, the home care aide may be assigned to assist with skin care and positioning, and to perform ADLs for the client.

Multiple Sclerosis (MS). Because MS is a progressive disease affecting the central nervous system, clients with MS may have widely varying abilities. Multiple sclerosis is usually diagnosed when a person is in their early twenties to thirties. It progresses slowly and unpredictably. During some periods, called remissions (ree-MI-shuns), it doesn't seem to progress. During other periods, called exacerbations (ex-a-ser-BAY-shuns), it progresses very quickly.

Care of the person with MS. The role of a home care aide may range from housekeeping and assistance with ADLs, to providing care for a client who is completely unable to care for him- or herself. Report observations on both physical and mental health for clients with physical disabilities.

Spinal Cord and Head Injuries. Injuries to the head, neck, and back can affect the central nervous system, causing problems that range from mild confusion or temporary memory loss to coma, paralysis, and death. Injuries may be caused by vehicle accidents, sports activities, falls, industrial accidents, war, and criminal violence.

Injuries to the head may cause damage to the scalp, skull, and/or brain. Trauma to the head from an accident, birth injury, or violence can cause hemorrhage within the brain and its surrounding structures. Skull fractures from trauma may tear or bruise brain tissue.

Because brain tissue does not regenerate (it cannot renew itself) as bone tissue does, most persons who have severe head injuries have some degree of permanent damage. Clients who have had a head injury may have the following problems: mental retardation, personality changes, breathing problems, seizures, coma, memory loss, loss of consciousness, paresis (pa-REE-sis), and paralysis (pa-RAL-a-sis). Paresis is paralysis, or loss of ability, that affects only part of the body. Often, paresis is used to mean a

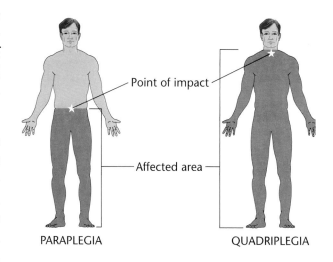

Fig. 17-6. Injuries in the cervical or neck area may lead to quadriplegia, or loss of muscle use from the neck down. Injuries in the lower or middle spinal cord may lead to paraplegia, or loss of muscle use in the lower body and lungs.

weakness or loss of ability on one side of the body.

The disability caused by a spinal cord injury depends on the severity of the trauma to the spinal cord and the level at which injury occurred. Paralysis or partial paralysis below the site of injury is usually the result. People who are injured in the cervical or neck region may lose the function of the muscles in their arms, chest, and lower body. This is called quadriplegia (kwad-ri-PLEE-jee-a) (**Fig. 17-6**). People who are injured in the middle or lower regions of the spinal cord may lose the function of their lower body and legs, a condition termed paraplegia (payr-a-PLEE-jee-a).

Rehabilitation is necessary for clients with spinal cord injuries to maintain the muscle function that remains and to help them live as independently as possible. Clients will need constant emotional support as they adjust to their disability and change in lifestyle. Their specific needs will vary, depending on the functions that have been lost and those that remain.

Care of the client with a head or spinal cord injury. Clients who have received rehabilitation for a head or spinal cord injury and are now in home care will continue to need emotional and psychological support as well as physical assistance. Frustration and anger may surface as they attempt to deal with the reality of their lives.

Safety in the home is very important. You will have to be very careful that clients with these disabilities do not fall or burn themselves. Because clients who are paralyzed have no sensation, they are unable to feel a burn or do anything to reduce its effects. Good skin care is essential to prevent decubitus ulcers, or pressure sores, when a client's mobility is limited. Clients must change positions every two hours to prevent pressure sores from developing.

In addition to personal care and home maintenance, you may assist with bowel and bladder training, range-of-motion and other physical therapy exercises, occupational therapy, and vocational training.

Hearing Impairment or Deafness. Persons who have impaired hearing or are deaf may have lost their hearing gradually, or they may have been born deaf. If they have a gradual hearing loss, they may not be conscious of it. Signs of hearing loss include the following:

- Speaking loudly
- Leaning forward when someone is speaking
- Cupping the ear to hear better
- Responding inappropriately
- Asking the speaker to repeat what has been said
- Failing in school or on the job
- Speaking in a monotone
- Avoiding social gatherings or acting irritable in the presence of people who are having a conversation
- Suspecting others of talking about them or of deliberately speaking softly

Care of clients who are hearing impaired. People who have hearing impairment may use a **hearing aid**, they may read lips, or use sign language. A hearing aid is a battery-operated device that amplifies sound. People with impaired hearing also closely observe the facial expressions and body language of others to add to their knowledge of what

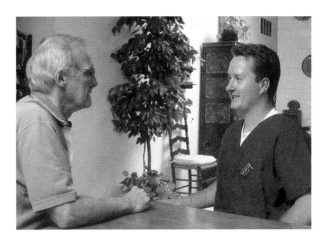

Fig. 17-7. Speak face-to-face, in good light.

is being said. The following suggestions offered by professionals who work with the deaf will make communicating with hearing-impaired clients more effective:

- Do not startle clients by approaching from behind. Walk in front of them so they can see you or touch them lightly on the arm to let them know you are near.
- Speak face-to-face, in good light (**Fig. 17-7**).
- Do not turn your face or move away in the middle of a conversation. If you plan to leave, announce it.
- If your client hears better out of one ear, communicate from that side.
- Speak slowly.
- Do not shout. Speak in your normal tone of voice.
- High-pitched voices are more difficult to hear. Use lower tones if possible.
- Do not have anything in your mouth while you are talking. Enunciate clearly and distinctly.
- Use short sentences and simple words.
- Get to the point early in the conversation.
- Ask if you should write down important words or names.
- Repeat words or rephrase sentences and ideas if you believe this will help.
- Avoid long, tiring conversations.

In addition, some hearing impaired clients have speech problems and may be difficult to understand. Do not pretend you understand if you do not. Ask your client to repeat what was said, and observe the lips, facial expressions, and body language. Then tell your client what you think you heard. You can also request that the client write down important words.

If your client uses a hearing aid and has difficulty understanding you, try the following:

▶ Check to see if the hearing aid is on.

▶ Adjust the hearing aid volume up or down.

▶ Check the batteries.

▶ Reduce background noise, as the hearing aid amplifies that too.

▶ Wash the external ear piece daily with soap and water, and dry it thoroughly.

▶ Make sure hearing aid is positioned correctly and placed in the correct ear.

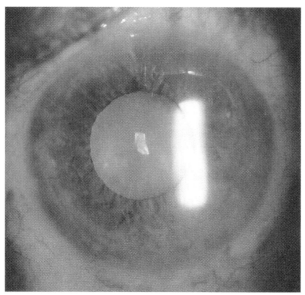

Fig. 17-8. When a cataract develops, the lens of the eye becomes cloudy, preventing light from entering the eye.

Vision Impairment. Like hearing impairment, vision impairment can affect people of all ages. It can exist at birth or develop gradually; it can occur in one eye or in both. Vision impairment can also be the result of injury, congenital problems, illness, or aging.

Some vision impairment caused by defects in the eye occurs in most people at some point in their lives, requiring them to wear corrective lenses, which can be contact lenses or eyeglasses. For example, **farsightedness**, the ability to see objects in the distance better than objects nearby, develops in most people as they age. **Nearsightedness**, the ability to see things near but not far, may occur in younger persons. Some people need to wear eyeglasses all the time; others only need them to read or for activities, such as driving, that require seeing distant objects.

People over the age of 40 are at risk for developing certain serious vision problems, including **cataracts**, **glaucoma**, and blindness. When a cataract develops, the lens of the eye becomes cloudy, pre-

venting light from entering the eye (**Fig. 17-8**). Vision blurs and dims initially, and is eventually lost entirely. This disease process can occur in one or both eyes and is corrected with surgery, in which a permanent lens implant is usually performed.

Glaucoma is a disease that causes the pressure in the eye to increase, eventually damaging the retina and the optic nerve and causing blindness. The chief cause of blindness, glaucoma can occur suddenly, causing severe pain, nausea, and vomiting, or it can occur gradually, with symptoms that include blurred vision, tunnel vision, and blue-green halos around lights. Glaucoma is treated with medication and sometimes surgery.

Caring for clients with vision impairment. Clients who are blind or have vision impairment must be treated with respect and acceptance as they make the necessary adjustments in their lives. The following are some suggestions from health care professionals who care for people who are blind:

▶ When you enter a room, identify yourself immediately. Do not touch your client until you've said your name.

▶ Do not leave a room without telling your client that you are going.

▶ Do not change the position of furniture and other objects.

▶ When you enter a new room with your client, orient him or her to where things are and allow time to walk about and touch the objects.

▶ Keep doors entirely open or entirely shut, never partly open.

▶ If your client needs guidance in getting around,

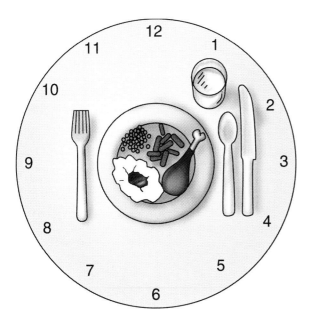

Fig. 17-9. Use the face of an imaginary clock as a guide to explain the position of objects that are in front of your client.

walk slightly ahead, letting the client touch or grasp your arm lightly.

▶ When guiding clients with vision impairment, tell them where obstacles, steps, and turns are.

▶ Use the face of an imaginary clock as a guide to explain the position of objects that are in front of your client (**Fig. 17-9**).

▶ Some clients may need assistance with cutting food and opening containers.

▶ Talking books (books on tape), large-print books, and braille books are available. Learning to read braille, however, takes a long time and requires special training.

▶ In caring for eyeglasses, clean glass lenses with water and soft tissue. Clean plastic lenses with a special cleaning fluid and lens cloth or tissues.

▶ Guard against losing, breaking, or scratching eyeglasses. Eyeglasses are expensive. Keep them in protective cases when not in use. Remember that plastic lenses scratch easily. Do not lay them on a hard surface.

▶ If the client is able, it is best to leave contact lens care to him or her.

Amputation. Amputation is the removal of some or all of a body part, usually a foot, hand, arm or leg. Amputation may be the result of an accident, or it may be done because the body part is badly diseased or badly damaged.

After amputation, some people feel that the limb is still there, or they complain of pain in the part that has been amputated. This is called **phantom limb pain,** and it may persist for a short time or for several years. The pain, which is caused by remaining nerve endings, is real and should not be ignored or ridiculed.

Caring for clients who have had an amputation. Clients who have had an extremity amputated must make many physical, psychological, social, and occupational adjustments to their disability. They will need support in adapting to the change in physical appearance and in performing their ADLs. You may also be trained by your supervisor to help clients use a **prosthesis,** or artificial limb, or perform exercises that will strengthen other muscles (**Fig. 17-10**). If a prosthesis is being used, observe the stump for signs of skin breakdown caused by pressure and abrasion.

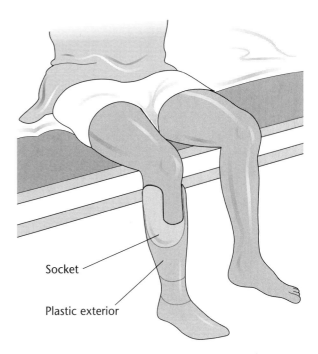

Socket

Plastic exterior

Fig. 17-10. Clients who have had a limb amputated will have many adjustments to make, often including the use of a prosthesis.

❏ 10. List important changes to report and document about the status of a client with disabilities

As discussed above, each client with a disability is an individual and will have different abilities. However, if a client is unable to perform a task that he or she was previously able to do, you should immediately report this to your supervisor and document it in your notes. For example, if a client with some vision impairment is suddenly unable to see anything, you should report the change immediately.

Be very careful to observe and report changes in the skin, particularly for clients with disabilities that affect mobility. Pressure sore prevention is an important role of the home care aide.

In addition to physical changes, emotional changes should be observed and reported. Because of the life changes a disability can bring, clients may be at risk for depression. Report any signs of depression, including moodiness, weight loss or gain, fatigue, or withdrawal.

Chapter 18

Understanding Mental Health and Mental Illness

❑ 1. Identify five characteristics of mental health

Mental health refers to the normal functioning of emotional and intellectual abilities. Characteristics of a person who is mentally healthy include the following:

▶ the ability to function and to interact effectively with others (**Fig. 18-1**)

▶ the ability to adapt to change, care for self and others, and give and accept love

▶ the ability to deal with situations that cause anxiety, disappointment, and frustration

▶ the ability to take responsibility for decisions, feelings, and actions

▶ the ability to control and fulfill desires and impulses in an appropriate manner

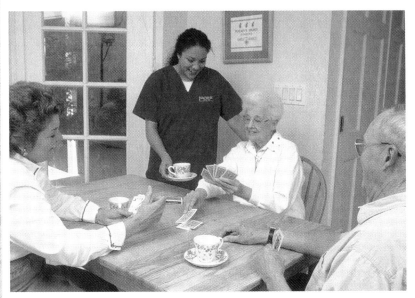

Fig. 18-1. The ability to interact well with other people is a characteristic of mental health.

❑ 2. Identify four causes of mental illness

Although it involves the emotions and mental functions, **mental illness** is a disease similar to any physical disease. It produces signs and symptoms, affects the body's ability to function, and responds to appropriate treatment and care. Mental illness disrupts a person's ability to function at a normal level in the family, home, or community, and it often produces inappropriate behavior. Some signs and symptoms of mental illness include confusion, disorientation, agitation, and anxiety.

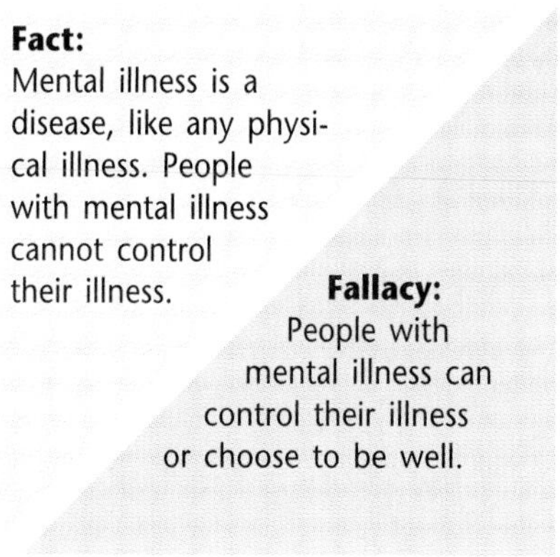

However, signs and symptoms like those seen with mental illness can occur as a response to certain situations when mental illness is not present. A personal crisis, temporary physical changes in the brain, side effects from medications, interactions among medications, and catastrophic change in the environment may cause what is called a **situation response**. In a situation response, the signs and symptoms are temporary, and they subside when the situation improves.

Mental illness can be caused or made worse by chronic stress from any of the following conditions:

1. Physical factors. Physical illness, disability, or aging can cause stress that may lead to mental illness, especially when these conditions bring physical limitations, frustration, and anxiety. Substance abuse or a chemical imbalance can also lead to mental illness. Self-respect and self-worth, the building blocks of mental health, are challenged when people who are ill or disabled have difficulty performing activities of daily living (ADLs). They may become fearful of the future and concerned about their dependency on others.

2. Environmental factors. Unusually weak interpersonal or family relationships, or traumatic early life experiences (such as suffering abuse as a child) can lead to mental illness.

3. Heredity. Either because of inherited traits or family influence, mental illness can occur repeatedly in some families.

4. Stress. Different people can tolerate different levels of stress. People have different ways of coping with stress. When the amount of stress becomes too great and a person is unable to cope with it, mental illness may arise.

❑ 3. Distinguish between fact and fallacy concerning mental illness

A fallacy (FAL-a-see) is a false belief. The greatest fallacy concerning mental illness is that people who are mentally ill can control their illness or even simply choose to be well. This is not true. As we said above, mental illness is a disease like cancer or diabetes or any other physical illness. Mentally healthy people may be able to control their emotions and their responses to people and situations. Mentally ill people usually do not have this control. Recognizing that mental illness is a disease much like any physical illness will help you work with clients who suffer from mental illness.

Fact:
Mental illness is a disease, like any physical illness. People with mental illness cannot control their illness.

Fallacy:
People with mental illness can control their illness or choose to be well.

Fig. 18-2. Separate fact from fallacy.

❑ 4. Explain the connection between mental and physical wellness

Mental health is important to physical health. The ability of mentally healthy people to reduce stress can help prevent some physical illnesses and can help them cope if illness or disability occur. Thus mental health can help protect and improve physical health. The reverse is also true: physical illness or disability can cause or worsen mental illness, because the stress these conditions create takes a toll on mental health.

❑ 5. List three guidelines for communicating with mentally ill clients

Different types of mental illness and different degrees of mental functioning will determine how well clients are able to communicate. As always, you must treat each client as an individual and tai-

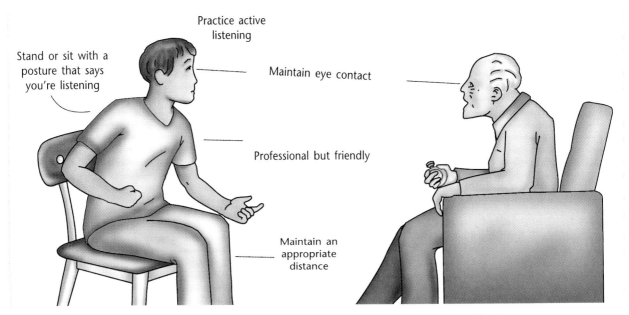

Stand or sit with a posture that says you're listening

Practice active listening

Maintain eye contact

Professional but friendly

Maintain an appropriate distance

Fig. 18-3. Practice good communication skills with mentally ill clients.

lor your style of communication to the situation. However, the following general guidelines apply when communicating with clients who are mentally ill (**Fig. 18-3**):

▷ Do not talk to adults as if they were children. Use simple, clear statements and a normal tone of voice.

▷ Be sure that what you say and how you say it communicate respect and concern for the client. Sit or stand at a normal distance from the client. Be aware of what your body language is saying.

▷ Be honest and straightforward, as you would with any client.

▷ Avoid arguments.

▷ Maintain eye contact.

▷ Listen carefully.

❑ 6. Identify and define common coping mechanisms

We all experience frustration at times. Frustrating experiences can create feelings of inferiority or a sense of failure. The physical response that accompanies frustration is what we call stress. One common reaction to stress and frustration is anger. Often we use other unconscious psychological mechanisms to cope as well. These techniques, called **coping**

mechanisms, reduce frustration, help us get through the crisis, and protect our sense of self-worth in the face of failure. Coping mechanisms generally fall into three categories:

1. withdrawal
2. aggression
3. substitution or compromise

Withdrawal. When we face a difficult or frightening situation, we may experience the "fight or flight" response, which is based in the nervous system. We either run from the situation or we fight it. One way to run from a frustrating and stressful psychological situation is to use withdrawal. Some forms of withdrawal include fantasy, denial, physical removal, or a psychological return to a more secure period of life.

Aggression. The use of aggression as a defense against a frustrating obstacle is a "fight" response. Although attacking a problem may sometimes eliminate it or overcome it, aggression is often counterproductive to living in social settings. In general, aggression is only a temporary means of reducing frustration. Aggression may be physical or verbal, and it often results in some form of punishment or retribution. Aggressive behavior is usually impulsive, destructive, and irrational.

Substitution or compromise reactions. When frustration is not reduced by withdrawal or aggression, substituting or compromising may give relief. A person who wants love may settle for a sexual relationship, or may substitute alcohol or drugs for love. This allows some feeling of satisfaction, but doesn't truly meet the person's original need.

All people occasionally resort to the use of coping mechanisms, but people who are mentally ill use them to a greater degree. This excessive use of unconscious coping mechanisms prevents a person from achieving a conscious understanding of their emotional problems and behaviors. If a person is unable to recognize their problems, he or she will not address the problems, and they may simply get worse.

❑ 7. Describe the symptoms of anxiety, depression, and schizophrenia

In many ways, we understand physical health much more than mental health. Even for doctors trained in mental illness (psychiatrists), diagnosis and treatment is very challenging.

There are many degrees of mental illness, from mild to severe. Severe mental illness is relatively easy to identify. A person may lose touch with reality and become unable to communicate or make everyday decisions. Some people with mild mental illness, however, may seem to function normally but sometimes become overwhelmed by stress or unreasonably emotional. Many of the signs and symptoms of mental illness are simply extreme cases of behaviors and feelings most people occasionally experience. Recognizing such behavior may make it easier to understand clients who are mentally ill.

1. Anxiety-related Disorders. Anxiety (ang-ZYE-i-tee) is uneasiness or fear, often about a situation or condition. When a mentally healthy person feels anxiety, he or she can usually identify the cause, and the anxiety fades once the cause is removed. A mentally ill person may feel anxiety all the time and for no known reason. Physical symptoms of anxiety-related disorders may include shakiness, muscle aches, sweating, cold and clammy hands, dizziness, fatigue, racing heart, cold or hot flashes, a choking or smothering sensation, or a dry mouth (**Fig. 18-4**).

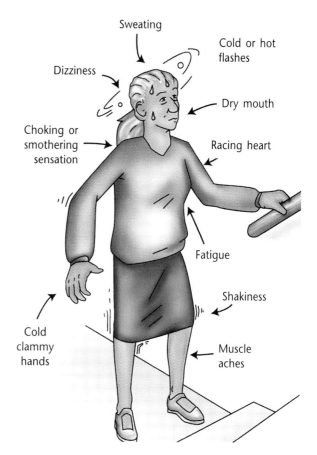

Fig. 18-4. Common symptoms of anxiety.

Phobias (FOH-bee-uhs) are an intense form of anxiety. Many people are intensely afraid of certain things (for example, dogs or snakes) or situations (like being in a confined space, or flying). For a mentally ill person, a phobia is a disabling terror that prevents the person from participating in normal, everyday activities. For example, the fear of being in a confined space, claustrophobia (claws-tro-FOH-bee-a), may make using an elevator or going into a public restroom a terrifying experience for a person with this type of phobia.

Other types of anxiety-related disorders include **panic disorder**, in which a person is overwhelmed with terror for no apparent reason. **Obsessive compulsive disorder** is the name for obsessive behavior a person uses as a coping mechanism for anxiety. For example, a person may wash his hands over and over again as a way of dealing with guilt. Anxiety-related disorders may also be brought on by a traumatic

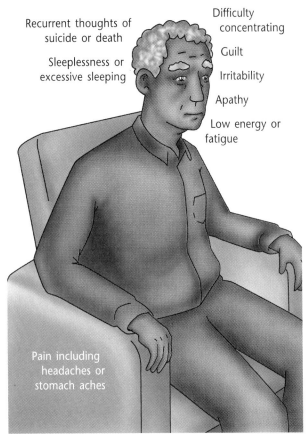

Recurrent thoughts of suicide or death

Difficulty concentrating

Guilt

Sleeplessness or excessive sleeping

Irritability

Apathy

Low energy or fatigue

Pain including headaches or stomach aches

Fig. 18-5. Common symptoms of clinical depression.

- low energy or fatigue

- apathy (A-pah-thee), or lack of interest in activities

- irritability

- anxiety

- problems with sexual functioning and desire

- sleeplessness, difficulty sleeping, or excessive sleeping

- guilt

- difficulty concentrating

- recurrent thoughts of suicide and death

Depression can occur in conjunction with other illnesses, most commonly cancer, HIV/AIDS, Alzheimer's disease, and diabetes. Occasionally, depression may be confused with a normal grief reaction. However, grief normally persists for two to three months and then steadily diminishes. Depression is very common in the elderly population.

There are different types and degrees of depression. **Major depression** may cause a person to lose interest in everything he once cared about and sink into complete apathy. **Manic depression** causes a person to swing from periods of profound depression to periods of extreme activity. These episodes of **mania** are characterized by excessive energy, little need for sleep, grandiose ideas and speeches, rapidly changing thoughts and moods, inflated self-esteem, overspending, and poor judgment.

Contrary to what many people think, people cannot overcome depression through sheer willpower. Depression is an illness like any other illness, and it can be treated. People who suffer from depression need compassion and support from family members, friends, and health care providers. You need to know the symptoms of depression so that you can recognize the onset (beginning) or worsening of depression in a client. Remember that any suicide threat should be taken seriously and reported immediately, not regarded as an attempt to get attention.

3. Schizophrenia (skit-zo-FRAY-nee-a). Contrary to popular belief, schizophrenia does not mean "split personality." Schizophrenia is a brain disorder that affects

experience such as violent crime. This type of anxiety is known as **post traumatic stress disorder**.

2. Depression. Clinical depression is a serious mental illness that may cause intense mental, emotional, and physical pain, and substantial disability. Depression also makes other illnesses worse, and if left untreated, it may result in suicide. An estimated eighty percent of suicide attempts are the result of depression.

Clinical depression is not a normal reaction to stress. Sadness is only one sign of this illness, and although sadness is frequently a major symptom of depression, not all people who have depression complain of sadness or appear sad. Other common symptoms of people who are clinically depressed include the following (**Fig. 18-5**):

- pain, including headaches, abdominal pain, and other body aches

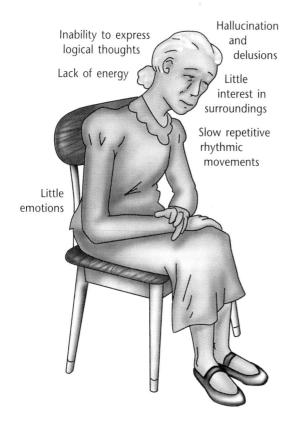

Inability to express logical thoughts

Lack of energy

Hallucination and delusions

Little interest in surroundings

Slow repetitive rhythmic movements

Little emotions

Fig. 18-6. Common symptoms of schizophrenia.

a person's ability to think and communicate clearly, manage emotions, make decisions, and understand reality. About two million Americans suffer from schizophrenia; however, treatment for the illness now makes it possible for many of its victims to lead relatively normal lives.

Some of the symptoms of schizophrenia are easy to observe (**Fig. 18-6**). Hallucinations (ha-loo-sin-AY-shuns) are illusions a person sees or hears. A person may see someone or something that is not really there, or hear a conversation that is not real. Delusions (de-LOO-zhuns) are persistent false beliefs. For example, a person may believe he or she can read or control other people's minds, or that other people are reading his or her thoughts. Paranoid (PAIR-a-noyd) schizophrenia, is a form of the disease that centers mainly on hallucinations and delusions. Not all cases of hallucinations or delusions, however, are related to schizophrenia.

Other symptoms of schizophrenia include disorganized thinking and speech, making a person unable to express logical thoughts. Disorganized behavior means a person moves slowly, repeating rhythmic gestures or movements. People with schizophrenia may also show less emotion, seem to have less interest in the things around them, and have a lack of energy or motivation.

❑ 8. Explain how medications can help a client who is mentally ill

As previously stated, it is extremely important to remember that mental illness can be treated. Medication and psychotherapy are common methods of treating mental illness. Medication can have a very positive effect for some people with mental illness, allowing them to function more completely than otherwise possible.

As with all medication, drugs used to treat mental illness must be dosed and taken precisely to maximize benefits and avoid side effects. Home care aides may be assigned to observe clients taking their medications. As always, be careful and conscientious.

❑ 9. Explain your role in caring for clients who are mentally ill

Personal care of clients who are mentally ill is similar to care for any client. As always, the care plan will tell you what kinds of care and what specific procedures you must perform. You will have some special responsibilities when caring for clients who are mentally ill, including the following:

▶ Observe clients carefully for changes in condition or abilities. Document and report your observations.

▶ Support the client and the family. Coping with mental illness can be extremely frustrating for everyone involved. Your positive, professional attitude and understanding will help encourage the client and the family. If you need help coping with the stress of caring for someone who is mentally ill, speak to your supervisor.

- Encourage clients to do as much for themselves as possible. Progress toward independence may be very slow, but if you don't expect progress, you probably will not see it.

- Help preserve the mentally ill client's role and authority in the family. Remember that you are not replacing the client, but only filling in until the client is well enough to resume his or her role in the family.

❏ 10. Identify important observations that should be made and reported

Carefully observe your clients and report any of the following:

- changes in ability

- positive or negative mood changes, especially withdrawal (**Fig. 18-7**)

- behavior changes, including changes in personality, extreme behavior, and behavior that does not seem appropriate to the situation

- comments, even jokes, about hurting self or others

- failure to take medicine or improper use of medicine

- real or imagined physical symptoms

- events, situations, or people that provoke certain reactions

Remember not to draw conclusions about the cause of the behavior. Report the facts of your observations, including what you saw or heard, how long the behavior lasted, and how frequently it occurred.

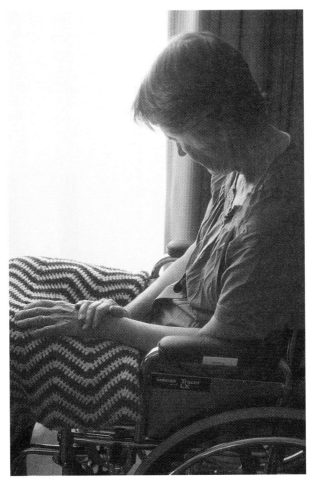

Fig. 18-7. Withdrawal is an important change to report.

❏ 11. List types of home management assistance often required for the client who is mentally ill

Abilities vary among people who are mentally ill, and clients should do as much as possible for themselves. However, a stable home environment is important in managing many forms of mental illness. By assisting the family with meeting their basic needs, you help the recovery process even if your care is not physically directed to the recovering person. For example, knowing that their children are being well cared for can greatly assist persons being treated for depression. You may be assigned to provide the following services:

- food shopping, meal planning, and preparation

- housecleaning and laundry

- assistance with ADLs and personal care such as bathing

- caring for children and other family members

❏ 12. List the signs of substance abuse

Substance abuse refers to the use of legal or illegal drugs, cigarettes, or alcohol in a way that is harmful to oneself or others. It is not necessary for a substance to be illegal for it to be abused (**Fig. 18-8**). Alcohol and cigarettes are legal for adults, but are often abused. Over-the-counter medications including diet aids and decongestants can

be addictive and harmful. Even household substances such as paint or glue are increasingly abused, causing injury and death.

As a home care aide, you may be in a position to observe the signs of substance abuse in your clients, their children, or other family members. It is important that you report these signs to your supervisor. You can report the signs you observe without actually accusing anyone of abuse. Simply report what you see, not what you think the cause may be.

Possible signs of substance abuse include the following:

▶ changes in personality, moodiness, strange

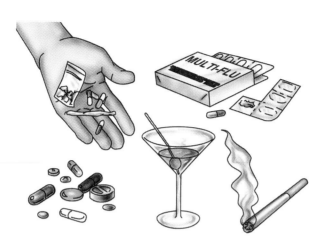

Fig. 18-8. Illegal drugs are not the only substances that are abused.

behavior, disruption of routines

▶ changes in physical appearance (red eyes, dilated pupils, weight loss)

▶ smell of cigarettes, liquor, or other substances on breath or clothes

▶ diminished sense of smell

▶ loss of appetite

▶ inability to function normally at school or work

▶ need for money, or money missing from the home

▶ alcohol or cigarettes missing from the home

▶ new friends or companions, strange phone calls

Chapter 19

Caring for New Mothers, Infants and Children

❑ **1. Explain the growth of home care for new mothers and infants**

It was once common for new mothers and their babies to stay in the hospital for several days after delivery. With the increasing popularity of natural childbirth techniques and new restrictions by insurers, many new mothers and their babies are sent home as early as 24 hours after an uncomplicated delivery. Thus, new mothers today are generally more tired and uncomfortable, and less confident feeding and handling their babies when they come home than women were in the past. Home care helps these women and babies make the transition from hospital to home and allows the mother to rest and recuperate.

Learning Objectives

In this chapter you will learn to:

Home cares aides are also called upon more frequently than in the past to assist with household management when an expectant mother is put on **bed rest** by her doctor. Bed rest is ordered if a woman shows signs of early labor, has a history of miscarriage or premature deliveries, or is extremely ill. Stopping all activity and staying in bed may help prevent labor from starting before the baby is ready to be born. An expectant mother may have to stay mostly in bed for a period of a few weeks up to a few months.

❑ 2. Identify common neonatal disorders

Neonatal (nee-oh-NAY-tal) is the medical term for newborn. Doctors who specialize in caring for newborn babies are called neonatologists (nee-o-nay-TAH-loh-jists). **Neonatal nurses** and **neonatal nurse practitioners** also specialize in caring for newborn babies. A newborn baby is sometimes referred to as a neonate (NEE-oh-nayt).

While most births are uncomplicated and most babies are born healthy, some babies are born with diseases or disorders that require special care. Babies born prematurely or at low birth weight, or who are injured during birth will also need special care (**Fig. 19-1**). Many of these special babies will have been in the hospital for some time before they are sent home.

The most common neonatal disorders are as follows:

▶ prematurity (birth more than three weeks before due date)

▶ low birth weight

▶ cerebral palsy

▶ cystic fibrosis

▶ Down's syndrome

▶ viral or bacterial infections

▶ susceptibility to sudden infant death syndrome (SIDS)

The effects of some of these disorders in older children and adults are described in Chapter 17, Assisting Clients with Disabilities.

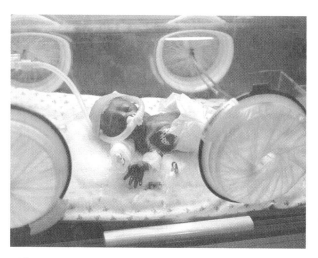

Fig. 19-1. Some babies need special attention at the hospital before they are sent home. For example, a baby born prematurely may need to spend time in a warm, controlled environment at the hospital.

❑ 3. Identify ways of assisting a new mother with her transition to the home

What you do to care for a new mother will be spelled out for you in the care plan and your assignment sheet. Each situation will be different. The care needed will depend on the mother's condition, the baby's condition, and the situation in the home. More care or different care will be needed depending on whether there are older children to care for and how much support the mother has from her husband, family, or others.

In general, a new mother making the transition from hospital to home may need the following assistance:

▶ basic care for the baby: feeding, diapering, bathing

▶ basic care for herself: rest, meal preparation, and comfort measures such as heat, ice, or sitz baths

▶ light housekeeping and laundry

▶ care of older children

▶ meal planning and shopping for the family

In some cases, special care for the mother or baby may be needed. You may be asked to assist the mother in caring for a caesarian section (se-SAYR-ee-an) incision or an episiotomy (e-pee-zee-AHT-o-mee).

A **caesarian section** is a birthing procedure in which the baby is delivered through an incision in the mother's abdomen. An **episiotomy** is an incision sometimes made in the perineal area during vaginal delivery.

If the baby is on a monitor (for pulse and respiration) or receiving oxygen, you may be asked to monitor the equipment. In some cases, the mother may need your help in establishing or continuing breastfeeding.

❑ 4. List important observations to report and document

Your supervisor should instruct you about observations to make. You may be documenting the baby's or the mother's vital signs regularly. You may also be documenting how much the baby eats, how long the baby nurses, how often the baby feeds, the baby's sleeping patterns, and how many wet or soiled diapers are changed.

Document and/or report any observations that seem important to you. In addition, pay attention to the following:

▶ The home: Is it a clean, healthy, and safe environment?

▶ The family: Are older children maintaining their regular routines? Do the husband and other family members know how they can help?

▶ The mother: Is she able to rest? Does she seem to be handling everything? Is she depressed, crying, or moody? Watch for signs of **postpartum** (after birth) **depression**, similar to signs of depression described in Chapter 18.

▶ The baby: Is the baby eating regularly, wetting and soiling the diapers, and sleeping well? Does the baby have good color?

▶ The baby's room or space: Is there a safe place

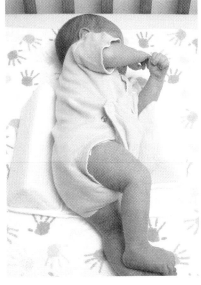

Fig. 19-2. After feeding, a baby should be laid down on its side, and a rolled towel or blanket should be placed behind the baby's back for support.

for the baby to sleep? Is the crib, bassinet, or bed free of pillows or excess bedding that could cause suffocation? Is the room temperature comfortably warm?

❑ 5. Explain guidelines for safely handling a baby

Wash your hands thoroughly before touching a baby or any baby supplies. Preventing the spread of germs is extremely important around a newborn baby. See that all visitors and family members wash their hands frequently, and especially before touching or holding the baby. People with colds or possible signs of illness or infection should stay away from the newborn, or wear a mask to prevent transmission of disease.

Always lift and hold a baby safely, according to the procedure below. Newborn babies cannot hold their heads up without assistance, and leaving the head unsupported can cause injury. Be sure all visitors and family members hold the baby safely.

Never leave a baby in an unsafe location or position. *The only safe place to leave a baby is in a crib with the side rails up or in an adult's arms.* Do not leave babies in swings, carriers, seats or on blankets on the floor unless you can see them at all times. Never put seats, swings or carriers on tables, chairs, or countertops. Even when changing a baby's diaper, never leave the baby on a table or countertop without keeping at least one hand on the baby at all times. Letting go, even for one second, can be dangerous. Never leave a baby or any child alone in a bath.

Never put a baby down in the prone position (on the abdomen) if the baby is too young to lift its head to breathe. Babies should be placed on their backs or propped on their sides with a rolled blanket or towel (**Fig. 19-2**). The side position is best after a feeding in case the baby vomits.

1. Wash your hands.

2. Reach one hand under the baby and behind his head and neck. Cradle the head and neck in your hand. Support the head at all times when lifting or holding a newborn.

3. With the other hand, support the baby's back and bottom (**Fig. 19-3**).

4. There are several ways to hold a baby safely, including the **cradle hold**, the **football hold**, and holding the baby **upright** against your chest (**Figs. 19-3 through 19-5**). Always be sure the baby's head and neck are supported.

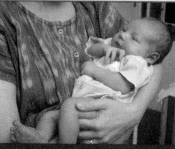

Fig. 19-3. The cradle hold is with the baby's head and neck resting in the crook of one elbow and the legs in the other arm. You must support the baby's back with one or both hands.

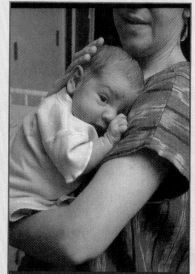

Fig. 19-5. When holding a baby upright against your chest, you must support the baby's head, neck, and back with one hand while keeping the other arm under the baby's bottom to support its weight.

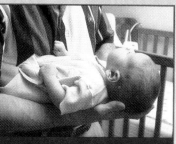

Fig. 19-4. The football hold is accomplished by holding the baby's head in one hand and supporting the baby's back with the arm on the same side of your body. The baby's body will lie along the side of your body.

Crib mattresses should be firm. Infants should not be placed on a blanket, comforter, pillow, or sheepskin. These items can cause suffocation and may contribute to SIDS, which occurs when a baby stops breathing and dies.

Supervise older children and pets around babies. Jealousy can cause even well-behaved children and pets to harm babies. Older children may not mean to hurt a baby, but may not know how to touch or handle a baby.

❑ 6. Describe guidelines for assisting with feeding a baby

Assisting with Breastfeeding

Many pediatricians encourage mothers to breastfeed, or nurse, their babies because breastfeeding has been shown to provide the perfect nutrition for infants. The decision to breast or bottle feed is a personal one that each mother must make for herself. If a mother chooses to try breastfeeding, she may need support while getting established and learning how to breastfeed. Many professionals recommend that women try breastfeeding for two weeks before deciding whether to continue or stop. The first two weeks may be challenging for the mother, and your support can help her get off to a good start.

Discuss with the mother how much help she wants or needs. Ask her questions to determine her experience with and knowledge of breastfeeding: Did you breastfeed your other children? If yes, for how long? If no, what made you decide to do so now? Did the nurses in the hospital teach you about breastfeeding? Did you take any newborn classes before delivery? The mother may only want you to help her get into position, or she may need your coaching throughout the process. Make sure she knows that breastfeeding consultants are usually available to help solve breastfeeding problems. Report any problems you observe or the client tells you.

Women have different breastfeeding styles. Some are very comfortable and will nurse anytime, in the presence of older children or family members. Others may want more privacy while nursing. Be sensitive to individual preferences. A calm setting where the mother can relax will help her body provide the most milk for the baby.

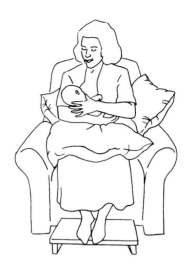

Fig. 19-6. A new mother usually prefers to nurse in an upright, sitting position. Provide support with pillows and a footrest.

Guidelines for helping the mother with breastfeeding

▶ Remind the mother to wash her hands. Help her get in position for breastfeeding, usually sitting upright in a comfortable chair or in bed supported by pillows. Provide a low footrest if possible, and a pillow for the mother's lap (**Fig. 19-6**). Some mothers are able to breastfeed while lying down, but many find this more difficult, especially with a newborn baby.

▶ Provide for privacy. Close the door and occupy older children if necessary.

▶ Change the baby's diaper if necessary before bringing him to the mother. Use the towel, shawl, or blanket to cover the mother's breast and baby's head after baby has latched on.

▶ If necessary, remind the mother how to hold the nipple and areola between thumb and forefinger to allow baby to latch on. If baby does not latch on right away, have the mother stroke his cheek with the nipple.

▶ Good nutrition and plenty of fluids are important for nursing mothers. Offer frequent drinks of water, juice, or milk, and snacks as needed. Instruct the mother not to eat spicy foods, chocolate, or caffeinated beverages, as they may affect the breast milk.

▶ Observe the baby nursing to be sure he stays latched on properly (**Fig. 19-7**). If necessary, have

the mother use one hand to hold the breast tissue away from the baby's nose.

▶ When it is time to switch from one breast to the other, the mother can break the suction by pressing down on the breast above the nipple or by gently putting her finger in the baby's mouth.

▶ Help the mother burp the baby when switching breasts and when finishing the feeding.

▶ Change the baby's diaper after the feeding, and help the mother lay the baby down safely.

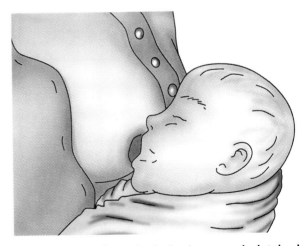

Fig. 19-7. When the baby is properly latched on to the mother's nipple, his mouth covers much of the areola and the nipple is sucked straight out rather than at an angle. Making sure the baby is latched on properly ensures the best milk flow and helps keep the mother's nipples from becoming very sore.

▶ Many women find it helpful to tie a ribbon or place a pin on the side the baby last fed on. This reminder helps them remember to start the baby's feeding on that side next time, so the breasts will be emptied more evenly.

Assisting with Bottle Feeding

Many women choose to bottle feed their babies some or all of the time. Infant formula is commercially prepared and provides the nutrition babies need. There are many brands and types of formula, so, if you are doing the shopping, be sure you know exactly which type you need to buy. The three most common types are ready-to-feed formula, concentrated liquid formula, and powdered formula (**Fig. 19-8**).

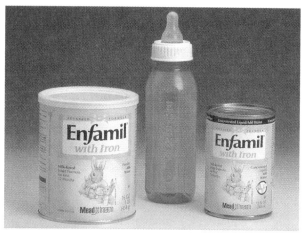

Fig. 19-8. Baby formula is available ready-to-feed in cans or bottles, concentrated in cans, or powdered in cans.

Ready-to-feed or prepared formula is sold in bottles or cans. This formula is ready to use and should not be diluted or mixed with water. If the formula comes in small bottles, simply shake, unscrew the cap, and screw on a standard nipple and ring. Discard any formula remaining in the bottle after feeding. If the ready-to-feed formula comes in a can, shake the can before opening it with a sterilized can opener. Pour into sterile bottles. Store remaining formula in the can, covered and refrigerated, for no more than two days. Ready-to-feed formula is the most convenient to use, but also the most expensive.

Concentrated formula is sold in small cans and must be mixed with sterile water before using. Shake

the can and open it with a sterile can opener. Measure an amount into a marked bottle and add an equal amount of sterile water. Screw on the nipple and ring, and shake to mix. Sterile water can be purchased in small bottles, or you can use water sold in gallon jugs. You can also make sterile water by bringing water to a boil and then cooling. Store unused concentrate in the can, covered and refrigerated, for no more than two days.

Powdered formula is sold in one- or two-pound cans and must be carefully measured and mixed with sterile water before feeding. A special scoop is included in the can for measuring. Mix the powder and sterile water in sterile bottles or a sterilized pitcher or covered container. Follow the directions on the package carefully. Once mixed, the formula can be stored for two days in the refrigerator. Shake before feeding. Powdered formula is the most difficult to use, but is usually the cheapest way to buy formula.

Before feeding, bottles should be warmed. To heat, immerse the bottle in warm tap water for several minutes. Bottles or formula just out of the refrigerator will take longer to warm. Never use the microwave to warm bottles, as this can create hot spots in the liquid that can burn the baby (**Fig. 19-9**). Always shake the bottle after warming and shake a few drops of formula from the bottle onto the inside of your wrist. It should feel warm, not hot or cold.

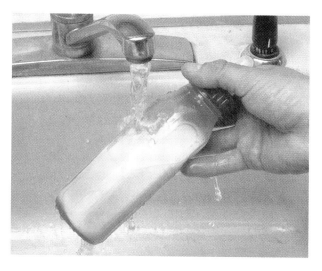

Fig. 19-9. Warm bottles in warm tap water—*not* in the microwave!

Procedure 2: Sterilizing bottles

1. Wash your hands.
2. Assemble equipment:
   - clean bottles, nipples, and rings to be sterilized: these should be washed in hot, soapy water using a bottle brush, and allowed to drain
   - large kettle filled halfway with water
   - tongs
   - clean dish or paper towels to set sterile bottles on
3. Bring water to a boil and put bottles, nipples, and rings in. Use tongs to push bottles under water.
4. Bring water to boil again and allow to boil for five minutes.
5. Using tongs, remove bottles, nipples, and rings, draining the water into the pot. Set everything on the clean towels. When dry, store in a clean, dry cabinet.
6. Discard water.

Procedure 3: Assisting with bottle feeding

1. Wash your hands.
2. Prepare bottle and formula as directed.
3. The person giving the bottle should sit in a comfortable chair and hold the baby safely in either the cradle hold or football hold.
4. Stroke the baby's lips with the bottle nipple until she opens her mouth. Put the bottle nipple in the baby's mouth.
5. Be sure the baby's head is higher than her body during feeding. Also make sure the nipple

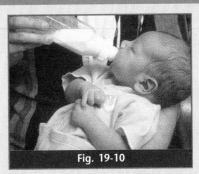
Fig. 19-10

stays full of milk so the baby does not swallow air (**Fig. 19-10**).
6. Talk or sing to the baby while feeding. Feedings are the high points of her days and should be special times.

7. When baby is through or has stopped sucking, burp her (see Procedure 4). Resume feeding, or, if finished, change the diaper (see Procedure 7) and put the baby down safely.
8. Wash your hands and document the feeding, how much was consumed, and any other observations.
9. Throw out unused formula left in bottle. Wash the bottle, nipple, and ring in hot soapy water with a bottle brush, and allow to dry. Sterilize before using again.

Procedure 4: Burping a baby

1. Wash your hands.
2. Assemble equipment: a clean towel, cloth diaper, or burp pad.
3. Pick up the baby safely. There are two different positions to use for burping. Most people like to hold the baby against the shoulder to burp (**Fig. 19-11**). However, babies who are very small, who have breathing problems, or who tend to choke or vomit should be held on the lap with the head supported by holding the baby's chin with the thumb and forefinger (**Fig. 19-12**). This

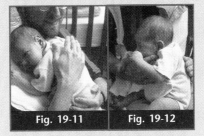
Fig. 19-11   Fig. 19-12

position allows you to watch the baby for signs of respiratory distress, especially color changes, or spit up. Whichever position you use, put the burp pad under the baby's chin to catch any spit up that may come up.
4. With the baby in a safe and

comfortable position, pat the baby's back gently with your flat hand, concentrating on the area between the shoulder blades. Some people like to pat up and down the baby's back. Others like to massage the back using an upward motion with the flat hand. Use any technique that works for you. The more relaxed and comfortable the baby is, the sooner the burp will come.
5. After the baby has burped, return him or her to a safe position or resume feeding.

1. Wash your hands.
2. Assemble equipment:
   - disposable gloves
   - clean basin
   - blanket or towel to pad surface
   - washcloth and towel
   - baby cleanser or mild soap
   - baby shampoo or other mild shampoo
   - cotton hat
   - lotion or oil
   - cotton ball or cotton-tipped swabs and alcohol
   - diaper ointment if used
   - clean diaper
   - clean clothes or sleeper
   - clean receiving blanket

3. Put on gloves. Be careful—gloves make the baby slippery!

4. Give the bath in a warm place. Use a blanket or towel to pad the countertop, changing table, or other surface the baby will lay on. Have all your supplies within reach, as you will need to keep one hand on the baby during the entire bath. Remove caps from shampoo and cleanser to make it easier.

5. Fill the basin with warm water. Test the temperature on the inside of your wrist. Put the bottle of lotion or oil in the warm water to warm it.

6. With the baby still dressed and wrapped in a blanket, hold him or her in the football hold. Wet the washcloth and gently wipe the eyes, from the inner corner to the outer (**Fig. 19-13**). Then clean the rest of the face, using no soap or cleanser, only

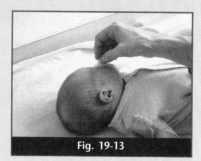
Fig. 19-13

warm water.

7. To wash hair, hold the baby in the football hold with the head over the basin. Use the washcloth to wet the hair. Using a small amount of shampoo, lather the baby's hair (**Fig. 19-14**). Rinse with the washcloth. Pat the head dry immediately with the towel and put a cotton hat over the baby's head. Much heat is lost through the head, so you must be careful to keep the head warm.

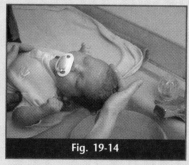
Fig. 19-14

8. Lay the baby down on the padded surface. *Always keep at least one hand on the baby.*

9. Undress the upper body and wash the neck, chest, back, arms and hands, using the washcloth and small amounts of cleanser or

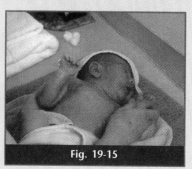
Fig. 19-15

soap. Rinse using the washcloth and water from the basin (**Fig. 19-15**). Pat dry and cover the upper body with a towel.

10. Undress the lower body, removing the diaper, and wash the baby's abdomen and legs. Rinse. Pat dry.

11. Wash the perineal area last. For a girl, wipe the perineal area from front to back. For a boy who is not circumcised, gently pull the foreskin of the penis back to clean the tip. For a boy who has recently been circumcised, do not wash the area of the circumcision. Follow special instructions to care for the circumcision (see guidelines for circumcision care).

12. Wash the baby's bottom thoroughly and dry the entire area completely with the towel. Moisture can contribute to diaper rash.

13. As gently and quickly as possible, rub lotion over the baby's body, avoiding the cord if it has not yet healed. Use lotion on the face only if skin is very dry, and be extremely careful not to get any lotion near the eyes. Keep the baby covered except for the part you are rubbing.

14. Diaper and dress the baby. Wrap baby in blanket and put him or her down safely.

15. Put used towels and washcloth in the laundry. Discard water. Clean basin and store. Store other supplies. Discard gloves.

16. Wash your hands.

17. Document the bath, including any observations.

Babies must be burped or "bubbled" after each feeding to release air swallowed during feeding. Burping prevents babies from developing gas, which can be very uncomfortable for them. Burping in the middle of a feeding may allow a baby to eat more.

❑ 7. Explain guidelines for bathing and changing a baby

Keeping a baby clean is important to his health. Follow the guidelines for safely handling a baby. In addition, remember the following:

▶ Because of the potential for coming into contact with body fluids, you should wear disposable gloves when bathing or changing a baby. Remember, however, that gloves can make a wet baby slippery! Be very careful when handling a baby during a bath.

▶ Whether bathing or changing a baby, be sure to keep one hand on the infant at all times. Have all supplies ready, so you never have to take both hands off the baby when he is on a changing table or padded counter.

▶ Keep the baby warm. Give baths in a warm place. Close doors and windows to prevent drafts. Dry the baby's head immediately after washing hair.

▶ Be very careful about bath temperature. Always test the temperature of the water (either on the inside of your wrist or with a bath thermometer).

▶ Keep the baby's bottom dry. Be sure the area is thoroughly dried after a bath (moisture contributes to diaper rash). Be sure to dry the bottom after changing a diaper. Leaving the diaper off for a few moments when changing the baby allows air to circulate and helps prevent diaper rash.

▶ Do not use powder unless directed to do so. Babies who are very small, premature, or who have breathing problems, can be harmed by inhaling baby powder.

Diapers catch the baby's urine and feces. Children wear diapers until they are toilet trained, generally between two and three years of age. Diapers are either cloth or disposable, made of paper and plastic. Cloth diapers are used with special waterproof diaper covers or with diaper pins and plastic pants.

Procedure 6: Giving an infant tub bath

In addition to the supplies listed in Procedure 5 for a sponge bath, you will need a large basin or baby bath tub. You may also bathe a baby in a clean sink. Follow the first seven steps in Procedure 5 for preparing the bath and washing the baby's face and hair.

1. Lay the baby down on the padded surface and undress him or her completely. Immerse baby in the tub or basin, supporting the head and neck above water with one hand at all times (**Fig. 19-16**).

2. Using the washcloth and small amounts of cleanser or soap, wash the baby from the neck down.

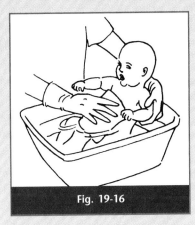

Fig. 19-16

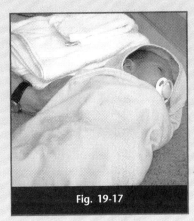

Fig. 19-17

3. Remove the baby from the bath and lay him or her down on the padded surface, keeping one hand on the baby at all times. Cover baby immediately with a towel and pat dry (**Fig. 19-17**).

4. Apply lotion, keeping the baby covered as much as possible.

5. Diaper, dress, and wrap the baby in a receiving blanket. Put him or her down safely.

6. Put used linens in the laundry. Discard bath water. Clean and store basin. Store all supplies. Discard gloves.

7. Wash your hands.

8. Document the bath, including any observations.

1. Wash your hands.

2. Assemble supplies:
   - clean disposable diaper or
   - clean cloth diaper, diaper cover or pins, and plastic pants
   - wipes or a washcloth wet with warm water
   - diaper ointment or oil if used
   - clean clothes if clothes are soiled or wet

3. Put on gloves.

4. Change the diaper in a warm place. You need a padded surface, which may be a special changing table or a countertop. Never turn your back on the baby, and always keep one hand on baby at all times. Have supplies within reach.

5. Undress the baby as necessary and remove wet or soiled diaper. Set it aside for handling later.

6. Clean the perineal area with wipes or washcloth. Remove all traces of feces. Spread the legs to clean thoroughly. For girls, wipe from front to back and spread the labia to clean as needed.

7. Let air circulate on the bottom for a moment. Exposure to air prevents diaper rash. Apply ointment or oil as directed.

8. **For disposable diapers:** Unfold the diaper and expose tapes. Place the diaper flat under the baby's bottom with the tapes in back. Bring the front of the diaper up between the baby's legs and bring the back sides around and over the front (**Fig. 19-18**). Peel tapes open and tape the side of the diaper securely to the front.

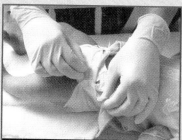

Fig. 19-18. A disposable diaper is fastened with adhesive or Velcro tape attached to the back sides of the diaper.

9. **For cloth diapers with diaper cover:** Fold the diaper in thirds lengthwise. Then open out the back corners about three inches (Fig. 19-19). Lay the back of the diaper inside the back of the diaper cover (the back of the diaper cover has the tabs extending from it). Place the diaper and cover underneath the baby's bottom. Bring the front of the diaper and cover up through the baby's legs. Bring the tabs around from the sides to the front of the diaper cover and use them to close the cover securely over the diaper. Check that all the edges of the diaper are tucked under the cover.

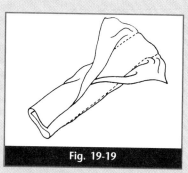

Fig. 19-19

10. **For cloth diapers with pins and plastic pants:** Fold the diaper lengthwise in thirds, then open out the back corners about three inches. Place the diaper

under the baby's bottom and bring the front of the diaper up between the baby's legs. Fold down the front of the diaper to the inside (next to baby's skin) so that the diaper covers the genitals and lower abdomen (**Fig. 19-20**). Bring the corners of the diaper around the baby's sides and pin them to the front of the diaper. Hold your fingers inside the diaper next to baby's skin when pinning, to avoid sticking the baby (**Fig. 19-20**). You do not need to pin through all layers, just enough to fasten the back of the diaper to the front. When diaper is securely pinned, put plastic pants over the diaper to keep urine from leaking onto baby's clothes.

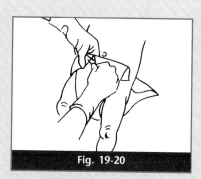

Fig. 19-20

11. Dress the baby in clean clothes and put him down safely.

12. Dispose of diaper properly. Disposable diapers can be rolled into a ball (dirty side in), sealed with tapes, and disposed of in a special trash bag in a sealed container to prevent odors. Cloth diapers may need to be soaked before washing or removal by a diaper service. Check with mother or supervisor for instructions.

13. Remove gloves.

14. Wash your hands.

15. Clean changing area and store supplies.

16. Wash hands again as needed.

17. Document any observations, including unusual color, consistency, or odor.

A newborn will need between six and ten diaper changes in 24 hours. As babies get older, they use fewer diapers each day. The appearance, consistency, and smell of a baby's feces will depend on what he or she is fed. Some newborn babies have loose bowel movements with every feeding, as many as eight a day. Others have different schedules. Babies must be changed frequently to avoid diaper rash or irritation.

❏ 8. Explain guidelines for special care

Umbilical Cord Care

At birth, the umbilical (um-BIL-i-kul) cord that connected the baby to the placenta (pla-SEN-ta) inside the mother's uterus (YOU-ter-us) is cut. The stump of the cord remains attached to a newborn's navel for up to three weeks. Proper care of the cord stump is necessary to prevent infection and allow healing.

▶ With every diaper change, the cord should be moistened with rubbing alcohol. Use a cotton ball

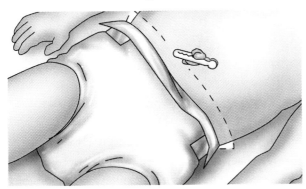

Fig. 19-21. Keep diapers folded down away from the cord to allow air to circulate and prevent irritation.

or cotton-tipped swabs soaked in rubbing alcohol to swab the area around the navel and cord. This helps the stump dry up and fall off.

▶ *Never* pull on or handle the cord; it will fall off by itself. The baby will feel no pain when the cord falls off.

▶ Keep diapers folded down away from the cord to allow air to circulate and prevent irritation (**Fig. 19-21**).

▶ Do not give an infant a tub bath until the cord has fallen off.

Procedure 8: Taking an infant's axillary or tympanic temperature

An infant's temperature is typically taken by the axillary or tympanic methods. Rectal temperatures are no longer recommended for infants because of the chance of damaging rectal tissue. Oral temperatures are never taken for infants because the method is too difficult and dangerous.

1. Wash your hands.

2. Assemble supplies:
   ▶ thermometer
   ▶ disposable probe cover, if needed

3. Be sure thermometer is clean. Put on disposable probe cover, if used. If using glass thermometer, shake down mercury.

4. **For axillary temperature:** Undress the upper body on one side. Lay the baby on a padded surface. Place the tip of the thermometer under the arm and hold the baby's arm close to his body, so the thermometer tip touches skin on all sides (**Fig. 19-22**). Keep thermometer in place for 3 to 5 minutes for a glass thermometer, or until the signal sounds for a digital thermometer.

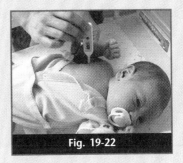

Fig. 19-22

Continued on page 256

Continued from page 255

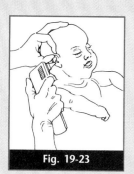

Fig. 19-23

5. For tympanic temperature: Lay the baby on his side. Pull the outside of the ear gently toward the back of the head. Insert the thermometer tip into the ear, pointing toward the opposite eye (**Fig. 19-23**). Be sure the ear is sealed by the thermometer. Press the button and hold for one second.

6. For all methods, remove the thermometer and read the temperature, keeping one hand on the baby at all times.

7. Dress the baby and put him down safely.

8. Clean and store thermometer and supplies.

9. Wash your hands.

10. Document temperature.

Circumcision care

Circumcision (SIR-kum-si-zyun) is the removal of part of the foreskin of the penis. It is commonly performed on male babies. Some religions require circumcision. Other parents choose to have their baby circumcised for hygienic or social reasons.

After the circumcision is performed, usually in the hospital or at the doctor's office when the baby is only days old, the circumcision site needs special care to heal. Usually this will include covering the tip of the penis with a gauze pad rubbed with petroleum jelly to prevent the diaper from irritating the site as it heals. However, some types of circumcision require different care. Follow your supervisor's instructions carefully.

Working around medical equipment

Some babies who need special care will have medical equipment in the home with them. You will probably not be responsible for operating or handling the equipment, but it may be helpful to be familiar with the purpose and use of various items. Always follow your supervisor's instructions before touching any medical equipment.

Apnea monitor. Apnea (AP-nee-a) is the state of not breathing. Some babies may stop breathing for periods of time due to immaturity of the lungs or other reasons. The apnea monitor alerts parents or caregivers if breathing has stopped. Many apnea monitors also monitor heart rate.

Ventilator or oxygen equipment. Some babies with breathing problems need to be given oxygen. Oxygen is considered a medication, and in most states it cannot be given by a home care aide. In addition, home care aides are not allowed to change the dose or amount of oxygen being given. As always, be careful when working around oxygen, as it is flammable. Follow your supervisor's instructions carefully when working in a home where oxygen is in use.

Part 2
Understanding and Caring for Children

As a home care aide, you may have contact with children in several ways. Most often, you may be assigned to care for the children of a client when the client is unable to care for the children him- or herself. In this case you are a substitute for the parent. In other cases, the child may be the client, suffering from a disease or disability that requires home care. In either case, it is important to understand some basic principles of caring for and working with children.

❑ 9. Identify special physical, mental, and emotional needs of children

Children have the same basic physical and emotional needs as adults (see Chapter 8, Basic Human Needs). However, because they are growing and developing at a faster pace, children have some special physical, mental, and emotional needs. Children's growing bodies need adequate and nutritious food and fluids, exercise, fresh air, and plenty of sleep. Their developing minds need to be stimulated by age-appropriate activities, opportunities for learning, and chances for increasing independence. Emotionally, children need love and affection, reassurance, encouragement, security and guidance, and consistent and constructive discipline. In addition, children need protection from injury and illness. Chapter 10, Understanding Human Development and Aging, describes child development in more detail.

In addition to their special needs, children with disabilities have the same physical and emotional needs as other children. Remember to treat these children as children first. Disabilities may make normal social contact with other children difficult, but it is essential that children with disabilities have time to interact with others their own age. Chapter 17, Assisting Clients with Disabilities, offers more information on caring for clients with special needs.

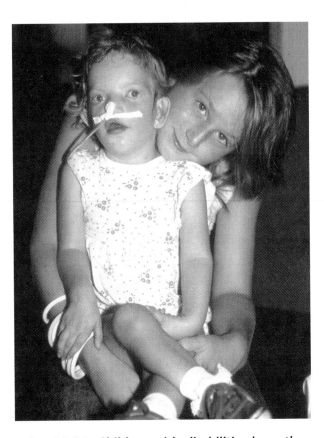

Fig. 19-24. Children with disabilities have the same emotional needs other children have: for love and acceptance, reassurance, encouragement, security and guidance, and consistent and constructive discipline.

❑ **10. List three symptoms of common childhood illnesses and the care they require**

Most childhood illnesses are caused by bacterial or viral infections. These include colds, flu, and various infections causing fever, diarrhea, vomiting, or coughs. You can help prevent illness by preventing the spread of infection in the home. Handwashing, cleaning, and disinfection are the best ways to control infection (see Chapter 5). Treatment for some of the most common symptoms of childhood illnesses is described below.

1. **Fever.** Fever may indicate serious illness in a child

and should always be reported to your supervisor. Rest and fluids are recommended for fevers. Treatment for a fever may also include acetaminophen, or a lukewarm bath or sponging. Although home care aides never give any medication, including over-the-counter medications, you can assist by making sure the family caregiver follows a doctor's dosage instructions for all medications. Because the strength of over-the-counter drugs varies in infant, children, and adult formulas, it is especially important to follow dosage instructions. For example, infant acetaminophen is *stronger* than children's acetaminophen, and the dosage is *much* smaller. Too much can cause liver damage or failure. In general, children should *not* be given aspirin, as it has been associated with some serious disorders.

2. **Diarrhea.** Diarrhea, or frequent loose or watery bowel movements, can have many causes. In children, it is often caused by a virus. Cramps and abdominal pain may accompany diarrhea. Children with diarrhea should rest and drink plenty of clear liquids, including water, broth, and diluted juices. Doctors may recommend electrolyte-replacement drinks to prevent dehydration. Usually, doctors recommend that children with diarrhea avoid solid foods until the problem subsides, and then that they follow the BRAT diet: **b**ananas, **r**ice, **a**pplesauce, and **t**oast. Other starchy foods, such as pasta or crackers, are also allowed. Milk products, fruits, vegetables, and fatty foods should be avoided until the bowels return to normal.

3. **Vomiting.** The treatment for vomiting is similar to the treatment for diarrhea, including rest and clear liquids, and later the BRAT diet.

Box 19-1. Some Practical Suggestions for Working with Children

Introduce yourself. Treat children in the homes you work in as important members of the family, and worthy of your notice. Be friendly, tell the children your name, and explain why you are there.

Maintain routine. As much as possible, stick with the family's regular schedule. The comfort of a routine can help ease the stress children may feel if someone in their household needs home care.

Give comfort. Children who are hurt, angry, or sad may need a hug, a pat, or soothing words to make them feel more secure (**Fig. 19-25**).

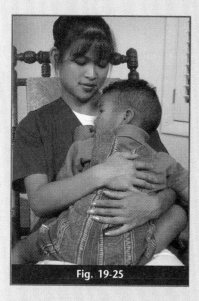
Fig. 19-25

Offer encouragement and praise. Encouragement and praise contribute to the child's sense of self-worth and build self-confidence. Word your praise so that it does not belittle other children.

Do not make comparisons. Children should not be compared or played against each other.

Use positive phrases. Children often respond better to guidance such as "Let's try it this way..." rather than "no" or "don't."

Listen. Pay attention when children attempt to communicate. Do not interrupt them or deny their feelings. Help them to express what they are feeling by using your communications skills (see Chapter 4).

Answer. Respond to children's questions immediately, willingly, and clearly. If you do not know the answer to a question or are not sure you are the right person to answer it, tell the child. Bring the child's question to the attention of the appropriate person.

Do not force children to eat. Like adults, children do not always feel like eating. Do not allow a meal to become a power struggle. Children are usually motivated to eat when meals are simple but attractive and contain their favorite foods.

Involve children in household activities. Children feel capable and responsible when they are given household tasks to perform (**Fig. 19-26**). Like all people, they like to feel they are making a contribution to the family.

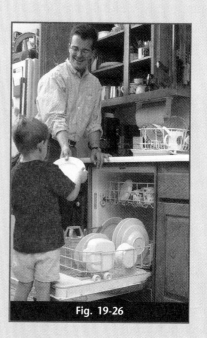
Fig. 19-26

Encourage children to play. Children need to exercise and socialize with other children. Playing helps children express themselves and be creative. Exercise is important for their growth and health. Socialization is important for all human beings, but especially for children who are learning social skills.

Recognize individual needs. Not all children are the same. They have different needs for sleep, food, and exercise, and they grow and develop at different paces.

Be nonjudgmental. As with any client, you must accept a child regardless of disabilities or problems.

Always call your supervisor if symptoms continue. As with all clients, follow instructions in the care plan or your assignment sheet carefully.

❑ 11. Identify five guidelines for working with children

The following suggestions by home health care professionals may help you establish a trusting and honest relationship with the children in your care. See **Box 9-1**, page 258.

❑ 12. List the signs of child abuse and neglect and know how to report them

Child abuse is the physical, sexual, or psychological mistreatment of a child. Children who are abused can range in age from infant to adolescent. Sexual abuse of children includes inappropriate touching of a child's body, sexual contact, or penetration. Psychological abuse includes verbal abuse, such as name calling, social isolation, and seclusion. **Child neglect** is the conscious or unconscious failure to provide for the needs of a child. Children who are neglected may not receive adequate food, water, medications, supervision, or shelter.

Children should never be harmed, threatened, or teased. They must be treated with respect and concern. Adults must talk to children calmly and quietly and give them positive comments, praise, and encouragement.

Child abuse or neglect can come from anyone who is responsible for a child's care, including parents, guardians, paid caregivers, teachers, friends, or relatives. Our society has become increasingly conscious of child abuse and neglect, and laws have been passed in many states requiring health pro-

Box 19-2.
Common Signs of Child Abuse

▶ Child has burns, cuts, bruises, abrasions, or fractured bones.

▶ Child stares vacantly or watches intensely.

▶ Child is extremely quiet.

▶ Child avoids eye contact. In some cultures, however, it is the norm to avoid eye contact.

▶ Child is afraid of adults.

▶ Child behaves aggressively.

▶ Child exhibits excessive activity or hyperactivity. Some hyperactive children, however, have a chemical imbalance that produces this behavior.

▶ Child tells you that someone is abusing him or her.

fessionals to report suspected child abuse. If you observe or suspect abuse or neglect, or if a child reports that someone has abused or neglected him or her, you must immediately report this to your supervisor. You and your agency can get into trouble for *not* reporting suspected child abuse or neglect.

If you observe any of these signs of child abuse or neglect, or if you suspect abuse or neglect, speak to your supervisor immediately. Your employer may have specific policies and procedures for reporting suspected abuse in the home. Follow these, or ask your supervisor how to handle the situation.

Chapter 20

Common Chronic and Acute Conditions

1. Define arthritis

Arthritis (ar-THRYE-tis) is a general term that refers to inflammation of the joints that causes stiffness, pain, and decreased mobility. Arthritis may be the result of aging, injury, or an **autoimmune illness,** in which the body's immune system attacks normal tissue in the body. There are several types of arthritis.

Osteoarthritis (AH-stee-oh-ar-thrye-tis). The more common type of arthritis, osteoarthritis affects many elderly clients to some extent. Osteoarthritis may occur with aging or as the result of joint injury. It commonly affects the hips and knees, which are weight-bearing joints. However, joints of the fingers, thumbs, and spine can also be affected. Pain and stiffness seem to increase in cold or damp weather.

Rheumatoid Arthritis (ROOM-a-toyd ar-THRYE-tis). Rheumatoid arthritis can affect people of all ages (**Fig. 20-1**). Physicians believe that an infection activates the immune system's inflammatory response, causing an attack on normal connective tissue in the joints and throughout the body. The joints become inflamed, red, swollen, and very painful, and movement is eventually restricted. Fever, fatigue, and weight loss are also symptoms. Rheumatoid arthritis usually affects the small joints first, then progresses to larger ones. Other parts of the body that may be affected are the heart, lungs, eyes, kidneys, and skin.

2. Identify common treatments for arthritis

Arthritis is generally treated with some or all of the following:

▶ anti-inflammatory medications such as aspirin or ibuprofen

▶ local applications of heat to reduce swelling and pain

▶ range of motion exercises

▶ a regular exercise and/or activity regimen

▶ diet to reduce weight or maintain strength

3. Identify five care guidelines for clients with arthritis

Keep the following guidelines in mind when caring for clients with arthritis:

1. **Watch for stomach irritation or heartburn caused by aspirin or ibuprofen.** Some clients cannot tolerate these medications. Report signs of stomach irritation immediately.

2. **Encourage activity.** Gentle activity can help reduce the effects of arthritis. Follow the care plan instructions and your assignment sheet carefully. Use canes or other walking aids as needed.

3. **Adapt activities of daily living (ADLs) to allow independence.** Many devices are available to allow clients to bathe, dress, and feed themselves even when arthritis has impaired their abilities. Choose clothing that is easy to put on and fasten. Suggest handrails and safety bars for the bathroom. Special utensils are available to make it easier for clients to feed themselves (**Fig. 20-2**).

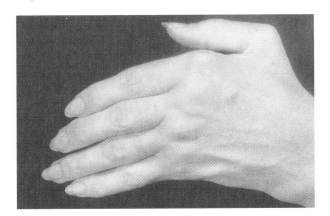

Fig. 20-1. Rheumatoid arthritis can affect people of all ages.

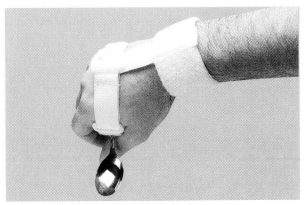

Fig. 20-2. Adaptive equipment can help a person with arthritis continue to perform ADLs independently.

4. Treat each client as an individual. Because arthritis is so common among elderly clients, you may be tempted to assume each client experiences the same symptoms and needs the same care. This is not true; the disease affects each person differently and the care plan may vary. Follow the care plan and your assignments for each individual.

5. Help maintain client's morale. Although arthritis is common, it is a chronic, painful, degenerative disease, the effects of which can be devastating for some clients. By encouraging self-care, maintaining a positive attitude, and listening to the client's feelings, you can help him or her manage the disease and remain independent for as long as possible.

Part 2
Caring for the Client with Cancer

❑ 4. Define cancer

Cancer is a general term used to describe many types of malignant tumors. A tumor (TOO-mer) is a cluster of abnormally growing cells. Benign (bee-NINE) tumors grow slowly in local areas and are considered noncancerous. Malignant (ma-LIG-nant) tumors grow rapidly and invade surrounding tissues.

Cancer can not only invade local tissue, but it can spread or metastasize (me-TAS-ta-size) to other parts of the body. When a cancer has metastasized, it has spread from the site where it first appeared, and now affects one or more other body systems. This process is called metastasis (me-TAS-ta-sis). In general, treatment is more difficult and cancer is more deadly after metastasis has occurred. Cancer often appears first in the breast, colon, rectum, uterus, prostate, lungs, or skin.

Although many advances in cancer research have been made in the past twenty years, there is no known cure for cancer. Cancer appears to overwhelm the body's immune system when tumors grow too large or develop in areas of the body that cannot be reached by the infection-fighting cells of the immune system. However, some treatments (discussed below) are effective.

❑ 5. List eight risk factors for cancer

Risk Factors. Although we do not know the exact cause of cancer, certain behaviors and environmental factors appear to contribute to cancer:

1. Smoking. Smoking is responsible for 83% of all cases of lung cancer: 85% among men and 75% among women. Approximately 174,000 cancer deaths in 1997 were related to tobacco use.

2. Sunlight. Approximately 900,000 cases of skin cancer were diagnosed in 1997. Many of these cancers could have been prevented by using protection from the sun's rays (**Fig. 20-3**).

3. Alcohol. Cancer of the mouth, throat, larynx, esophagus, and liver is diagnosed more commonly among persons who drink heavily. Approximately 19,000 cancer deaths in 1997 were linked to excessive alcohol use.

4. Chemicals and industrial agents. Asbestos, vinyl chloride, large quantities of pesticides and herbicides, and other substances increase the risk of certain cancers.

5. Food additives. Esophageal and stomach cancer have been linked to foods that are smoked, salt-cured, or that contain nitrites.

6. Radiation. Excessive exposure to high doses of radiation can cause cancer. Diagnostic x-rays have been adjusted so that optimal imaging can be obtained with minimal doses. Radon (RAY-don), a natural source of radiation in the environment, is also a risk factor for

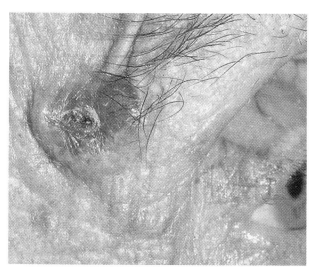

Fig. 20-3. Excessive exposure to sun can lead to skin cancer.

lung cancer. Homes should be tested for radon and proper action should be taken if levels are high.

7. Nutrition. Diets that are low in fiber and high in fat appear to contribute to cancer of the breast, colon, and prostate. Obese people are at risk for colon, breast, and uterine cancer.

8. Estrogen. Estrogen replacement in menopausal women increases the risk for cancer of the lining of the uterus.

❏ 6. List seven warning signs of cancer

When diagnosed early, cancer can often be treated and controlled. The American Cancer Society has identified seven warning signs of cancer.

The American Cancer Society's Seven Warning Signs of Cancer:

1. change in bowel or bladder habits

2. a sore that does not heal

3. unusual bleeding or discharge from a body opening

4. a thickening or lump in the breast or elsewhere

5. persistent indigestion or difficulty swallowing

6. an obvious change in a wart or mole

7. persistent hoarseness or a nagging cough

❏ 7. Identify the three common treatments for cancer and list their side effects

People with cancer can often live longer and can sometimes recover from cancer if they are treated using the following methods. These treatments are most effective when tumors are discovered early. Often these treatments are used in combination.

1. Surgery. Surgery is the front line of defense for most forms of cancer and is the key treatment for malignant tumors of the skin, breast, bladder, colon, rectum, stomach, and muscle. Surgeons attempt to remove as much of the tumor as possible to prevent cancer from spreading.

2. Chemotherapy. Chemotherapy refers to medications given to fight cancer. Certain drugs have been developed to destroy cancer cells and limit the rate of cell growth. However, many of these drugs are toxic to the body and destroy healthy cells as well as cancer cells. Chemotherapy can have severe side effects, including nausea, vomiting, diarrhea, hair loss, and decreased resistance to infection.

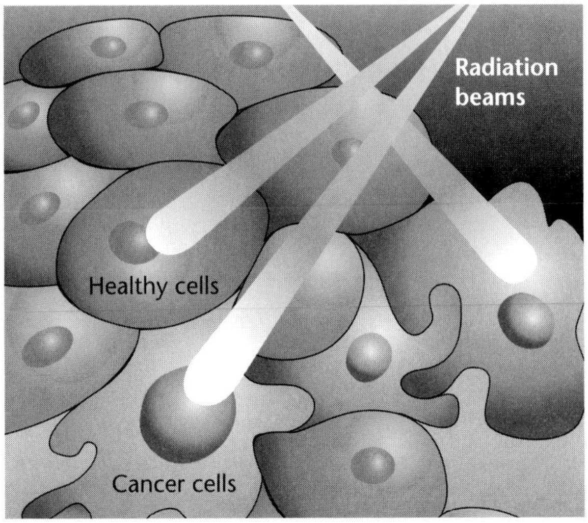

Fig. 20-4. Radiation is targeted at cancer cells, but it also destroys some healthy cells in its path.

3. Radiation. Radiation kills normal as well as abnormal cells. Radiation therapy directs radiation to a limited area to kill only cancer cells, but other cells in its path are also destroyed (**Fig. 20-4**). By controlling cell growth, radiation can reduce pain. Radiation can cause the same side effects as chemotherapy. The skin of the area exposed to radiation may become sore, irritated, and sometimes burned.

❏ 8. Discuss four guidelines for effective communication with the client who has cancer

Coping with cancer can be a tremendous challenge. Keep the following guidelines in mind when working with clients who have cancer.

1. Each case is different. Cancer is a general term and refers to many separate situations. Clients may expect to live many years or only several months. Treatment affects each person differently. Don't make assumptions about a client's condition.

2. Clients may want to talk or may avoid talking. Respect each client's needs. Listen if a client wants to share feelings or experiences with you, but never push a client to talk. If you think a client needs to talk but is not comfortable talking to you, report this to your supervisor.

3. Be honest. Never tell a client everything will be okay. You do not know that it will, and for many people with cancer, it will not. Discussing the client's prognosis or outlook is not within the scope of your practice. Instead, maintain a positive attitude and focus on concrete details. For example, comment if a client seems stronger today, or notice that the sun is shining outside.

4. Be sensitive. Remember that cancer is a disease, and we do not know its cause. Some people believe that cancer is caused in part by negative thoughts or emotions and can be cured by eliminating negativity and focusing on love and faith. While a positive attitude may contribute to good health in general, this way of looking at cancer can also lead to feelings of responsibility and guilt about the disease if the condition worsens. Never discuss the causes of a client's cancer.

❑ 9. Describe ways to help clients with cancer

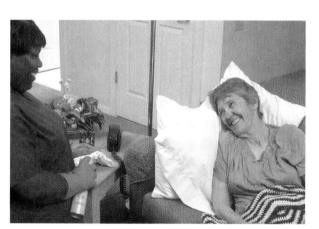

Fig. 20-5. Distractions such as conversation or music can help a client with cancer deal with pain.

Nutrition. Good nutrition is extremely important for clients with cancer. Follow the care plan instructions and your assignments carefully. In general, clients need many calories and should be served four to six meals a day. Serve favorite foods that are high in nutrition. Some doctors recommend serving fluids between meals so clients can eat more at meals. Liquid nutrition supplements may also be used in addition to, not in place of, meals. If nausea or swallowing is a problem, try to find foods such as soups, gelatin, or starches that may appeal to the client.

Pain control. Cancer can cause terrible pain, especially in the late stages. Watch your client for signs of pain. Observe the client's use of pain medication. Assist with comfort measures, including repositioning and providing distractions such as conversation, music, or reading materials (**Fig. 20-5**). Report to your supervisor if pain seems to be uncontrolled.

Skin care. Use lotion regularly on dry or delicate skin. Do not apply lotion to areas receiving radiation therapy. Offer back rubs to provide comfort and increase circulation. For clients who spend many hours in bed, egg crate mattress covers or sheepskins may be more comfortable. Moving to a chair for some period of time may improve comfort as well. Clients who are very weak or immobile need to be repositioned every two hours.

Oral care. Help clients brush and floss teeth regularly. Medications, nausea, vomiting, or mouth infections such as thrush may cause a bad taste in the mouth. If the client is receiving chemotherapy, he is at risk for oral discomfort. Using a soft-bristled toothbrush or a Toothette, rinsing with baking soda and water, or using a prescribed rinse, can all help ease discomfort. Do *not* use a commercial mouthwash, as the alcohol in it can further irritate the client's mouth.

Odor control. People suffering from cancer, especially in the late stages, may have an unpleasant odor at times. You can use a room deodorizer to mask any odor you notice. However, you should check with the client before using a deodorizer, as a new smell may trigger or worsen nausea.

Self-image. People with cancer may suffer from a low self-image because they are weak and their appearance has changed (for example, hair loss is a common side effect of chemotherapy). Help your client feel more attractive by bathing and dressing, and using hats or scarves to cover the head. Assist with makeup if the client desires. Your concern and interest can help improve self-image.

Psychosocial needs. If visitors help cheer your client, encourage them and do not intrude. If some times of day are better than others, suggest this to the client's friends or family. Support groups exist for people with cancer and their families. Check with your supervisor for referrals in your area. It may help a person with cancer to think of something besides cancer and treatment for a while. Pursue other topics and get to know what interests your clients have. As always, report any signs of depression immediately (Chapter 18 describes the signs of depression).

Family assistance. Caring for a person with cancer at home can be very difficult for family members. Be alert to needs that are not being met or stresses created by the illness. Report your observations. Know the resources available in your area.

❏ 10. Identify community resources available to people with cancer and their families

Numerous services and support groups are available for people with cancer and their families or caregivers. Hospitals, hospice programs, churches, and synagogues offer many resources, including meal services, transportation to doctors' offices or hospitals, counseling, and support groups. Check the local yellow pages under "cancer," or call the local or state chapter of the American Cancer Society.

Part 3
Caring for the Client with Diabetes

❏ 11. Define diabetes and name two types

Diabetes mellitus (dye-a-BEE-tees mel-EYE-tus), commonly called diabetes, is a metabolic (met-a-BOL-ic) disease of the endocrine (EN-doh-krin) system (see Chapter 9 for more on the endocrine system). The pancreas (PAN-kree-as) does not produce a sufficient supply of insulin (IN-su-lin). Insulin is the substance the body needs to convert glucose (GLOO-kohs), or natural sugar, into energy for the body. If insulin is not present to process the glucose, it accumulates in the blood, causing problems with circulation and possibly damaging vital organs.

Diabetes commonly occurs in people with a family history of the illness, the elderly, and people who are obese. Two types of diabetes have been identified:

Type I, or insulin-dependent diabetes mellitus (IDDM), is often called juvenile diabetes because it typically appears before age twenty and continues throughout a person's life. However, a person can develop Type I diabetes up to age 40. Type I diabetes is treated with insulin and a special diet.

Type II, or noninsulin dependent diabetes mellitus (NIDDM) appears in adults and can usually be controlled with diet and/or oral medications. This type is also called adult-onset diabetes. Type II diabetes usually has a gradual onset and is the milder form of diabetes mellitus. It typically develops around age 35, and often occurs in obese individuals.

❏ 12. Recognize signs of diabetes

People with diabetes mellitus may have the following signs and symptoms:

Box 20-1.
Observing and Reporting:
Clients with Cancer

Report any of the following to your supervisor:

▶ increased weakness or fatigue

▶ weight loss

▶ nausea, vomiting, diarrhea

▶ changes in appetite

▶ fainting

▶ signs of depression (see Chapter 18 for a discussion of these signs)

▶ confusion

▶ blood in stool or urine

▶ change in mental status

▶ changes in skin integrity

▶ new lumps, sores, or rashes

▶ increase in pain, or pain unrelieved by current measures

Report any of the following to your supervisor:

▶ any breakdown in the skin

▶ change in appetite (client overeating or not eating enough)

▶ weight changes

▶ changes in mental status

▶ increase or decrease in urine output

▶ visual changes

▶ change in mobility

▶ change in sensation

▶ increased thirst

▶ increased hunger

▶ weight loss

▶ elevated levels of blood sugar

▶ presence of sugar in the urine

▶ increased frequency of urination

❑ 13. Recognize complications of diabetes

Diabetes can lead to the following complications:

▶ Changes in the circulatory system can cause heart attack and stroke, reduced circulation to the extremities, poor wound healing, and kidney and nerve damage.

▶ Damage to the eye can cause impaired vision and blindness.

▶ Poor circulation and impaired wound healing may result in leg and foot ulcers, infected wounds, and gangrene. Gangrene can lead to amputation. Good foot care is vitally important for people with diabetes (see Procedure 1).

❑ 14. Describe the differences between insulin shock and diabetic coma, and list care for each

Insulin shock and **diabetic coma** are complications of diabetes that can be life-threatening. Discuss each individual client's status with your supervisor.

Insulin shock, or hypoglycemia (hye-poh-glye-SEE-mee-a), can result from either too much insulin or too little food. It frequently occurs when a dose of insulin is administered and the person with the illness skips a meal or does not eat all the food required. Even when a regular amount of food is eaten, excessive physical activity may rapidly metabolize the food so that the amount of insulin in the body is excessive. Vomiting and diarrhea may also lead to insulin shock in people with diabetes.

The first signs of insulin shock include feeling weak or "different," nervousness, dizziness, and perspiration (see list below for further signs). These are signals that the client needs food in a form that can be rapidly absorbed. A lump of sugar, a hard candy, or a glass of orange juice should be consumed right away. The client who is diabetic should always have a quick source of sugar handy. Contact your supervisor if the client has shown early signs of insulin shock.

The following are signs and symptoms of insulin shock:

▶ hunger

▶ weakness

▶ rapid pulse

▶ headache

▶ low blood pressure

▶ perspiration

▶ cold, clammy skin

▶ confusion

▶ trembling

▶ nervousness

▶ blurred vision

▶ numbness of the lips and tongue

▶ unconsciousness

Diabetic coma, also known as acidosis (a-sid-OH-sis) or hyperglycemia (high-per-glye-SEE-mee-a), is caused by having too little insulin. It can result from undiagnosed diabetes, going without insulin or not taking enough, eating too much food, not getting enough exercise, and physical or emotional stress.

The signs of diabetic coma include increased thirst or urination, abdominal pain, deep or labored breathing, and breath that smells sweet or fruity (see complete list of symptoms below). Call your supervisor immediately if you suspect your client is experiencing diabetic coma or insulin shock. Know and follow your agency's policies and procedures for when to call emergency services.

Other signs and symptoms of diabetic coma include the following:

- hunger
- weakness
- rapid, weak pulse
- headache
- low blood pressure
- dry skin
- flushed cheeks
- drowsiness
- slow, deep, and labored breathing
- nausea and vomiting
- abdominal pain
- sweet, fruity breath odor
- air hunger, or client gasping for air and being unable to catch his breath
- unconsciousness

❏ 15. List five guidelines for care of the client with diabetes

Diabetes must be carefully controlled to prevent complications and severe illness. When working with clients with diabetes, follow care plan instructions and your assignments to the letter, paying special attention to the following guidelines:

1. **Follow diet instructions exactly.** The intake of **carbohydrates**, including breads, potatoes, grains, pasta, and sugars, must be regulated. Meals must be eaten at the same time each day, and the client must eat everything that is served. If a client refuses to eat what is directed, or if you suspect that he or she is not following the diet when you leave, report this to your supervisor. More information on diet for a person with diabetes is provided in learning objective 16 in this chapter.

2. **Be sure client follows exercise program.** Because exercise affects the body's rate of metabolism and the amount of insulin produced by the pancreas, a regular exercise program is important. Exercise also helps improve circulation. Exercises may include walking or other active exercise, or passive range of motion exercises. Encourage the client to perform the exercises provided in the client care plan, and assist as necessary. Try to make it fun. A walk can be a chore or it can be the highlight of the day.

3. **Observe the client's management of insulin doses.** Doses are calculated exactly and should be administered at the same time each day, or exactly according to instructions in the care plan. *Home care aides are not permitted to inject insulin.* However, you may be asked to bring the insulin and supplies to the client, to check the expiration date, to store the insulin (usually in the refrigerator), and/or to keep a record of where on the body the insulin was injected.

4. **Perform urine and blood tests as directed.** Sometimes the care plan will specify that a client's blood or urine be tested daily to determine sugar or insulin levels. Home care aides are sometimes assigned to perform these tests; however, not all states allow home care aides to do this. Your agency will train you, and you will be tested for competency before you are asked to perform this procedure.

5. **Perform foot care only as directed.** Because circulation may be decreased in people with diabetes, they are susceptible to ulcers and sores that may not heal. Even a small sore on the leg or foot can grow into a large wound that could result in amputation. Careful foot care, including inspection, monitoring, and prevention, is very important for diabetic clients. The goals of diabetic foot care are to check for signs of irritation or sores, to stimulate blood circulation, and to prevent infection.

Procedure 1: Providing foot care for the diabetic client

1. Wash your hands.

2. Explain what you will do.

3. Assemble supplies:

- basin of warm water
- mild soap
- gloves
- washcloth
- soft towel
- lotion
- cotton balls
- cotton socks
- shoes or slipper

4. Put on gloves.

5. Using the washcloth and soap, wash the feet gently. Rinse with the warm water.

6. Pat the feet dry gently, wiping between the toes.

7. Starting at the toes and working up to the ankles, gently rub lotion into the feet with circular strokes. Your goal is to increase circulation, so take several minutes on each foot.

8. Observe the feet, ankles, and legs for dry skin, irritation, blisters, redness, sores, corns, discoloration, or swelling.

9. Help client put on socks and shoes or slippers.

10. Put used linens in the laundry. Pour water into the toilet. Clean and store basin and supplies.

11. Remove gloves.

12. Wash your hands.

13. Document the procedure, including any abnormalities you observed on the feet or legs.

Box 20-3.
Using Meal Plans and Exchange Lists to Control Diet

The following is a sample meal plan and a partial exchange list a person with diabetes might use. Keep in mind that this is only an example. A client's diet may also be under other restrictions, and the diet will vary according to the client's daily calorie needs. Exchange lists contain many more choices than the sample below.

Sample Meal Plan

Breakfast (to be eaten between 7:30 and 8:30 am): two starches, one milk, one fruit, one fat

Snack (to be eaten between 10 and 11 am): one milk

Lunch (12:30 to 1:30 pm): one meat, one milk, two starches, one vegetable, one fruit

Snack (3:00 to 4:00 pm): one vegetable, one milk

Dinner (5:30 to 6:30 pm): three meats, one starch, two vegetables, one milk, two fats

Snack (7:30 to 8:30 pm): one milk, one starch

Following the meal plan for what types of food and how many servings to eat, the person chooses specific foods and determines serving size using the exchange lists.

Exchange List Sample Items

Starch list: 1 slice of bread, ½ bagel, ½ cup cereal, ½ cup pasta, ½ cup rice, 1 baked potato, 3 cups popcorn, 15-20 fat-free potato chips

Milk list: 1 cup milk (skim, 1%, 2%, or whole, depending on other dietary guidelines), ¾ cup yogurt

Fruit list: ½ cup unsweetened applesauce, 1 small banana, ½ cup orange juice, 2 tablespoons raisins, 1 small orange, ½ cup canned pears

Vegetable list: ½ cup cooked vegetables or vegetable juice, 1 cup raw vegetables (not included are corn, potatoes, and peas, which are on the starch exchange list instead)

Meat list: 1 oz. meat, fish, poultry, or cheese, 1 egg, or ½ cup dried beans

Fat list: 1 teaspoon margarine or butter, 2 teaspoons peanut butter, 2 tablespoons sour cream, 1 tsp mayonnaise, 10 peanuts

In addition to daily foot care, people with diabetes should be encouraged to wear comfortable, well-fitting shoes that do not irritate or hurt the feet. To avoid cuts or injuries to the feet, diabetics should never go barefoot. Cotton socks are best because they absorb perspiration. *Home care aides should never cut any client's toenails, but especially not a diabetic client's toenails.* Only a nurse or physician should cut the toenails of a person with diabetes because, as explained before, even a small cut on the foot can lead to a very serious wound.

❑ 16. Describe a meal plan for the client with diabetes

People with diabetes must be very careful about what they eat. In order to keep their blood glucose levels near normal, they must eat the right amount of the right type of food at the right time. To make it easier to keep track of what they should be eating, people with diabetes are usually taught to follow **meal plans** and use **exchange lists**.

A dietitian, working closely with the client, will make up a meal plan that includes all the right types and amounts of food for each day. Then the client uses exchange lists, or lists of similar foods that can substitute for one another, to make up a menu for each day. For example, the meal plan might call for one starch and one fruit to be eaten as a snack. Looking at the exchange list, the client may choose *which* starch and fruit he wants to eat. The list has many choices, from bagels to biscuits to pretzels. The equivalent serving size for each food is also given, so the person will get the right amount of carbohydrates, protein, and fat to meet the meal plan requirements. Using meal plans and exchange lists, a person with diabetes can control his diet while still making his own food choices.

Home care aides are not responsible for making up meal plans. A dietitian will create meal plans, provide exchange lists, and train the client to use them. If you are assigned to prepare food for the client, however, you should follow the diet exactly. If you observe the client not following his or her diet, report it to your supervisor.

❑ 17. Define cerebral vascular accident (CVA) and list common warning signs

The medical term for a stroke is a cerebral vascular accident (ser-EE-bral VAS-kyoo-lar AK- si-dent; or CVA). The term indicates that CVA has something to do with the brain (cerebrum) and something to do with the blood vessels (vascular). CVA, or stroke, is caused when blood supply to the brain is cut off suddenly by a clot or a ruptured blood vessel (**Fig. 20-6**). The section of the brain that was fed by the damaged blood vessel no longer receives oxygen, and cells die. Brain tissue is further damaged by leaking blood, clots, and swelling that cause pressure on surrounding areas of healthy tissue.

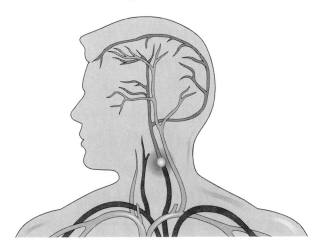

Fig. 20-6. CVA, or stroke, is caused when blood supply to the brain is cut off suddenly by a clot or a ruptured blood vessel.

A transient ischemic attack (TRAN-see-ent is-KEE-mik a-TAK), or **TIA**, is a warning sign of a CVA. It is the result of a temporary lack of oxygen in the brain and may last several days, weeks, or months. Symptoms include tingling, weakness, or some loss of movement in an extremity. These symptoms should not be ignored. Report any of these symptoms to your supervisor immediately.

A stroke may be preceded by symptoms that signal the oncoming hemorrhage or blockage. These symptoms may include dizziness, ringing in the ears, headache, nausea, vomiting, slurring of words, and loss of memory. These symptoms should also be reported immediately.

Signs that a stroke is occurring include any of the following: loss of consciousness, redness in the face, noisy breathing, seizures, loss of bowel and bladder control, hemiplegia (hem-i-PLEE-jee-a), hemiparesis (hem-i-pa-REE-sis), aphasia (a-FAY-see-a), use of inappropriate words, elevated blood pressure, and slow pulse rate. Hemiplegia refers to paralysis on one side of the body. Hemiparesis refers to weakness on one side of the body. Aphasia is the inability to speak or to speak clearly.

Because the two sides of the brain control different functions, symptoms will indicate the side of the brain in which the stroke occurred. Weaknesses on the right side of the body indicate that the *left* side of the brain was affected. Weaknesses on the left side of the body indicate that the *right* side of the brain was affected.

❑ 18. Describe six common physical changes in CVA clients

Strokes can be mild or severe. After a stroke, a client may experience any of the following:

▶ weakness or paralysis on one side of the body

▶ difficulty speaking or inability to speak

▶ loss of sensations such as temperature or touch

▶ loss of bowel or bladder control

▶ confusion

▶ poor judgment

▶ memory loss

▶ loss of cognitive abilities

▶ tendency to ignore one side of the body

However, in the case of a mild stroke the client may experience few, if any, of these effects. Physical therapy may help stroke victims regain physical abilities. Speech therapy and occupational therapy can also be useful in helping a person who has had a stroke learn to communicate and perform ADLs again.

❑ 19. Describe guidelines for care of the CVA client

Clients who have had a stroke will need care that is specific to their disabilities. A client with hemiplegia will need different care than a client with speech loss. Follow the care plan and your assignments for each client, but keep the following general guidelines in mind.

Paralysis, weakness, or loss of movement. Clients with these effects will usually be receiving physical therapy or occupational therapy. You may be asked to participate in the therapy by helping clients perform exercises or try to use their limbs. range of motion exercises will help strengthen muscles and keep joints mobile. Clients may also be instructed to perform leg exercises to improve circulation. Safety is always the most important when post-CVA clients are exercising.

When providing personal care for clients with one-sided paralysis or weakness, you will need to adapt procedures. When helping with transfers or walking, stand on the weaker side. Always use a gait belt for safety.

Never refer to the weaker side as the "bad side," or talk about the "bad" leg or arm. Use the terms **weaker** or **involved** to refer to the side with paralysis or paresis. Or, focus on the **uninvolved** side, the side without weakness or paralysis.

Speech loss or communication problems. If a client is receiving speech therapy, you may be asked to help with exercises. These may include helping clients recognize written words or speak words.

Use verbal and nonverbal communication to express your positive attitude. Let the client know you have confidence in his or her abilities through your smiles, touches, and gestures. Gestures and pointing can also help you convey practical information or allow the client to speak to you. For more ideas for communicating with CVA clients, see learning objective 20 in this chapter.

Confusion or memory loss. In some clients, a stroke will result in changes in thinking and emotions. In some cases, multiple strokes can cause a form of dementia, similar to the changes that occur in people with Alzheimer's disease. Working with clients who are confused or forgetful requires a lot of patience. Again, your positive attitude will be important. Establishing a routine of care will also help make the client feel more secure. More information on working with clients with dementia can be found in Part 7 of this chapter, Caring for the Client with Alzheimer's Disease or Other Dementias.

Safety. Monitoring the home safety of clients who have had a stroke is essential. Clients who are unsteady, weak, or confused are at risk of falling. Clients with loss of sensation are at risk of burning themselves in the bathroom or at the stove. Some safety tips include:

▶ Remove any hazards from the home, including unnecessary clutter or throw rugs.

▶ Unplug appliances like toasters and coffee makers when not in use.

▶ Check the refrigerator and cabinets for spoiled food. A stroke may impair the senses of smell and taste.

▶ Report any suspected safety hazards to your supervisor.

▶ Follow instructions for safe client transfers using good body mechanics (see Chapters 6 and 12).

▶ Always check on the client's body alignment. Sometimes an arm or leg can be caught and the client is unaware.

▶ Pay special attention to skin care and observing for changes in the skin if a client is unable to move.

Box 20-4.
Assisting in Rehabilitation of the Client Who Has Had a Stroke

You will often be called upon to help in the rehabilitation of a person who has suffered a stroke. Depending on where in the brain the stroke occurred, these clients commonly have weakness or paralysis on one side, difficulty with speaking and swallowing, and occasionally, loss of half of the visual field in one or both eyes.

People who have had a stroke typically have a long recovery period. Therefore, it is important to work with them in stages or steps that allow them to master simple goals first, such as strengthening a weak arm. By doing this you will help them gain confidence in their difficult fight to regain strength and ability.

Many people who have had strokes have one-sided weakness of the arm and hand or leg and

foot. Encourage the client to use and exercise the weaker side. Instruct him or her to use the strong arm or leg to assist the range of motion exercises on the weak side. Rolling over onto the strong side first is recommended for changing positions. Remind recovering stroke clients to place the strong foot under the involved ankle when crossing the legs in preparation for rolling over or moving the leg (**Fig. 20-7**). If the client is in the sitting position, place the elbow on an armrest to support the involved shoulder (**Fig. 20-8**). Ninety-

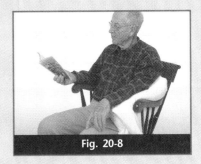
Fig. 20-8

degree flexion is a good position for the weak hip and knee. It is very important for you to remember to position the involved side correctly, because often a person who has had a stroke cannot feel that one side of the body is weaker than the other (**Fig. 20-9**).

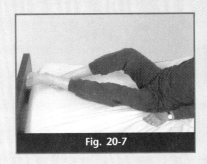
Fig. 20-7

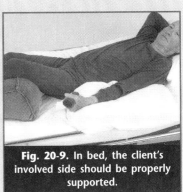
Fig. 20-9. In bed, the client's involved side should be properly supported.

Encouraging independence and self-esteem. Whatever the effects of the stroke, clients should be encouraged to learn to care for themselves again as much as possible. Let the client do things for him or herself whenever possible, even if you could do a better or faster job. Appreciate and acknowledge clients' efforts to do things for themselves even when they are unsuccessful. Praise even the smallest successes to build confidence.

Guidelines for assisting the client with one-sided weakness with transfers, dressing, and eating.

Many CVA clients will have some degree of weakness on one side of the body. The basic procedures for assisting with transfers (Chapters 12 and 13) can still be used when assisting a client who has a one-sided weakness. However, some additional guidelines must be remembered, for the client's safety and for yours.

When assisting with a transfer for a client with one-sided weakness, remember the following:

▶ Support the involved side.

▶ Lead with the uninvolved (stronger) side (**Fig. 20-10**).

▶ For your safety as well as your client's, follow the principles of good body mechanics (discussed in Chapter 6, Safety and Body Mechanics).

When assisting a client with one-sided weakness in getting dressed, remember the following:

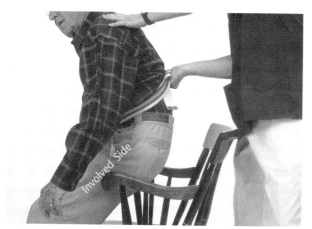

Fig. 20-10. When helping a CVA client with a transfer, stand on the client's weaker side and have the client lead with his stronger side.

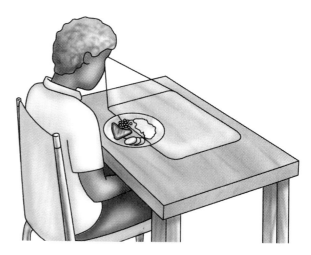

Fig. 20-11. The field of vision may be limited in a client who has had a CVA. Be sure the client can see what you place in front of him.

▶ Dress *involved* side first. Placing the weaker arm or leg into the clothing first prevents unnecessary bending and stretching of the limb to get it into arm- or legholes.

▶ Undress *uninvolved* side first. Leading with the stronger side and then removing the weaker arm or leg from clothing last prevents the limb from being stretched and twisted to remove the clothing.

▶ Use adaptive equipment to help client dress himself (see Chapters 13 and 15).

▶ Encourage self-care.

When assisting a client who has a one-sided weakness with eating, remember the following:

▶ Be sure to place food in the client's field of vision (**Fig. 20-11**).

▶ Use assistive devices such as silverware with built-up handle grips, plate guards, and drinking cups (see Chapter 15).

▶ Watch for signs of choking.

▶ Serve soft foods if swallowing is difficult.

❑ 20. Describe techniques for communicating with the CVA client

Depending on the severity of the stroke and the degree of speech loss or confusion, the following tips may be helpful:

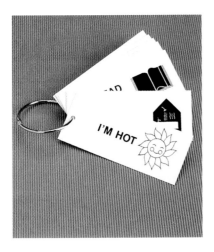

Fig. 20-12. Picture cards can help a post-CVA client communicate.

▶ Keep your questions and directions simple.

▶ Phrase questions so they can be answered with a yes or no.

▶ Agree on signals, such as shaking or nodding the head, or raising a hand or finger to indicate yes or no.

▶ Use pictures, gestures, or pointing. A simple set of pictures, including a bathroom, a glass of water, food, a person walking, a person in a bed or a chair, and so on, can allow a client to express needs without words (**Fig. 20-12**).

▶ Use a pencil and paper if a client is able to write. A pencil or pen with a thick grip or with tape wrapped around it may help the client hold it more easily.

▶ Use a bell or other call signal so client can let you know you are needed.

▶ Never talk about a client as if he or she were not there. Speak to all clients with respect.

sclerosis (ath-er-oh-skle-ROH-sis), or hardening and narrowing of the blood vessels (**Fig. 20-13**). Hypertension can also result from kidney disease, tumors of the adrenal gland, complications of pregnancy, and head injury. Hypertension can develop in persons of any age.

Symptoms. Signs and symptoms of hypertension are not always obvious, especially in the early stages of the disease. Often the illness is only discovered when a blood pressure measurement is taken in the doctor's office. Persons with the disease may complain of headache, blurred vision, and dizziness.

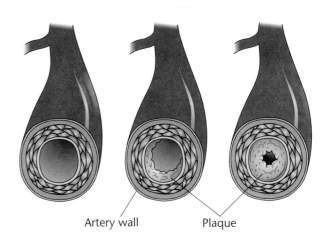

Artery wall   Plaque

Fig. 20-13. Arteries may become hardened, or narrower, because of a buildup of plaque on the walls of the blood vessels. Hardened arteries cause hypertension, or high blood pressure.

Part 5
Caring for the Client with Circulatory Disorders

❏ **21. Identify common circulatory disorders, their symptoms, and care guidelines**

Hypertension or High Blood Pressure

When blood pressure consistently measures higher than 140/90, a person is diagnosed as having hypertension (high-per-TEN-shun). The major cause of hypertension, or high blood pressure, is athero-

Care of a client with hypertension. Because hypertension can lead to serious conditions such as CVA, MI, kidney disease, or blindness, treatment to control high blood pressure is essential. Clients with hypertension will probably be taking medication such as cholesterol-lowering drugs and diuretics (dye-you-RET-iks). Diuretics are drugs that reduce fluid accumulation in the body. Clients with hypertension may also have a prescribed exercise program or be on a special low fat, low sodium diet. You will probably be required to take frequent, accurate blood pressure measurements. You can also help these clients by encouraging them to follow their diet and exercise programs.

Coronary Artery Disease (CAD)

Coronary artery disease occurs when atherosclerosis narrows the blood vessels in the coronary arteries, reducing the supply of blood to the heart muscle and depriving it of oxygen and nutrients. Over time, as fatty deposits block the artery, the muscle that was supplied by the blood vessel dies. CAD can lead to heart attack or stroke.

Angina Pectoris (an-JYE-na PEK-tor-is), or chest pain, originates from heart muscle that is not getting enough oxygen. The heart's need for oxygen is increased during exercise or exertion, stress, excitement, or a heavy meal. In coronary artery disease, constricted blood vessels prevent the extra blood with oxygen from getting to the heart (**Fig. 20-14**).

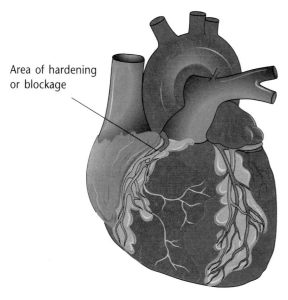

Area of hardening or blockage

Fig. 20-14. Angina pectoris results from the heart not getting enough oxygen.

Symptoms. The pain of angina pectoris is usually described as pressure or tightness in the left side of the chest or in the center behind the sternum or breastbone. Some people complain of the pain radiating or extending down the inside of the left arm or to the neck and left side of the jaw. A person suffering from angina pectoris may perspire or appear pale or grayish. The person may feel dizzy and have difficulty breathing.

Care of a person with angina pectoris. Rest is an extremely important aspect of care for a client who is having an episode of angina pectoris. Rest reduces the heart's need for extra oxygen, helping the blood flow return to a normal rate, often within three to fifteen minutes. Medication is also necessary to relax the walls of the coronary arteries, allowing them to dilate (DYE-late) or open to allow increased blood flow to the heart muscle. This medication, nitroglycerin (nite-roh-GLIS-er-in), comes as a small tablet that the client places under the tongue, where it is dissolved and rapidly absorbed into the circulatory system. Clients who have angina pectoris should keep nitroglycerin at hand to use as soon as symptoms arise. Clients may also be required to avoid heavy meals, overeating, overexertion, and exposure to cold or hot and humid weather.

Myocardial Infarction (MI) or Heart Attack

When blood flow to the heart muscle is completely blocked, oxygen and important nutrients fail to reach the cells in that region (**Fig. 20-15**). Waste products are not removed and the muscle cell dies. This is called a myocardial infarction (mye-oh-KAR-dee-al in-FARK-shun) or **MI**, coronary thrombosis (KOR-oh-nayr-ee throm-BOH-sis), or heart attack. The area of dead tissue may be large or small, depending on the artery involved.

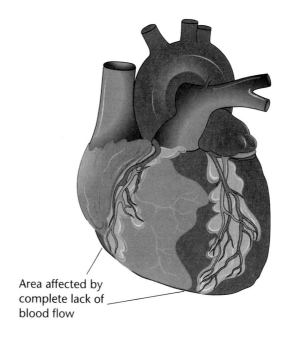

Area affected by complete lack of blood flow

Fig. 20-15. A heart attack occurs when blood flow to the heart or a portion of the heart is cut off completely.

Symptoms. A myocardial infarction is an emergency that can result in serious heart damage or death. The following are signs and symptoms of MI:

▶ sudden, severe pain in the chest, usually on the left side or in the center behind the sternum

▶ a feeling of indigestion or heartburn

▶ nausea and vomiting

▶ dyspnea (DISP-nee-a) or difficulty breathing

▶ dizziness

▶ skin color may be pale, grey, or cyanotic (sye-a-NOT-ik), a bluish color indicating lack of oxygen

▶ perspiration

▶ skin may feel cold and clammy

▶ weak and irregular pulse rate

▶ low blood pressure

▶ anxiety and a sense of impending doom

▶ denial

The pain of a heart attack is commonly described as a crushing, pressing, squeezing, stabbing, piercing, vise-like pain, or "like someone is sitting on my chest." It may radiate down the inside of the left arm. A person having a heart attack may also feel it in the neck and/or in the jaw. The pain does not go away, even when the person rests or takes nitroglycerin.

Care of a person who is having or recovering from a heart attack. Someone having a heart attack must receive emergency treatment from medical personnel to minimize damage and prevent further illness or death. Call 911 for emergency medical assistance immediately if a client is having a heart attack. If you are trained to perform cardiopulmonary resuscitation (CPR), do so if necessary when help is not available or until help arrives. Contact your supervisor after medical personnel arrive to take over care of the client.

The care of a client recovering from a heart attack will depend on the extent of the damage, whether they have had any complications, and how long it has been since the attack occurred. In general, clients who have had a heart attack will be placed on a regular exercise program and a diet that is low in fat and cholesterol. A low sodium diet and other changes in lifestyle may also be prescribed. Medications may be prescribed to regulate heart rate and blood pressure. Clients recovering from a heart attack may be cautioned to avoid exposure to cold temperatures.

Congestive Heart Failure (CHF)

When heart muscle has been severely damaged by coronary artery disease, heart attack, hypertension, or other disorders, the heart fails to pump effectively. Blood backs up into the heart instead of circulating. This failure of the heart muscle to pump effectively is called **congestive heart failure**, and it can occur on one or both sides of the heart.

Symptoms. Signs and symptoms of congestive heart failure include:

▶ difficulty breathing; coughing or gurgling with breathing

▶ dizziness, confusion, and fainting

▶ skin appears pale or cyanotic

▶ low blood pressure

▶ swelling of the feet and ankles

▶ bulging veins in the neck

▶ weight gain

Care of a client with congestive heart failure. Although congestive heart failure is a serious illness, it can be successfully treated and controlled. Medications are prescribed to strengthen the heart muscle and improve its pumping action. A low sodium diet may also be recommended. Home health care of clients with congestive heart failure may include the following:

▶ limited activity: a weakened heart pump may make it difficult for clients to walk, carry groceries, or climb stairs

▶ measurements of intake of fluids and output of urine (see Chapter 14)

▶ weight measurement to monitor accumulation of fluids (see Chapter 14)

- fluid reduction
- low sodium diet
- application of elastic stockings to reduce swelling in feet and ankles (see Chapter 14)
- range of motion exercises to improve muscle tone when activity and exercise are limited (see Chapter 15)
- assistance with personal care and ADLs (see Chapters 13 and 14)
- more frequent trips to the bathroom: many clients with congestive heart failure are on diuretics, in addition to heart medication
- observance for side effects of medications

A common side effect of medications for congestive heart failure is dizziness, which may result from a lack of potassium. This can easily be remedied by eating high-potassium foods and drinks such as bananas or raisins, orange juice, or other citrus juices. These foods should be eaten as a preventive measure as well. The client care plan should mention the possible side effects of drugs, and what signs or symptoms to report to your supervisor (also see Chapter 16).

> ### Part 6
> ### Caring for the Client with HIV/AIDS

❑ 22. Define HIV and AIDS and recognize their symptoms

Acquired immunodeficiency (im-YOU-noh-de-FISH-en-see) syndrome, or **AIDS**, is an illness caused by the **human immunodeficiency virus**, or **HIV**. HIV attacks the body's immune system and gradually disables it. Eventually the HIV-infected person has weakened resistance to other infections, and death is the result. HIV is a sexually transmitted disease, but it can also be spread through the blood, from infected needles, or to the fetus from its mother. More information on high-risk behaviors for contracting HIV, avoiding HIV, and transmission of HIV is provided in Chapter 9, The Human Body in Health and Disease.

Symptoms of HIV and AIDS. In general, HIV affects the body in stages. The first stage involves symptoms similar to flu, with fever, muscle aches, cough, and fatigue. These are symptoms of the body's immune system fighting the infection. As the infection worsens, the immune system overreacts and attacks not only the virus, but also normal tissue.

When the virus weakens the immune system in later stages, a cluster of problems may appear, including opportunistic infections, tumors, and central nervous system symptoms that would not occur if the immune system were healthy. This stage of the disease is known as AIDS.

In the late stages of AIDS, damage to the central nervous system may cause symptoms including memory loss, poor coordination, paralysis, and confusion. These symptoms together are known as **AIDS dementia complex**.

The following are the signs and symptoms of HIV infection and AIDS:

- appetite loss
- involuntary weight loss of 10 pounds or more
- vague, flu-like symptoms, including fever, cough, weakness, and severe or constant fatigue
- night sweats
- swollen lymph nodes in the neck, underarms, or groin
- excessive diarrhea
- dry cough
- skin rashes
- painful white spots in the mouth or on the tongue
- cold sores or fever blisters on the lips and flat, white ulcers on a reddened base in the mouth
- cauliflower-like warts, caused by the **human papilloma virus**, on the skin and in the mouth
- inflamed and bleeding gums
- bruising that does not go away
- susceptibility to infection, particularly pneumonia, but also tuberculosis, herpes, bacterial infections, and hepatitis
- **Kaposi's sarcoma**, a rare form of skin cancer that appears as purple or red skin lesions (**Fig. 20-16**)
- pneumocystis pneumonia (new-moh-SIS-tis new-MOH-nee-a), a lung infection
- AIDS dementia complex

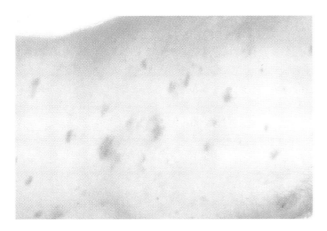

Fig. 20-16. Another sign of AIDS is a purple or red skin lesion called Kaposi's sarcoma.

Opportunistic infections, such as pneumonia, tuberculosis, and hepatitis, invade the body because the immune system is weak and unable to mount a vigorous defense. These illnesses complicate AIDS, may hasten immune deficiency, and are frequently the cause of death in people with AIDS.

AIDS-related complex or **ARC** is a combination of illnesses that is similar to AIDS. However, the symptoms of ARC are not as severe as AIDS symptoms. ARC may eventually lead to AIDS.

Persons who are infected with HIV are treated with antiviral drugs that slow the progress of the disease, but do not cure it. Other aspects of HIV treatment include relief of symptoms and prevention and treatment of opportunistic infection.

❑ 23. Define standard precautions and explain why you must follow them

You can help prevent the spread of HIV/AIDS by carefully following **standard precautions**. Standard precautions are described in detail in Chapter 5, but in short they mean treating blood and all body fluids as if they carried an infectious disease. Of course you will want to take special care when working with clients who have known HIV/AIDS. But the symptoms of HIV/AIDS may not appear for months or years after the infection is present. *This means that you and even the client him- or herself may not know the infection is present, and you could be infected accidentally.* But if you follow standard precautions

and other infection control procedures, and take the same care when working with all your clients, you will be safe from contracting HIV from clients.

❑ 24. List guidelines for care of the client with HIV/AIDS

You can provide valuable care for your clients who have HIV or AIDS. Their home health care will focus on the relief of symptoms and prevention of complications.

Weight Loss. Involuntary weight loss occurs in almost all people who develop AIDS. One goal of care is to preserve lean body mass with high protein, high calorie, and high nutrient meals and with fortified nutritional supplements.

Some people with HIV/AIDS lose their appetites and have difficulty eating. These clients should be encouraged to relax before meals and to eat in a pleasant setting. Serve familiar and favorite foods. Report appetite loss or difficulty eating to your supervisor. If appetite loss continues to be a problem, the physician may prescribe an appetite stimulant.

Food Handling. It is extremely important to carefully follow guidelines for safe food preparation and storage when working with a client who has HIV/AIDS. Food-borne illnesses caused by improperly cooking or storing food can cause death for someone with HIV/AIDS.

Chapter 23, Meal Planning, Shopping, Preparation, and Storage, discusses safe food handling in detail. In short, wash your hands frequently, keep everything clean (especially countertops, cutting boards, and knives after they have been used to cut meat), thaw food in the refrigerator, and wash and cook foods thoroughly. When storing food, keep cold foods cold and hot foods hot, use small containers that seal tightly, check expiration dates, and remember "when in doubt, throw it out."

Mouth Infections and Painful Swallowing. Clients who have infections of the mouth and esophagus may require food that is low in acid and neither cold nor hot. Spicy seasonings should be eliminated. Soft or pureed foods may be easier to swallow.

Drinking liquid meals and fortified drinks, such as milk shakes, may help ease the pain of chewing. If loose stools result from this regimen, liquid supplements that are high in fiber may be prescribed. Painful lesions of the mucous membranes of the mouth may be relieved with frequent rinses of warm salt water or other rinses prescribed by the doctor. Good mouth care is essential.

Nausea and Vomiting. Someone who has nausea or vomiting should eat small frequent meals, if they are tolerated, and eat slowly. The person should avoid high-fat and spicy foods, and eat a soft, bland diet of foods such as mashed potatoes, noodles, rice, crackers, pretzels, toast, gelatin, and clear soups. Cold foods that have little odor are usually easier to eat than hot foods. When nausea and vomiting persist or are severe, liquids and salty foods should be encouraged, including clear soups, clear juices, ginger ale and colas, saltines, and pretzels. Clients should eat small, frequent meals and drink fluids in between meals. Care must be taken to maintain an adequate intake of fluids.

Diarrhea. Clients who are experiencing mild diarrhea will most likely be placed on frequent small meals and a diet that is low in fat, fiber, and milk products. If diarrhea is severe, the client's physician may order a "BRAT" diet (a diet consisting of **b**ananas, **r**ice, **a**pples, and **t**oast). This diet, although nutritionally incomplete, is helpful for short-term use, and after several days, can be followed with other foods.

Because diarrhea rapidly depletes the body of fluids, rehydration or fluid replacement is necessary. Good rehydration fluids include water, juice, soda, and broth. Clients with diarrhea should avoid high fiber foods, including seeds, nuts, wheat brans, whole wheat bread, and the skins of fruits and vegetable. They should also avoid fats, milk, cheese, ice cream, beans, cabbage, spicy foods, and caffeine.

Neuropathy. Neuropathy (NOOR-oh-path-ee), or numbness, tingling, and pain in the feet and legs is usually treated with pain medications. Going without shoes or wearing loose, soft slippers may be helpful. If blankets and sheets cause pain, construct

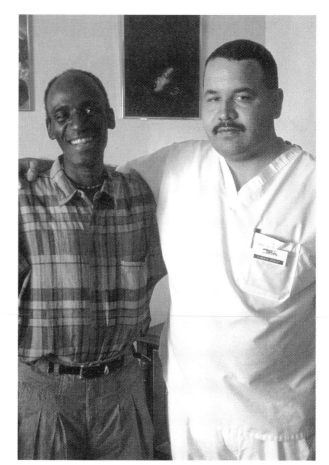

Fig. 20-17. Many people with AIDS have already lost family members or friends to the disease.

a bed cradle from a cardboard box and use it to keep sheets and blankets from resting on the legs and feet (see Chapter 12).

Emotional Problems. Clients with HIV/AIDS may suffer from anxiety and depression caused by having an incurable illness. In addition, they must deal with the perceptions of family, friends, and society. Some people may blame them for their illness. People with HIV/AIDS may experience tremendous stress due to uncertainty over the course of their illness, loss of significant numbers of people in their social support network of friends and family, difficulty in obtaining adequate health care, and finances (**Fig. 20-17**).

Clients with HIV/AIDS need support from others. This support may come from family, friends, religious and community groups, and support groups, as well as the health care team. Treat all your clients with respect and help provide the emotional support they need.

Central nervous system damage and AIDS dementia complex. Some symptoms of central nervous system damage show up early in HIV infection, including withdrawal, apathy, avoidance of complex tasks, and mental slowness. In addition, medications may cause side effects of this type.

Later in the course of the disease, AIDS dementia complex may develop, causing further apathy, withdrawal, and mental symptoms. There may also be muscle weakness and loss of muscle control, making falls a risk. Clients in this stage of the disease will need a safe environment and close supervision in their ADLs.

Part 7
Caring for the Client with Alzheimer's Disease or Other Dementias

---

❑ 25. Describe normal changes of aging in the brain

As we age, we typically lose some of our ability to think logically and quickly. This ability is called cognition (kog-NI-shun), and when we lose some of this ability we are said to have cognitive impairment (KOG-ni-tiv im-PAYR-ment). Cognitive impairment affects concentration and memory. Elderly clients may lose their memories of recent events, which can be frustrating for them. Home care aides can help elderly clients by encouraging them to make lists of things to remember, write down names and phone numbers, or use other simple methods to make up for memory loss.

Other normal changes of aging in the brain include slower reaction time, difficulty finding or using the right words, and sleeping less and being more wakeful at night.

❑ 26. Define dementia and recognize its causes

Dementia (di-MEN-shee-a) is a loss of mental abilities such as thinking, remembering, reasoning, and

communicating. This loss of ability makes it difficult to perform ADLs such as eating, bathing, dressing, and toileting. Dementia is *not* a normal part of aging.

The following are some of the causes of dementia (**Fig. 20-18**):

▶ Alzheimer's disease
▶ Multi-infarct dementia (a series of strokes causing damage to the brain)
▶ Parkinson's disease
▶ Huntington's disease
▶ AIDS
▶ metabolic imbalances
▶ circulatory disorders (e.g., CVA)

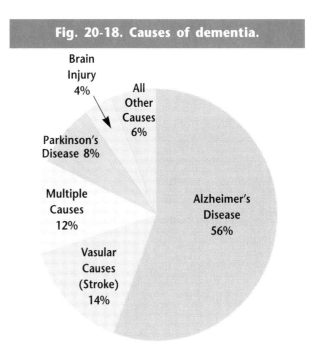

Fig. 20-18. Causes of dementia.

Brain Injury 4%
All Other Causes 6%
Parkinson's Disease 8%
Multiple Causes 12%
Vasular Causes (Stroke) 14%
Alzheimer's Disease 56%

❑ 27. Describe Alzheimer's disease

Alzheimer's disease is a **progressive, degenerative, irreversible** disease that causes tangled nerve fibers and protein deposits to form in the brain, eventually causing dementia. Progressive and degenerative mean the disease gets worse, causing greater and greater loss of health and abilities. Irreversible means the disease cannot be cured. Thus, clients with Alzheimer's disease will never recover and will need more and more care as the disease progresses.

As people in our society live to be older and older, more will develop Alzheimer's disease in their later years. One in fourteen people over age sixty-five have Alzheimer's disease, but one in *four* people over age eighty-five have Alzheimer's disease. Thus there is a growing need for care of people with Alzheimer's. Because 70% of people with Alzheimer's disease live at home, much of this care will be performed by home care aides.

❑ 28. Identify the stages of Alzheimer's and list the related behaviors

Alzheimer's disease generally begins with forgetfulness and confusion and progresses to complete loss of all ability to care for oneself. Each person with Alzheimer's will show different symptoms at different times, so it is difficult to divide the disease into stages. For example, one person with Alzheimer's may be able to read, but may be unable to use the phone or remember her own address. Another person with Alzheimer's may have lost the ability to

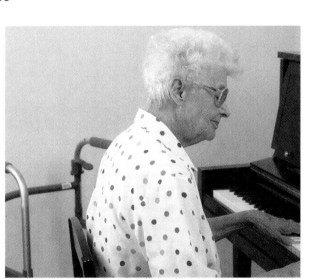

Fig. 20-19. A person with Alzheimer's disease may retain skills she has used her whole lifetime, even when much of her memory has been lost.

read, but may still be able to do simple math. Skills a person has used constantly over a long lifetime are usually kept longer. Thus some people with Alzheimer's can cook or play a musical instrument with some help long after they have lost a great deal of their memory. Look for these "preserved skills" and help your clients use and enjoy them as long as possible (**Fig. 20-19**).

Clients with Alzheimer's disease should also be encouraged to perform ADLs and keep their minds and bodies as active as possible. Working, socializing, reading, problem solving, and exercising should all be encouraged. Having clients with Alzheimer's do as much as possible for themselves may even

help slow the progression of the disease. Look for tasks that are challenging but not frustrating, and help your clients succeed in performing them.

❑ 29. Identify personal attitudes helpful in caring for people with Alzheimer's disease or any dementia

The following attitudes will help you give the best possible care to your clients with Alzheimer's disease:

Don't take it personally. Always remember that people with Alzheimer's do not have control over their words and actions. They may often be unaware of what they say or do. If a client with Alzheimer's doesn't recognize you, doesn't do what you say, ignores you, accuses you, or insults you, remember that it's the disease and not the person.

Put yourself in their shoes. Think about what it would be like to have Alzheimer's disease. Imagine being unable to perform ADLs. Treat clients with Alzheimer's disease with dignity and respect, as you would want to be treated.

Work with the symptoms and behaviors you see. Because each person with Alzheimer's disease is an individual, your clients with Alzheimer's will not all show the same symptoms at the same times. Each client with Alzheimer's will do some things that others will never do. So the best strategy is to work with the behaviors you see today. For example, an Alzheimer's client may want to go for a walk today, when yesterday she didn't seem able to get to the bathroom without help. If allowed by the care plan or your assignment, by all means try to take her for a walk.

Box 20-5.
General Progression of Alzheimer's Disease

Stage I

- recent (short term) memory loss
- disorientation to time
- lack of interest in doing things, including work, dress, recreation
- inability to concentrate
- mood swings
- irritability
- petulance: peevish, ill-humored, rude behavior
- tendency to blame others
- carelessness in personal habits
- poor judgment

Stage II

- increased memory loss, may forget family members and friends
- slurred speech
- difficulty finding right word, finishing thoughts, or following directions
- tendency to make statements that are illogical
- inability to read, write, or do math
- inability to care for self or perform ADLs without assistance
- incontinence
- dulled senses (for example, cannot distinguish between hot and cold)
- restlessness, wandering, and/or agitation (increase of these in the evening is called "sundowning")
- sleep problems
- lack of impulse control (for example swears excessively or is sexually aggressive or rude)
- obsessive repetition of movements, behavior, or words
- temper tantrums
- hallucinations or delusions

Stage III

- total disorientation to time, place, and person
- apathy
- total dependence on others for care
- total incontinence
- inability to speak or communicate, except for grunting, groaning, or screaming
- total immobility/confined to bed
- inability to recognize family members or self
- increased sleep disturbances
- difficulty swallowing, which produces risk of choking
- seizures
- coma
- death

Work as a team. As with all your clients, it is very important that you always report and document your observations about Alzheimer's clients to your supervisor. Because the symptoms and behavior of Alzheimer's clients can change from day to day, you are in an excellent position to give details about your clients' cases. Being with your clients frequently and regularly allows you to be the expert on each case. Make the most of this opportunity and you will be helping to give your clients the best possible care.

Take care of yourself. Caring for someone with dementia can be exhausting — both emotionally and physically. You need to take care of yourself in order to be able to continue giving Alzheimer's clients the best possible care.

Work with family members. Family members can be a wonderful resource, helping you learn more about your client and providing familiarity and comfort to the person with Alzheimer's. Try to build relationships with family members and keep the lines of communication open. Home care aides are a big support to family members. You need to serve as a role model for appropriate behavior to assist the family in caring for the client.

Remember the goals of the client care plan. In addition to the practical tasks you will perform for your clients with Alzheimer's, the client care plan will also call for maintaining clients' dignity and self-esteem and helping them to be as independent as possible.

❏ 30. List three strategies for better communication with Alzheimer's clients

1. Speak in a low, calm voice, in a room with little background noise and distraction. Because many clients with Alzheimer's become agitated easily, it is important to do everything you can to keep them calm. This means speaking in a quiet, slow manner. It also means eliminating noise and distractions, such as televisions or radios, and children or family members who are noisy.

2. Repeat yourself, using the same words and phrases as often as needed. When an Alzheimer's client does not seem to understand what you are saying or asks questions over and over, repeat yourself using the same words. Remember that a person with Alzheimer's literally has tangles in the brain. It may take several repetitions for a message to get through. Keep messages simple, and break complex tasks into smaller, simpler ones.

Repetition can also be reassuring for a person with Alzheimer's. In fact, many clients with Alzheimer's will repeat words, phrases, questions, or actions frequently. This is called **perseveration**. If your client perseverates, do not try to stop him. Instead, answer his questions, using the same words each time, until he stops.

3. Use pictures or gestures to communicate. With some clients or at some point in the progression of Alzheimer's, it may be more effective to use nonverbal communication. This means using pictures, such as a drawing of a toilet on the bathroom door, and gestures, such as pointing to the closet or holding up a dress when you want to help your client dress. Usually it is most effective to combine verbal and nonverbal communication, saying for example, "Let's get dressed now," as you hold up clothes.

❏ 31. Describe a safe and well-organized environment for a client with Alzheimer's

Before you visit a client with Alzheimer's, a nurse should have already been to the home to assess its safety. She will have indicated changes to be made, such as using gates on stairways, putting locks on certain doors, and removing clutter or throw rugs. On your visits to the home, you should be aware of how these safety measures are working and report and document your observations.

When the client's condition changes, report this to your supervisor and another visit will be made to reassess the home and make further changes as needed. For example, if a client is no longer able to find the bathroom easily, signs can be posted on doors to indicate which room is which. If a client begins to wander, locks can be put on all doors and labels attached to clothing to identify the client who wanders away.

If you think additional changes need to be made in the home, speak to your supervisor. When a client displays a new behavior, such as wandering, report it immediately so that the environment can be adapted as necessary.

❏ 32. Explain how to assist with personal care and activities of daily living for the client with Alzheimer's disease

You will use the same procedures for personal care and ADLs for clients with Alzheimer's disease as you will with other clients. However, there are some guidelines to keep in mind when assisting with personal care and ADLs for clients with Alzheimer's. Two general principles will help you give your clients the best care:

Box 20-6.
Organizing the Home For a Client with Alzheimer's Disease

For disoriented clients:

- Use signs to mark rooms, including stop signs on rooms that should not be entered.

- Use calendars and other reminders of day, date, and location.

- Put bells on the door to indicate when someone is coming or going.

- Keep pictures and familiar objects around.

- Put stickers or brightly colored tape on glass doors, large windows, or glass furniture (**Fig. 20-20**).

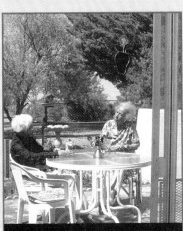

Fig. 20-20. Put stickers or brightly colored tape on glass doors, large windows, or glass furniture.

For the client who wanders:

- Use locks on doors. These can be installed low or high, so the client won't see them.

- Install alarms that go off when exit doors are opened.

- Have clients wear identification. Sew labels into clothes.

- Alert neighbors that client may wander. Show them a recent photo of the client.

- Keep a recent photo handy, as well as a piece of clothing the client has worn. These can help police and police dogs track a client who has wandered away.

For clients who pace:

- Remove clutter and throw rugs.
- Do not rearrange furniture.
- Do not wax floors.
- Be sure shoes and slippers fit and have nonslip soles.

For clients who have difficulty walking:

- Keep areas well lit, even at night.

- Block access to stairs with a gate placed at hip height (**Fig. 20-21**).

- Clear walkways of electrical cords.

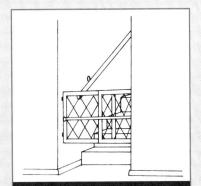

Fig. 20-21. A gate at the foot or head of stairs will help prevent an Alzheimer's client from injuring himself trying to walk up or down stairs. Place the gate at hip height to prevent the client from falling over it.

General tips:

- Keep medications and other chemicals out of reach.

- Display emergency numbers, including poison control, and home address near the phone.

- Use red tape around radiators or heating vents to prevent burns.

- Check refrigerator and "hiding places" for spoiled food.

- Prevent kitchen accidents by removing knobs on stove, unplugging toasters and other small appliances, and supervising kitchen visits.

1. Develop a routine and stick to it. Being consistent is very important when working with clients who are confused and easily agitated.

2. Promote self-care. Helping your clients to care for themselves as much as possible will help them cope with this difficult disease.

More specific guidelines for assisting Alzheimer's clients with performing ADLs and personal care, and maintaining physical and mental health are listed below:

Bathing, grooming, and dressing. The following guidelines can help make grooming less stressful for you and the client:

- Ensure safety by using nonslip mats, tub seats, and hand holds.

- Schedule bathing when the client is least agitated. Be organized so the complete bath can be quick. Give sponge baths if the client resists a shower or tub bath.

- Always use the same steps, explaining in the same way every time.

- Assist with grooming. Help the people in your care feel attractive and dignified.

- Lay out clothes in the order in which they should be put on. Choose clothes that are simple to put on (Fig. 20-22).

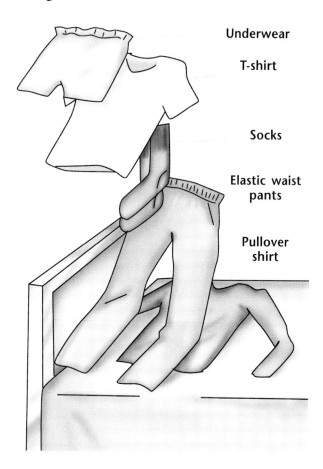

Underwear

T-shirt

Socks

Elastic waist pants

Pullover shirt

Fig. 20-22. Lay out clothes in the order in which they should be put on. Choose clothes that are simple to put on.

Toileting. Follow the care plan and your assignments to prevent toileting problems. Never withhold or discourage fluids because a person is incontinent. Though most people with Alzheimer's will eventually experience incontinence, they may remain continent longer if the following guidelines are followed:

- Set up a regular schedule for toileting and follow it.

- Mark the restroom with a sign as a reminder to use it and where it is.

- Do not discourage fluids *except* just before bed if that is when incontinence occurs.

- Check skin regularly for signs of irritation.

- Document bowel movements.

Physical health. Performing the tasks you have been assigned, as you would for any client, will help maintain health for a client with Alzheimer's disease. As always, observe, record, and report any changes in physical health.

- Prevent infections by following proper procedures for food preparation and storage, household management, and standard precautions.

- Observe the person's physical health and report any potential problems. People with dementia may not recognize their own health problems.

- Maintain a daily exercise routine.

Nutrition. Follow the instructions in the client care plan and your assignments.

- Maintain optimal nutrition.

- Schedule meals at the same time each day and serve familiar foods. If restlessness prevents getting through an entire meal, try smaller, more frequent meals. Finger foods can allow eating while moving around.

- Offer one course at a time using one utensil at a time. If a client needs to be fed, do so slowly, offering small pieces of food (Chapter 23 explains the procedure for feeding a client).

- Encourage fluids.

- Keep nutritious snacks nearby, especially favorites.

- Observe and report changes or problems in eating habits. Monitor weight accurately and frequently to discover potential problems as soon as possible.

Mental health.

- Maintain self-esteem by encouraging independence in ADLs.

- Assist with personal grooming to increase self-esteem.

- Provide a daily calendar to encourage activities.

- Share in enjoyable activities, looking at pictures, talking, and reminiscing.

- Reward positive and independent behavior with smiles, hugs, warm touches, and thank yous (**Fig. 20-23**).

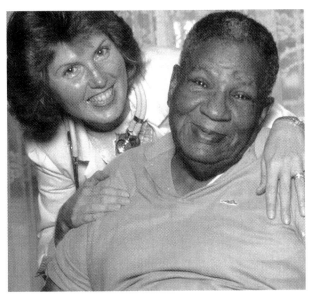

Fig. 20-23. Reward positive and independent behavior with smiles, hugs, warm touches, and thank yous.

❏ 33. List eight difficult behaviors common in clients with Alzheimer's and describe ways to manage each

Below are some common difficult behaviors that you may face when working with Alzheimer's clients. Remember that each client is different; one client may show all these behaviors, another may only show one or two. Work with each client as an individual and report behavior in detail to your supervisor.

1. Agitation. A client who is excited, restless, or troubled is said to be **agitated**. Situations that lead to agitation are said to be triggers, and may include change of routine or caregiver, new or frustrating experiences, or even violent television. Responses that may help calm a person who is agitated include the following:

- Try to eliminate triggers, keep routine constant, avoid frustration.

- Help client focus on a soothing, familiar activity, such as sorting things or looking at pictures.

- Remain calm and use a low, soothing voice to speak to and reassure the client.

- An arm around the shoulder, patting, or stroking may be soothing for some clients.

2. Pacing and Wandering. A client who walks back and forth in the same area is **pacing**. A client who walks aimlessly around the house or neighborhood is **wandering**. Pacing and wandering may have some of the following causes:

- restlessness

- hunger

- disorientation

- need for toileting

- forgetting how or where to sit down

- too much daytime napping

- need for exercise

Responses to pacing and wandering could include the following:

- Let clients pace or wander in a safe and secure (locked) area where you can keep an eye on them, such as in a level, fenced yard (**Fig. 20-24**).

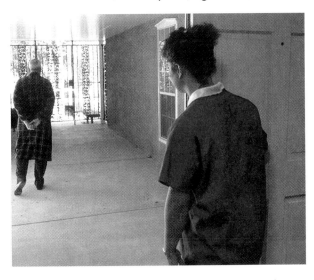

Fig. 20-24. If you cannot keep the client from pacing or wandering, provide a safe area for him to pace or wander in.

- Eliminate causes when you can, for example, by providing nutritious snacks, encouraging an exercise routine, or maintaining a toileting schedule.

- Suggest another activity, such as going for a walk together.

3. Hallucinations or Delusions. A client who sees things that are not there is having **hallucinations**. A client who believes things that are not true is having **delusions**. You can respond to delusions in the following ways:

- Ignore harmless hallucinations and delusions.

- Reassure a client who seems agitated or worried.

- Do not argue with a client who is imagining things. Remember that the feelings are real to him or her. Redirect client to other activities or thoughts.

- Be calm and reassure client that you are there to help.

4. Sundowning. When a person becomes restless and agitated in the late afternoon, evening, or night, it is called **sundowning**. Sundowning may be triggered by hunger or fatigue, a change in routine or caregiver, or any new or frustrating situation. Following are some effective responses to sundowning:

- Eliminate triggers, providing snacks or encouraging rest.

- Avoid stressful situations during this time, limit activities, appointments, trips, and visits.

- Play soft music.

- Set a bedtime routine and keep it.

- Recognize when sundowning occurs and plan a calming activity just before.

- Eliminate caffeine from the diet.

- Give a soothing back massage.

- Redirect the behavior or distract the client with a simple, calm activity like looking at a magazine.

- Maintain a daily exercise routine.

- Avoid using physical restraints.

5. Catastrophic Reactions. When a person with Alzheimer's overreacts to something in an unreasonable way it is called a catastrophic (kat-a-STRAH-fik) reaction. It may be triggered by any of the following:

- fatigue

- change of routine, environment, or caregiver

- overstimulation: too much noise or activity

- difficult choices or tasks

- physical pain

- hunger

- need for toileting

You can respond to catastrophic reactions as you would to agitation or sundowning. For example, eliminate triggers and help the client focus on a soothing activity.

6. Depression. When clients become withdrawn, have no energy, do not want to eat or do things they used to enjoy, they may be **depressed**. Chapter 18, Understanding Mental Health and Mental Illness, provides more information on depression and its symptoms. Depression may have many causes, including:

- loss of independence

- inability to cope

- feelings of failure, fear

- reality of facing a progressive, degenerative illness

You can respond to depression in a number of ways:

- Report signs of depression to your supervisor immediately. It is an illness that can be treated with medication.

- Encourage independence, self-care, and activity.

- Talk about moods and feelings if your client is willing. Be a good listener.

- Encourage social interaction.

7. Perseveration or Repetitive Phrasing. A client who repeats a word, phrase, question, or activity over and over is perseverating (per-SEV-er-ayt-ing). Repeating a word or phrase is also called **repetitive phrasing**. Such behavior may be caused by several factors, including disorientation or confusion. Respond to perseveration with patience. Do not try to silence or stop the client. Answer questions each time they are asked, using the same words each time.

8. Violent Behavior. A client who attacks, hits, or threatens someone is **violent**. Violence may be triggered by many situations, including frustration, overstimulation, or a change in routine, environment, or caregiver.

The following are appropriate responses to violent clients:

- Block blows but never hit back.

- Step out of reach.
- Call for help if needed.
- Do not leave client in the home alone.
- Try to eliminate triggers.
- Use techniques to calm client as you would for agitation or sundowning.

☐ 34. Describe creative therapies for clients with Alzheimer's

Although Alzheimer's is an irreversible disease, meaning it cannot be cured, there are many techniques that can improve the quality of life for clients with Alzheimer's. Follow the instructions in the client care plan and your assignments regarding creative therapies.

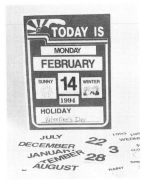

Fig. 20-25. Reality orientation involves frequently reminding the client of her identity and surroundings.

Reality Orientation

What is it? Using calendars, clocks, signs, and lists to reorient your client and help her remember who and where she is (Fig. 20-25).

When is it useful? In the early stages of Alzheimer's, when clients are confused but not totally disoriented. In later stages, reality orientation may only frustrate clients.

Example: Each day when you arrive at Mrs. Elkin's house, you show her the calendar and point out what day of the week it is. On the calendar or another piece of paper, you list all the things you will do today, for example, take a bath, go for a walk, eat lunch, and play cards. Whenever you speak to her, you call the client by her name, Mrs. Elkin. When assisting with tasks, you explain why you do things as you do, for example, "We use a tub seat in the shower so you don't have to stand up for so long, Mrs. Elkin."

Benefits: Using the calendar, making lists, and using names frequently all help your client stay in touch with the world around her. This will help her feel more in control of her life. It will also allow her to do as much as possible for herself. Explaining what you do and why you do it as you assist her will make her feel more like a participant in her care and less like an invalid.

Validation Therapy

What is it? Letting a client believe he lives in the past or in imaginary circumstances. Exploring and validating the client's beliefs. **Validating** means giving value to or approving, and making no attempt to reorient the client to actual circumstances.

When is it useful? In cases of moderate to severe disorientation.

Example: Mr. Baldwin tells you he does not want to eat lunch today because he is going out to a restaurant later with his wife. You know his wife has been dead for many years and that Mr. Baldwin can no longer eat out in restaurants. Instead of telling him that he is not going out to eat, you ask what restaurant he is going to, what he will have, and what time he is going. You suggest that he eat a good lunch now because sometimes the service is slow in restaurants and he might get hungry while waiting (Fig. 20-26).

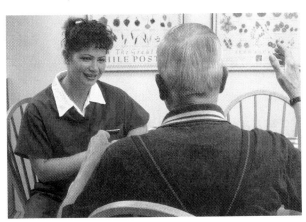

Fig. 20-26. Validation therapy is accepting a client's fantasies without attempting to reorient him to reality.

Benefits: By "playing along" with Mr. Baldwin's fantasy, you let him know that you take him seriously. You do not think of him as a crazy person or a child who does not know what is happening in his own life. You also learned more about your client: he used to enjoy eating out in restaurants, he liked to order certain dishes, and eating out is something he probably associates with being with his wife. These things can help you give Mr. Baldwin better care in the future.

Reminiscence Therapy

What is it? Encouraging your client to **reminisce**, to remember and talk about the past. Exploring his memories by asking about details. Focusing on a time of life that was more pleasant for him, or working through feelings about a difficult time in the past.

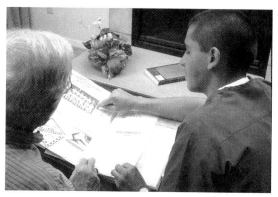

Fig. 20-27. Reminiscence therapy is encouraging a client to remember and talk about an important time in his past.

When is it useful? In many stages of Alzheimer's, but especially with moderate to severe confusion.

Example: Mr. Benavidez, a 77-year-old man with Alzheimer's, fought in World War II. In his home are many mementos of the war — pictures of his war buddies, a medal he was given, and more. You ask him to tell you where he was sent in the war, and he tells you a little bit about being in the

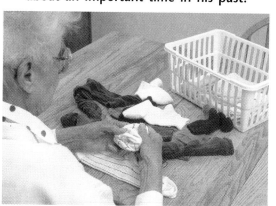

Fig. 20-28. Activity therapy allows a client with Alzheimer's to enjoy activities that help fight frustration and boost self-esteem.

Pacific. You ask him more detailed questions about his experiences, and eventually he tells you a lot: the friends he made in the service, why he was given the medal, times when he was scared and how much he missed his wife and oldest daughter (**Fig. 20-27**).

Benefits: By asking questions about Mr. Benavidez' experiences in the war, you show an interest in him as a person, not just a client. You also let him show you that he was once a person who was competent, social, responsible, and brave. This boosts his self-esteem. Furthermore, you learn that Mr.

Benavidez cared very much for his wife and daughter, and probably would enjoy visits from his daughter now that he cannot get out as much.

Activity Therapy

What is it? Using activities, especially those the client enjoys, to prevent boredom and frustration and promote self-esteem. Helping the client to take walks, do puzzles, listen to music, cook, read, or do other activities he or she enjoys (**Fig. 20-28**).

When is it useful? Throughout most stages of Alzheimer's, depending on the activity.

Example: Mrs. Hoebel, a 70-year-old woman with Alzheimer's, raised four children and ran a household for almost 50 years before being diagnosed with Alzheimer's. She loves cooking and baking, and misses being in the kitchen now that she cannot cook for herself. You learn that she always used to bake cookies at Christmas and would love to be able to bake cookies this year. You purchase some pre-made cookie dough and roll out the dough. Mrs. Hoebel uses her old cookie cutters to cut out the shapes. You bake the cookies for her, and another day she can decorate them.

Benefits: Mrs. Hoebel can enjoy an activity that always brought her pleasure. She feels competent, because you gave her small tasks, such as cutting out the cookies, that she could handle. You showed her that you care about her by taking the time to help her bake the cookies. She will associate positive feelings with you, which will make caring for her much easier.

SECTION VI
Practical Knowledge and Skills in Home Management

Chapter 21

Maintaining a Clean, Safe and Healthy Environment

❏ *1. Describe the contributions of housekeeping to physical and psychological well-being*

An important job you will do as a home care aide is household management. Establishing and maintaining order and cleanliness

---

Learning Objectives

In this chapter you will learn to:

are vital parts of home health care. Illness and disability cause great stress, and a household that is disorganized can add to the stress.

Providing a safe, clean, and orderly environment has always been an essential part of home health care. Clients feel better physically and psychologically and recover more quickly when their homes and families receive care and support. Infection and accidents are prevented. In addition, families who lack some of the skills and knowledge to manage their homes can be taught valuable household management skills. These skills include sanitation, safety, personal hygiene, nutrition, meal planning, shopping, food preparation, child care, communications skills, and specific health care techniques. You will be a role model for your clients and their families, helping them learn to accept greater responsibility.

❑ 2. *List qualities needed to effectively manage a home*

Efficiency and Planning. It takes efficiency and planning as well as knowledge and skills to manage a household. You will need to know how to use your time and energy well, so that you do not neglect your primary responsibility, the personal care of the client.

Sensitivity. Sensitivity is another important quality for you to have and to express when caring for your client's homes. As with all your duties, you must respect the customs, beliefs, and feelings of your clients and their families. How would you feel if a stranger were to handle your personal items and valuable possessions or assume your responsibilities in the home? How would you feel if you could no longer care for your home yourself?

Be sensitive when you ask members of the household for help with housekeeping as well. Know when it is appropriate to ask for their assistance and how to ask for it in an appropriate way. Some family members may be experiencing such stress that they are unable to help at all.

The home maintenance assignments that you can expect to receive may include simple cleaning and organizing of the client's room, general cleaning throughout the house, or management of all household functions including finances. You may be required to dust, straighten, vacuum, sweep, wash dishes, clean the bathroom and kitchen, and do laundry. Your assignments will outline the specific duties to be performed (**Fig. 21-1**).

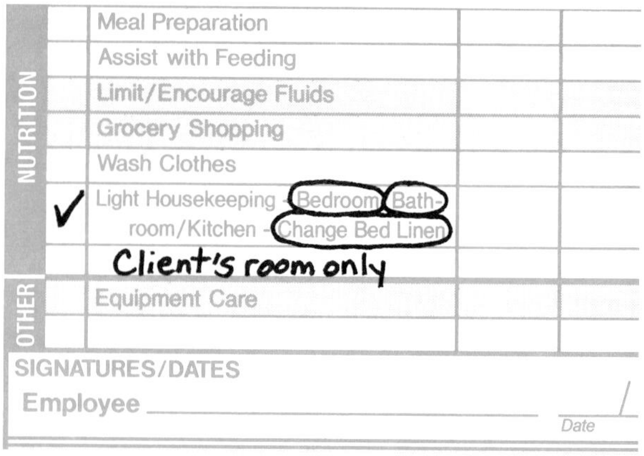
NUTRITION
Meal Preparation
Assist with Feeding
Limit/Encourage Fluids
Grocery Shopping
Wash Clothes
✓ Light Housekeeping - Bedroom Bathroom/Kitchen - Change Bed Linen
Client's room only
OTHER
Equipment Care
SIGNATURES/DATES
Employee ______ /
Date

Fig. 21-1. Your assignments will outline any home maintenance tasks you are to perform.

As with all other home health care activities, home maintenance activities are determined by the supervisor or the home care team and are written in the client's care plan and your assignments. Your assignments may indicate the days on which the specific tasks should be performed or they may indicate just the types of activities that must be done, allowing you to make your own schedule. Flexibility may be important depending on the client's and family's needs. If problems arise regarding housecleaning and home maintenance tasks, such as requests for services not listed in your assignments or frequent complaints about how tasks are done, contact your supervisor. Chapter 24 discusses in more detail how to handle criticism and complaints.

❑ 3. *Describe general guidelines for housekeeping*

Most home care agencies require home care aides to perform light housekeeping. Light housekeeping assigned by home care agencies usually focuses on the client's immediate environment and involves dusting, straightening, vacuuming or sweeping floors and floor coverings, cleaning bathrooms and the kitchen, and disposing of garbage and trash. These activities are an important part of maintaining a clean, safe, and healthy environment for clients and their families. Light housekeeping does *not* involve activities such as moving heavy furniture, washing windows, taking down drapes, cleaning the attic and basement, or mowing the lawn.

Keep the following guidelines in mind:

▶ **Invite family participation.** Depending on their abilities and availability, clients and family members may be asked to participate in housekeeping tasks.

▶ **Invite family and client input** when you determine the tasks that need to be done and the methods that will be used. Use cleaning materials and methods that are acceptable to and approved by clients and their families. Any efforts you make toward improving the home environment should coincide with the client's choices, lifestyle, and values.

▶ **Be organized** when performing home health care and home maintenance tasks. Being organized will help you conserve time and energy and provide more satisfying service to your client.

▶ **Write out detailed daily and weekly schedules** and seek feedback from your supervisor and the client and family. These schedules will be useful guides until a routine is established. Priority may need to be given to certain activities at certain times.

▶ **Build some flexibility in the schedule** to allow for changes in the client's condition, needs, appointments, or social activities.

▶ **Organize cleaning materials and equipment** by locating them in one closet. Place cleaning materials in a pail, a carrying bin that has a handle, a laundry basket, or a shopping bag (**Fig. 21-2**).

▶ **Familiarize yourself with the cleaning materials and equipment.** Read the labels and instruction booklets. Ask the client, family members, or your supervisor how the equipment works if you are unfamiliar with it.

▶ **Maintain a safe environment** as well as a clean and healthy one. Do not wax floors if your client is unsteady. Mop up spills immediately. Do not leave cleaning equipment around.

▶ **Use housekeeping procedures and methods that promote good health.** Many diseases may be trans-

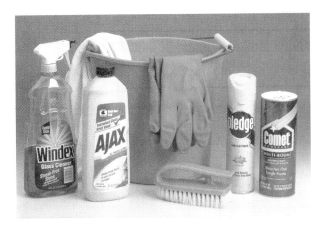

Fig. 21-2. Organize cleaning materials and equipment by locating them in one closet, for example, and placing cleaning materials in a pail, a carrying bin that has a handle, a laundry basket, or a shopping bag.

mitted through improper food handling, dishwashing, handwashing, and unclean bathrooms and kitchens.

▶ **Observe the home environment for signs of infestation** by roaches, rats, mice, lice, and fleas. These insects and animals are common carriers of disease. Controlling them is vital to family health and cleanliness.

▶ **Use good body mechanics** in performing home maintenance activities to prevent injury and undue fatigue. Review the principles of body mechanics in Chapter 6. House cleaning can require a great deal of bending, standing, stooping, and lifting. Watch your posture. Kneel instead of stooping for long periods.

▶ **Clean up and straighten up after every activity.** Spills that have dried are difficult to remove later.

▶ **Carry paper and a small pencil** to make note of items that must be purchased or replaced. Maintain a shopping list on a bulletin board, refrigerator door, or other convenient location, and encourage family members to use the list.

▶ **Use your time wisely and efficiently.** For example, prepare food while a load of wash is being done.

❏ 4. Describe cleaning products and equipment

Cleaning Products. Four basic types of home cleaning products are available in the market:

1. All-purpose cleaning agents can be used for many purposes and on several types of surfaces, for example, countertops, walls, floors, and baseboards.

2. Soaps and detergents are used for bathing, laundering, and dishwashing.

3. Abrasive cleansers are used mostly to scour hard-to-clean surfaces.

4. Specialty cleaners are used to clean special surfaces, such as glass, metal, or ovens.

All cleaning products must be used properly, not only to clean effectively, but also to protect surfaces, materials, and people. Cleaning products are chemicals, which can be irritating and can even cause burns. Some chemicals are poisonous when swallowed.

Keep the following precautions in mind when using household cleaning products:

▸ Read and follow the directions on the label of every product you use. For example, rinse or dilute when the directions say to, and use only the amount recommended on the label.

▸ Do not mix cleaning products. This can cause a dangerous chemical reaction that may harm you or others. In particular, *never mix bleach or products containing bleach with ammonia.* The fumes are toxic and can be fatal.

▸ If possible, open windows when cleaning to provide fresh air. Some cleaning products may have fumes that are unpleasant or even harmful if exposure is prolonged.

▸ Do not leave cleaning products on surfaces more than the recommended time, and do not scrub too vigorously on some surfaces. Cleaning products can harm the materials you are trying to clean.

Cleaning Equipment. A basic set of cleaning tools generally includes two types:

1. Wet mops, pails, toilet brushes, and sponges are tools for softening and removing soil that has dried and hardened on washable surfaces.

2. A vacuum cleaner and attachments, carpet sweeper, dust mop, dust cloths, broom, and brush and dustpan are tools for removing dry dirt and dust.

Remember to exercise caution with equipment.

Replacements can be expensive. Become familiar with the purpose and use of each piece of equipment. Keep it clean and in its proper place. Check the brushes and bags of vacuum cleaners frequently.

❑ 5. Describe proper cleaning methods for living areas, kitchens, bathrooms, and storage areas

Not all housekeeping tasks must be performed daily. Some tasks may be done weekly, and others only need to be done once a month or seasonally. Space out the special tasks, for example, food shopping, vacuuming, laundry, and floor washing, so that you do not have too many of them to do in one day. Conserve your time and energy. Do each cleaning job properly and efficiently, without taking a lot of steps and without reaching, bending, and stooping unnecessarily. Experiment a little to find the most comfortable and effective way to do a job. Cleaning can be done when your client is resting, sleeping, or doing another activity. Care of the client is your primary responsibility; however, housekeeping should not be neglected.

Straightening and Cleaning Living Areas. Keep the house orderly, organized, and safe by clearing up clutter and putting objects in their correct places. Pick up newspapers, magazines, and toys as needed. Empty wastebaskets and ashtrays daily. Make the beds each day. Straightening frequently is done for your client's benefit as well as your own. Much time and energy can be wasted looking for important objects that are lost in clutter.

Many clients with limited or restricted mobility spend much of their time in certain places, such as a favorite chair or in bed. Keep essential and frequently used items, such as eyeglasses, tissues, a wastebasket, newspaper, magazines, and books, within easy reach of this area. Organize them on an accessible table, magazine rack, or hanging organizer (**Fig. 21-3**).

Dust once a week or when necessary. If your client has allergies, you may need to dust daily. Dust mites are microscopic insects that live in dust, and their droppings cause allergic reactions, such as asthma, in some people.

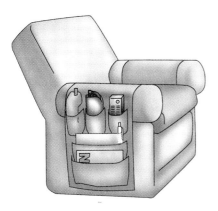

Fig. 21-3. A hanging organizer can help eliminate clutter while keeping frequently used items handy for clients with restricted mobility.

Vacuum floors and rugs once a week or more often if indicated. When vacuuming rugs, use long strokes and go over each area repeatedly, using a back and forth motion, especially if it is heavily soiled. If the home does not have a vacuum, use a broom to sweep the floors and rugs clean. Take care not to raise much dust.

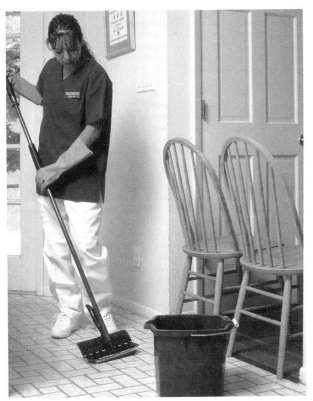

Fig. 21-4. Close off the area for the time it takes for the floor to dry.

Washing floors will make the house feel and smell clean. Do not wash wood floors. Floors covered with vinyl, ceramic tile, and linoleum may be washed. Some floor coverings should be cleaned with water only, so it is important to check with the client or family members before you begin. After removing loose dirt or crumbs with a vacuum or broom, wash floors with a cloth or mop dipped in warm sudsy water. Dry the floor after you have washed it or close off the area for the time it takes for the floor to dry (**Fig. 21-4**). Wet or waxed floors are slippery and are frequent causes of falls and accidents in the home.

Cleaning the Kitchen. Cleaning the kitchen prevents disease and injury. Many diseases may be transmitted by handling food on contaminated surfaces, improper dishwashing, and contaminated food storage areas. A kitchen infested by roaches, rats, and mice may be the source of disease and allergy, through the contamination of food by their saliva or through their droppings. Pest control is vital to health and cleanliness. Always report pest control problems to your supervisor.

Clean the kitchen after every use and ask family members to do the same. Do not wait until the end of the day to clean up. Daily kitchen cleaning tasks include washing dishes, wiping surfaces, taking out garbage, and storing leftover food. Weekly tasks include cleaning the refrigerator and washing the floor. Cleaning cabinets, drawers, and other storage areas is usually done a few times a year.

Wash dishes in hot soapy water using liquid dish detergent. Rinse them in hot water. When working with clients who have an infectious disease or a cold, use boiling water for rinsing and add a tablespoon of chlorine bleach to the soapy water. The combination of heat and chlorine will kill pathogens (PATH-o-jens), or harmful microorganisms. Wash glasses and cups first, then silverware, plates, and bowls. Pots and pans are washed last. Rinse with hot water and dry on a rack or drainer. Air drying dishes is more sanitary than drying them with a dish towel.

If the household has a dishwasher, ask a family member to demonstrate how to correctly load and start it. Dishwashers are not only time-saving, they also sterilize dishes because of the high temperature used in washing and drying. When using an automatic dishwasher, scrape dishes to remove large food particles, and empty cups and glasses. Do not place dishes, cups, and flatware too close together; this will keep them from being washed thoroughly. When you position them, place dishes, cups, and glasses so that their eating or drinking surfaces are facing the water source. For example, most dishwashers clean best when the dirty sides of the plates are facing inward and cups are upside down on the top rack, because the water source is on the floor of the dishwasher, toward the center of the machine.

Do not wash the following items in the dishwasher: electrical appliances, certain plastic materials, wooden pieces or utensils, hand-painted or antique dishes, delicate china, crystal, cast iron, most pots and pans, and sharp or carbon steel knives. Use only a dishwasher detergent and fill the well with only the amount recommended on the label.

Clean the outside of the stove, the trays, and burners with hot, sudsy water or an all-purpose cleaner, and rinse. Ovens should be cleaned according to manufacturer's recommendations; oven cleaners cannot be used on all ovens. Be sure to follow the directions; oven cleaners are caustic and can emit an irritating gas. Do not spray the light bulb inside the oven with cleanser, or it may break. Remember to soak the broiler pan immediately after use. Broiler pans are difficult to clean if food has been allowed to bake on them many times over without thorough cleaning.

The refrigerator should be totally cleaned once a week, but you should wipe it out more frequently (**Fig. 21-5**). The freezer should be defrosted whenever necessary. One half inch of frost is usually a good indicator that the freezer should be defrosted. To defrost a freezer, turn the dial to the "off" position and remove all food. Wrap frozen foods in newspapers to keep them from defrosting. Defrosting the freezer may be accomplished more quickly by placing pans of hot water in it. Do not use a knife to chip off the frost; this could damage the freezing unit.

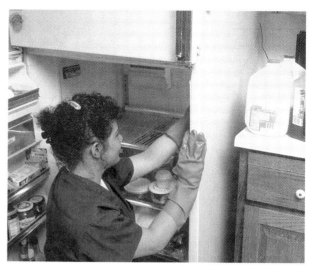

Fig. 21-5. The refrigerator should be totally cleaned once a week, but you should wipe it out more frequently.

Mix two tablespoons of baking soda in one quart of warm water and wipe the inside walls of the refrigerator and freezer. Baking soda will remove odors. Wash the shelves and trays with warm, soapy water.

Clean countertops, tables, and the stove each time they are used. Clean cabinet and drawer fronts and the refrigerator once a week. Use a sponge or dishcloth that has been moistened with water and a detergent. If a cutting board or other surface has been used to cut fresh meat, scrub the surface thoroughly with soap and bleach, and rinse well. An all-purpose cleaner may be needed to remove grease and cooked foods that have spilled or splashed on surfaces. Clean the sink with a cleanser such as scouring powder or cream.

Never place food on soiled work or storage areas or in unclean containers. Keep food covered. Close lids of cartons and cover food storage containers to prevent contamination or infestation by insects and rodents. Place leftovers in covered containers and store them in the refrigerator immediately. Use them in two to three days. Chapter 23 contains more information about food preparation and storage.

Vacuum, sweep, or dry mop the floor daily. Damp mop uncarpeted floors at least once a week, using hot water and a floor cleaner. Be sure to rinse the floor if the label recommends doing so. Dry the floor or close off the area until the floor dries to prevent accidents.

Procedure 1: Cleaning a bathroom

1. Assemble supplies:
   - disinfectant (a cleaning product that kills germs)
   - scouring powder or scouring cream with bleach
   - sponge
   - toilet brush
   - glass cleaner
   - paper towels
   - disposable gloves

2. Put on gloves.

3. Using the disinfectant and sponge, wipe all surfaces and rinse as needed. Be sure to clean the sides, walls, and curtain or door of the shower or tub; the towel racks; holders for toilet paper, toothbrushes, and soap; and window sills.

4. Rinse sponge well or use a different sponge to wipe the outside of toilet bowl, seat, and lid. As a general cleaning rule, start with the cleanest surface first, then move to dirtier areas.

5. Use a different sponge to clean the bathtub, shower stall, and sink. Use scouring powder or cream for tile and porcelain, and disinfectant or all-purpose cleaner on other surfaces. Remember that scouring powder can scratch, so check with the client or a family member before using it. Be sure to scrub the sides, edges, and bottoms of all these areas. Clean faucets and scrub around their bases.

6. Scrub the inside of the toilet bowl with a brush and scouring powder containing bleach. Be sure to scrub under the rim. If you use a second, stronger toilet cleaner, flush the first cleaning product down the drain first to avoid possible chemical reactions. Wash the toilet brush with a disinfectant solution and store it in a plastic bag or holder after letting it air dry.

7. Vacuum or dry mop the floor first, then wash if the floor is tile or linoleum. Use an all-purpose floor cleaner in hot water. Wash the floor with a cloth or mop, taking special care to clean the area at the base of the toilet and sink. Do not leave the floor wet. Dry it carefully to avoid accidents.

8. Clean the mirror and any glass or chrome surfaces using glass cleaner and paper towels or clean rags.

9. Place dry, soiled towels in the laundry hamper. Empty the waste can into a plastic or paper garbage bag and dispose of it. Replace toilet tissue and facial tissue when needed. Open the bathroom window for a short time, if possible, to air the room out. Once a week, wash out the waste can and laundry hamper, and launder the bath mats and rugs.

10. Store supplies.

11. Remove and dispose of gloves.

12. Wash hands.

13. Document the cleaning.

Dispose of garbage daily. Drain off any liquid from waste items into the sink before putting it into a paper or plastic-lined pail. Place securely closed garbage bags outside in a large, covered garbage can or down the incinerator chute. If the kitchen has a garbage disposal, do not put hard or stringy, fibrous foods (like celery) into it. To prevent odor and discourage insects and rodents, rinse out tin cans and bottles before placing them in the garbage pail or recycling bin. Follow the recycling procedures for your client's community. Periodically wash wastebaskets and trash cans with hot, soapy water.

The kitchen is the site of many accidents in the home. It should be carefully checked for safety hazards. *All* cleaning materials should be stored away from food, food preparation utensils, food preparation areas, and out of reach of children and confused clients.

Cleaning and Organizing the Bathroom. A clean, organized, and odor-free bathroom is an important part of improving a family's hygiene and safety. Because it is moist and warm, the bathroom is a reservoir for the growth of microorganisms, mold, and mildew. Mold and mildew may grow around the bathtub and shower, particularly in the grout between tiles, and especially during the summer. A poorly cleaned toilet is another source of microorganisms and odors.

Involve the entire family in keeping the bathroom clean (**Fig. 21-6**). Teach all family members basic bathroom hygiene:

- flush the toilet each time it is used
- clean toothbrushes and toothbrush holders
- scrub the tub and shower after use
- remove hair from drain strainers
- pick up and hang up all used towels to dry
- put away toiletries
- rinse the sink after brushing teeth, shaving, and washing
- place soiled towels in the laundry hamper after they are dry

The bathroom is the location of many home accidents. Make sure that all bathroom rugs have non-skid undersides. Wipe up puddles of water immediately. If grab bars are not present and your client has difficulty moving about in the bathroom safely, report this to your supervisor.

Cleaning and Organizing Storage Areas. Cleaning and organizing storage areas will contribute to the order and organization of the home. Every item in the home should have a storage place that is convenient for use, that is, as close as possible to where they are used (**Fig. 21-7**). For example, bath towels should be stored in or near the bathroom, frequently used pots and pans and cooking utensils near the stove, eating utensils and dishes near the dining table, and food near the preparation area. Less frequently used items, such as waffle irons or popcorn poppers, should be stored in the less accessible storage places.

Items that are frequently used should be easily seen and reached. When they are used, they should be immediately replaced. Items that are used together should be stored near each other to save steps and time when cooking or performing other household tasks (for example, the broom and dustpan should be stored together). Arrange food on shelves according to category to save time in searching for items. Dangerous materials such as cleaning products should be stored out of reach of children and where they will not be mistaken for food or medicine by adults.

Some storage areas only need to be cleaned occa-

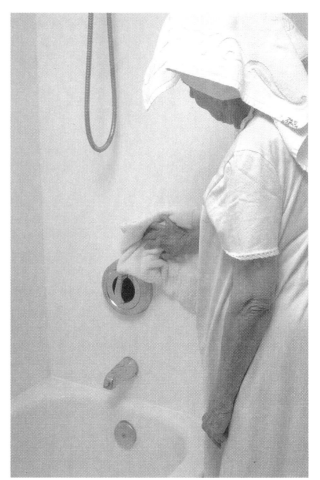

Fig. 21-6. If possible, help clients and their family members develop good habits of hygiene, like wiping out the shower after each use.

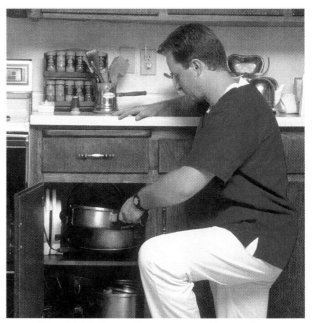

Fig. 21-7. Store items near where they will be used.

sionally. Remove the stored items and any shelf or drawer liners. Wipe the shelves and drawers with a damp cloth and all-purpose cleaner. Replace the liners or wipe them if they can be cleaned. Food storage areas and other storage areas that are used frequently should be cleaned more often.

Do not change the client's or the family's storage arrangements without consulting with them. If you think changes are needed, discuss your ideas with the family.

Several types of cleaning solutions can be prepared from common household items when supplies are not available or when the family budget is restricted.

▶ Baking soda can be used instead of scouring powder. Baking soda can also be diluted with warm water to make a solution that will eliminate odors when used to clean surfaces.

▶ White vinegar can be used to remove lime or other mineral deposits on sinks, toilets, or chrome fixtures. White vinegar diluted with water can be used instead of glass cleaner.

> Never mix different cleaning products together. Dangerous or even fatal chemical reactions can occur. In particular, never mix bleach and ammonia, or products containing either. The resulting fumes are toxic.

▶ Household bleach, diluted with four parts water, makes a strong disinfectant solution to clean bathroom surfaces. Diluted with ten parts water and stored in a spray bottle, bleach makes a milder disinfectant to use on kitchen counters. Be careful not to spill or splash undiluted bleach or bleach solutions on carpets, clothing, or other surfaces that might be discolored.

❏ 6. Describe how to prepare a cleaning schedule

Most house cleaning tasks should be done either immediately, daily, weekly, monthly, or less often. Taking into account the care plan, your assigned tasks, how much help is needed, and how much time you have in a particular home, you should prepare a cleaning schedule. You may not always stick to the schedule exactly, but it will guide your work and help you get essential cleaning done regularly. Establishing a schedule for your cleaning can also help the family maintain a housekeeping routine after your care has ended.

> **Box 21-1.**
> **Creating a Cleaning Schedule**
>
> Below is a sample cleaning schedule. The client can do almost nothing around the house. Her daughter comes in several times a week, but no family members live with the client to provide help.
>
> **Cleaning Schedule for Mrs. Fontine**
>
> **Immediately:** Wipe counters, wash dishes, store food, clean spills, put away supplies.
>
> **Daily:** Straighten up: make bed, sort mail, remove clutter, empty trash, etc. Clean bathroom. (One hour.)
>
> **Weekly:** Wash kitchen floors, wipe refrigerator, scrub sink, vacuum other floors, dust all surfaces, scrub bathtub. (Two to three hours.)
>
> **Monthly:** Clean out refrigerator, defrost freezer. (One hour.)
>
> **Less often:** Clean oven when needed. (One hour.)
>
> Cleaning schedules will be different for each client. Be flexible; you will need to adapt your schedule after you make it. Remember that client care is your first priority.

7. List special housekeeping procedures to use when infection is present

You must follow standard or universal precautions with every client, since you cannot always know when infection is present (see Chapter 5, Infection Control and Standard Precautions). However, when a client has a known infectious disease such as influenza, or one that weakens the immune system, such as AIDS or cancer, you need to take special precautions in housecleaning:

▶ Use disinfectant when cleaning countertops and surfaces in the kitchen and bathroom.

▶ Clean the client's bathroom daily, and have other family members use a different bathroom if possible.

▶ Use separate dishes and utensils for the infected client. In some cases, disposable dishes and utensils will be ordered.

▶ Wash dishes and utensils in the dishwasher or wash dishes in hot soapy water with bleach, rinse in boiling water, and allow to air dry.

▶ Disinfect any surfaces that contact body fluids, such as bedpans, urinals and toilets.

▶ Frequently remove trash containing used tissues.

▶ Keep any specimens of urine, stool, or sputum in double bags and away from food or food preparation areas.

Part 2
Laundry and Clothes Care

---

8. Explain how to do laundry and care for clothes

You may be expected to do hand or machine washing as part of an assignment. Clean clothes, bed linens, and towels are important for hygiene and comfort.

Laundry Products and Equipment. To do the laundry you will need laundry detergent, a washing machine or a basin for handwashing clothes, and a dryer or a clothesline and pins. The instructions for using washing machines are usually located on the inside of the washing machine lid.

In general, you will use all-purpose detergent. Some delicate fabrics, underwear, or stockings may require a special detergent. Some clients may prefer a non-detergent soap for use on baby clothes and diapers. Bleach, color brighteners, stain removers, and fabric softeners may also be used. Ask the client and family members about their preferences for laundry products.

Pretreating. Pretreating means that before washing is done certain laundry items and parts of items that have heavy soil, spots, and stains are given special treatment. Spots and stains should be treated immediately. The sooner they are treated, the easier they are to remove. Some oily stains harden with age and cannot be removed. Washing and ironing may set some stains, making them difficult or impossible to remove. Many stains are also difficult to see when the fabric is wet. If you can, identify the source of the stain and treat it according to a stain guide on the pretreating solution.

Bleach. Bleach is used with detergent and complements it, but bleach cannot be used on all fabrics. You must be familiar with the type of bleach and the fabric that is being washed. Three types of bleach are used in laundry: liquid chlorine, powdered chlorine, and oxygen or all-fabric bleach. Each type of bleach should be used with caution. Read the instructions on the container thoroughly.

Liquid chlorine bleaches are excellent stain removers and they whiten clothing. However, they can be very damaging. Bleach should always be diluted in water. Fill the washer, then add liquid bleach and stir the water before adding clothing. Never use liquid chlorine bleach on silk, spandex, wool, or any item that contains these fibers. Be careful not to spray or splash liquid chlorine bleach as it will remove color or damage fabric. Powdered chlorine bleach is more gentle than liquid, but it can also damage clothing. Either type of chlorine bleach is also an excellent disinfectant. Oxygen or all-fabric bleach is used on washable fabrics, but it is effective only in hot water.

Water Temperature. Read the washing instructions for all materials and garments (**Fig. 21-8**). Warm

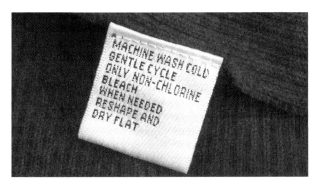

Fig. 21-8. A garment care tag that gives washing and drying instructions can be found on most clothing.

water is the safest temperature for most garments, but some must be washed in cold to prevent shrinking or colors fading. Hot water is generally used for towels, bed linens, and white or colorfast cottons. Warm is usually used for permanent press, knit, synthetic, sheer, lace, acetate, fabric blends, washable rayons, and plastic. Cold water is used for brightly-colored fabrics or fabrics that are not colorfast.

Washing Action or Cycle. Use the normal setting on the washer for cottons, linens, rayons, sturdy permanent press, knits, synthetics, blends, and most other items. Set the washer on the slow or gentle setting for washable woolens, old quilts, curtains, and delicate or fragile items.

Drying Clothes. Most homes have a clothes dryer. Settings on the dryer vary according to the model. Most dryers have a permanent press setting and a delicate setting. The more delicate a fabric the lower the drying temperature and the shorter the time in the dryer. Heavy items such as towels need higher temperature settings and a longer time in the dryer. Clean the lint filter each time you use the dryer.

Procedure 2: Doing the laundry

1. Sort clothes carefully, making separate piles of whites, colors, and bright colors. Check clothing labels for special washing instructions. Do not wash anything labeled "Dry Clean Only." If handwashing is recommended, do not wash in the machine.

2. As you sort laundry, check pockets and remove tissues, money, pens, and other items. Remove belts with buckles, trims, and nonwashable ornaments. Close zippers, buttons, and other fasteners. Check garments for stains and areas of heavy soil. If appropriate, mend or repair any holes, snags, rips, tears, pulled seams, and weak spots in garments and other items.

3. Pretreat spots and stains before washing. A small amount of liquid detergent or dry detergent dissolved in water can be

worked in with an old toothbrush (**Fig. 21-9**). Pretreat or soak clothing as soon as possible for best results. If you know something is spotted, don't let it sit in the laundry hamper all week until you do the laundry.

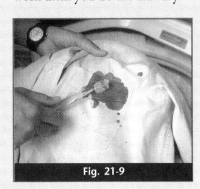
Fig. 21-9

4. Use the correct water temperature: hot for whites, warm for colors, cold for bright colors.

5. Use the appropriate laundry product(s) and follow the washing instructions on the container.

6. Follow written instructions or client or family instructions for using the washer. Use the correct washing cycle for the load you are laundering.

7. Dry clothes completely either in a dryer or on a clothesline. If using an automatic dryer, follow the drying instructions on clothing labels. Some fabrics require cooler temperatures.

8. Hand wash items in warm or cool water, depending on the fabric and instructions, using a mild detergent or special handwashing liquid. Line dry or lay flat on towels to preserve the shape of the garment.

9. Fold or hang clean laundry and sort into categories. Store in drawers or closets.

If your client does not have a clothes dryer, hang clothes on a clothesline using clothespins.

Folding. To reduce the amount of wrinkling, remove all clothes from the dryer immediately, and fold them neatly or place them on hangers. Set aside those that need to be ironed, and return other items to their drawers or closet.

Ironing. Before you begin to iron, check the label of the item for the recommended temperature. If the label does not recommend a particular setting or the fabric is a blend, use the lowest temperature on the iron. Take special care with pile fabrics, such as velvets and corduroy. They will keep their texture better if ironed on the wrong side over a terry cloth towel. Dark fabrics, silks, acetates, rayons, linens, and some wools must be pressed on the wrong side to prevent them from becoming shiny. Use a pressing cloth to protect the fabric.

To prevent stretching, iron all fabrics lengthwise. Iron collars, cuffs, and garment facings first. Next, iron the sleeves, then the front and back. Hang or fold clothes immediately, and fasten all hooks and buttons and close zippers. Be sure clothes are completely dry before putting them away.

Maintaining Clothing. You may need to help your clients and their families by doing basic mending or sewing occasionally, especially if you are taking care of a family, an older person with impaired vision, or people who may not have the time or the ability to keep clothing and household linens repaired. Some clients who can do their own mending may just need you to thread the needle.

❑ 9. List special laundry precautions to use when infection is present

When a client has a known infectious disease, you must take special precautions when handling laundry:

▶ Keep client's laundry separate from other family members.

▶ Handle dirty laundry as little as possible. Sort it and put it in plastic bags in the client's room or bathroom and take it immediately to the laundry area.

▶ Wear gloves and hold laundry away from your clothes and body when you are handling it.

▶ Use liquid bleach when fabrics allow.

▶ Use Lysol™ or other agency-approved disinfectants in all loads.

▶ Use hot water.

Part 3
Involving Family Members in Household Management

❑ 10. List five guidelines for teaching housekeeping skills to clients' family members

In some assignments, you will be asked to teach housekeeping skills to family members, preparing them to take over housekeeping and care when home care agency service is discontinued. By teaching household management skills, you can help families meet their daily needs and become more self-reliant. See the **Box 21-2** for tips to keep in mind when working with family members.

Part 4
Bedmaking

❑ 11. List three reasons careful bedmaking is important

When clients spend much or all of their time in bed, careful bedmaking is essential to their comfort, cleanliness, and health. Linens should always be changed after personal care procedures such as sponge baths, or any time bedding or sheets are damp, soiled, or in need of straightening. The following are three major reasons why it is important that clients' bed linens be changed frequently.

1. Sheets that are damp, wrinkled, or bunched up under a client are uncomfortable and may prevent the client from resting or sleeping well.

2. Microorganisms thrive in moist, warm environments, so bedding that is damp or unclean may encourage infection and disease.

3. Clients who spend long hours in bed are at risk for pressure sores caused by irritation from bedding. Sheets that do not lie flat under the client's body increase the risk of pressure sores because they cut off circulation.

Box 21-2. Points to Remember When Teaching Family Members

- Individualize your teaching for family members and their cultural patterns.
- Establish a relationship with family members before you begin to teach. Become acquainted with them and the nature and extent of their problems before you begin teaching.
- Allow people time to learn new habits and ways of doing things. They will not do things perfectly the first time.
- Limit the amount of time teaching at any one session.
- Demonstrate and explain how to do each task.
- Break down tasks into simple steps that can be easily learned.
- Answer every question as completely as possible. If someone wants to know why a particular product is used or why a task needs to be done in a certain way, take time to explain.
- Be flexible but set limits. When you can, set a time that is convenient for all for teaching and performing tasks.
- Give praise for tasks done well.
- Assist those who are having difficulty with tasks, but not without giving them a chance to work out their difficulties. Do not do the task or a part of the task for them.
- Point out how doing the task helps the home look better or the people in it feel better. Be careful not to talk down to people or treat them like children.

Adapted from the *Model Curriculum and Teaching Guide for the Instruction of the Homemaker-Home Health Aide*, National HomeCaring Council, Foundation for Hospice and Homecare, Washington, D.C.

**Box 21-3.
Maintaining Good Body Mechanics When Working in the Home**

Review the principles of body mechanics you learned in Chapter 6. Always use good body mechanics, and remember the following additional tips when working in a home:

- Bend the knees, not the back, when lifting things from the floor or when kneeling to pick up objects. Many people develop backaches because they strain muscles by bending their backs when lifting and stooping.
- Carry heavy objects close to the body and distribute the weight evenly (for example, when carrying a basket of clothes, hold it directly in front of the body, as shown in **Fig. 21-10**).
- Stand close to the work area. When possible, raise the work area to a comfortable level so

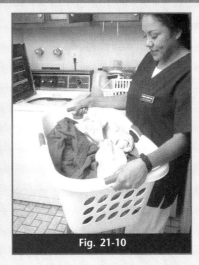

Fig. 21-10

you don't have to bend your back and neck to do the work.
- Try not to lift heavy objects. If you must move heavy objects such as furniture, try pushing, pulling, or rolling, using the entire body.
- Avoid lifting heavy objects from the floor (for example,

put the clothes basket on a chair before filling it, as in **Fig. 21-11**).

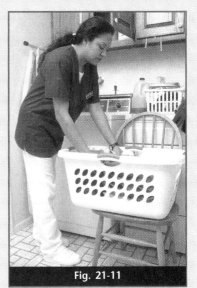

Fig. 21-11

- Stand erect when doing tasks like washing dishes. Your knees may be slightly bent.

1. Explain what you will do. Ask for the client's cooperation. It is useful to have a family member available to help you if possible.

2. Wash hands.

3. Assemble supplies. You will generally use the client's own bedding. Do not use torn linens, and do not use pins on bed linens. Notify your supervisor if the client does not have adequate bed linens.

- mattress pad
- fitted or flat bottom sheet
- waterproof bed protector or pad if needed
- flat draw sheet (see description below)
- flat top sheet
- blanket(s)
- pillowcase(s)
- laundry basket, hamper, or bag
- disposable gloves

4. Put on gloves.

5. If the bed is adjustable, raise it to a comfortable working height.

6. Cover the client with a cotton bath blanket or the loosened top sheet already on the bed. Ask client to roll to one side of the bed. You will make the bed one side at a time. If the client cannot roll to the side without assistance, roll him or her as explained in Chapter 12, Procedure 9. Make sure the client is comfortable and cannot roll off the bed. Raise the side rail if the bed has one, or use pillows, chair backs, or a family member to protect the client from falling out of the bed while you are making it.

7. On the opposite side of the bed, with the client's back to you, loosen the bottom sheet, mattress pad, and protector if present. Fanfold these toward the client like an accordion, tucking them under client's body.

8. Open the clean mattress pad and place it on the mattress. Do the same with the bottom sheet. If you are using a fitted bottom sheet, tuck the corners under the mattress corners.

9. If you are using a flat bottom sheet, leave enough overlap on each end to tuck under the mattress. If the sheet is only long enough to tuck in at one end, tuck it in securely at the top of the bed. The bottom sheet must be without wrinkles. Make a square or hospital corner (**Fig. 21-12**) at each corner and tuck the sides of the bottom sheet under the mattress.

10. Smooth the bottom sheet out toward the client. Be sure there are no wrinkles in the mattress pad. Fanfold the extra material toward the client and tuck it under the client's body.

11. If using a waterproof pad, unfold it and center it on the bed. Tuck the side near you under the mattress. Smooth it out toward the client, fanfold and tuck as you did with the sheet.

12. Place a **draw sheet** on the bed, tuck in on your side, and smooth, fanfold and tuck as you did with the other bedding (**Fig. 21-13**). A draw sheet is a small

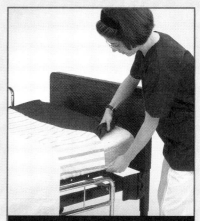

Fig. 21-13. Multiple layers of bedding, including a draw sheet, are often used for clients who spend a lot of time in bed.

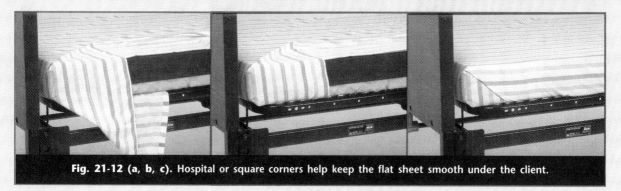

Fig. 21-12 (a, b, c). Hospital or square corners help keep the flat sheet smooth under the client.

sheet placed under the client (usually from shoulder blade to mid-thigh) to protect the bed and make it easier to move the client. Draw sheets can be made of plastic, rubber, or cotton. A regular sheet folded in half can also serve as a draw sheet. Never place plastic or rubber directly under the client's skin. It should always be covered by a layer of cloth.

13. Explain to the client that there is a lump in the middle of the bed. Ask client to turn toward you, over the lump. If client cannot move, roll client back over the lump onto the clean side of the bed. It is useful to have a family member assist you with this. Protect the client from any soiled matter on the old linens.

14. Make sure the client is comfortable and cannot roll off the bed. Raise side rail if available. Go to the other side of the bed and remove the soiled linens. Hold them away from your clothes and body and put them in the laundry hamper, basket, or bag. Never put them on the floor or furniture, and never shake them. Soiled bed linens are full of microorganisms that should not be spread to other parts of the room.

15. Pull the clean linens over the mattress and smooth them toward you. Be sure there are no wrinkles or lumps. Tuck bedding under, making square corners if you are using a flat bottom sheet.

16. Ask your client to turn onto his or her back. Keep client covered and comfortable, with a pillow under the head.

17. Unfold the top sheet and place it over the client. Ask the client to hold the top sheet. Slip the blanket or old sheet out from underneath and put it in the laundry hamper.

18. Place a blanket over the top sheet, matching the top edges. Tuck the bottom edges of top sheet and blanket under the bottom of the mattress, making square corners on each side. Loosen the top linens slightly over the client's toes for comfort.

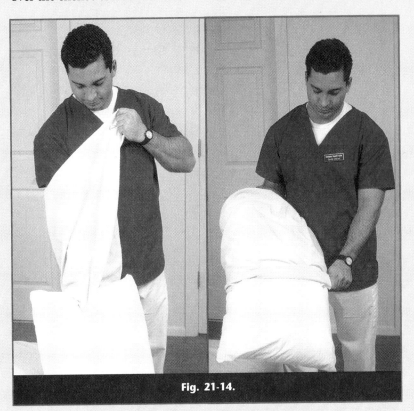

Fig. 21-14.

At the top of the bed, fold the top sheet over the blanket about six inches.

19. Remove the pillow under the client's head. Because it probably contains microorganisms from the client's mouth and nose, do not hold the pillow near your face. Remove the soiled pil-

lowcase by turning it inside out, and place it in the laundry hamper. Remove your gloves.

20. With one hand, grasp the clean pillowcase at the closed end and turn it inside out over your arm. Next, using the same hand that has the pillowcase over it, grasp one narrow edge of the pillow and pull the pillowcase over it with your free hand (**Fig. 21-14**). Do the same for any other pillows, and place them under your client's head or as desired.

21. If the client uses a bell or call signal, place it within reach. Make sure the client is comfortable. Take the laundry hamper to the laundry area.

22. Wash your hands.

23. Document the procedure and any observations.

Procedure 4: Making an unoccupied bed

1. Explain what you will do. Ask for the client's cooperation. It is useful to have a family member available to help you if possible.

2. Wash hands.

3. Assemble supplies:
- mattress pad
- fitted or flat bottom sheet
- waterproof bed protector or pad if needed
- flat draw sheet
- flat top sheet
- blanket(s)
- pillowcase(s)
- laundry basket, hamper, or bag
- disposable gloves

4. Put on gloves.

5. Remove soiled linens, rolling them into themselves in the center of the bed. Remove pillows and soiled pillowcases as well. Holding linens away from your clothes and body, put them in the laundry hamper or directly into the washing machine. Remove your gloves.

6. Remake the bed, spreading mattress pad and bottom sheet, tucking under and making square or "mitered" corners if using a flat bottom sheet. Put on mattress protector and draw sheet, smooth, and tuck under sides of bed.

7. Place top sheet and blanket over bed. Center these, tuck under end of bed and make square corners. Fold down the top sheet over the blanket about six inches. Fold both top sheet and blanket down so client can easily get into bed. If client will not be returning to bed immediately, leave bedding up.

8. Put on clean pillowcases (as described in Procedure 3), and replace pillows.

9. Carry laundry hamper to laundry area or the appropriate place.

10. Wash your hands.

11. Help the client back into bed, if desired. If the client uses a bell or call signal, place it within reach.

12. Document the procedure and any observations.

A correctly and comfortably made bed is an essential part of good care for clients who spend a great deal of time in bed. Remembering the following guidelines will help you make a comfortable and safe bed for clients.

1. If a client cannot get out of bed, you must change the linens with the client in bed. When making the bed, be careful to use a wide stance with knees bent. Avoid bending from the waist, especially when tucking sheets or blankets under the mattress. Mattresses can be heavy, so remember to bend your knees to avoid injury.

2. It is easier to make an unoccupied bed than one with a client in it. If the client can be moved temporarily to a chair or other comfortable spot, your job will be easier. As when making an occupied bed, be careful to use a wide stance with knees bent. Avoid bending from the waist, especially when tucking sheets or blankets under the mattress. Mattresses can be heavy, so remember to bend your knees to avoid injury.

Part 5
Additional Safety Measures

❏ 12. Identify hazardous household materials

Any of the following household materials can have harmful effects:

- household bleach
- cleaning products
- aerosol or spray cans
- paint
- chemicals such as turpentine or paint thinner
- medicines, both prescription and over-the-counter
- hair spray
- nail polish remover

These products should be kept in separate cabinets with childproof latches or locks, or up out of the reach of children. If a client is confused, mark these cabinets with signs that indicate danger.

Chapter 22

Understanding the Nutritional Needs of Your Clients

Part 1
Basic Nutrition

❑ **1. Describe the importance of good nutrition and list the six basic nutrients**

The importance of good nutrition can never be underestimated. For the human body to grow new cells, maintain normal functioning of all systems, and have energy for activities, it needs a well-balanced diet containing essential nutrients and adequate fluids.

Good nutrition in childhood and early adulthood helps ensure good health later in life. For those who are ill or elderly, a well-balanced, nutritious diet helps maintain muscle and skin tissues and prevent pressure sores. A good diet also promotes the healing of wounds and helps us cope with physical and emotional stress.

The Six Basic Nutrients

The body needs the following nutrients for growth and development:

1. **Protein.** Proteins are part of every body cell, and are essential for tissue growth and repair. Proteins also function as **hormones** or **enzymes**, combining with body fluids to assist with chemical reactions in the body. They help form **antibodies**, or chemicals that defend the body against disease. Proteins are also an alternate supply of energy for the body. Excess proteins are excreted by the kidneys or stored as body fat.

Good sources of protein are fish, seafood, poultry, meat, eggs, milk, cheese, nuts, peas, and dried beans or legumes (**Fig. 22-1**). Whole grain cereals, pastas, rice, and breads con-

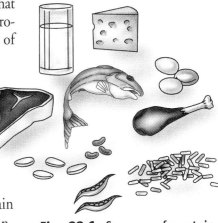

Fig. 22-1. Sources of protein.

Table 22-1. Source and Function of Essential Vitamins

VITAMIN	SOURCE	FUNCTION
Vitamin A	dark green and yellow vegetables, such as broccoli and turnips	assists with skin and eye development, keeps the skin healthy and helps the eyes adjust to dim light, helps the linings of the respiratory and digestive tracts resist infection
Vitamin C	fruits such as oranges, strawberries, grapefruit, and cantaloupe; and vegetables such as broccoli, cabbage, brussel sprouts, and green peppers	assists with healing wounds and building bones and teeth, holds cells together, strengthens the walls of blood vessels, and helps the body absorb iron
Vitamin B_2 or riboflavin	milk, milk products, lean meat, green leafy vegetables, eggs, breads, and cereals	helps cells use oxygen, which allows them to release energy from food; important for protein and carbohydrate metabolism; needed for growth, healthy eyes, skin, and mucous membranes
Vitamin B_3 or niacin	lean meat, poultry, fish, peanuts and peanut butter, whole grain breads and cereals, peas, beans, and eggs	important for protein, carbohydrate and fat metabolism, appetite, and the functioning of the skin, tongue, nervous system, and digestive system; helps cells use oxygen for energy
Vitamin D	milk, butter, liver, and fish liver oils, but it is also obtained by exposing the body to direct sunlight, which interacts with the cholesterol in the skin	responsible for the body's absorption of the minerals calcium and phosphorus and contributes to the formation of healthy bones; especially important to growing children, and women who are pregnant or breastfeeding
Thiamin	lean pork, dried beans, peas, whole grain and enriched breads and cereals, and certain types of nuts	helps the body obtain energy from foods

tain some proteins of lower quality, which must be complemented by a small quantity of the more complete proteins. Beans and rice, or cereal and milk, are examples of complementary proteins.

2. Carbohydrates. Carbohydrates (kar-boh-HIGH-drayts) supply the fuel for the body's energy needs at the cell and organ level. Carbohydrates supply extra protein and help the body use fat efficiently. During digestion, carbohydrates are broken down into sugars that are absorbed into the blood. Carbohydrates also provide **fiber**, which is necessary for bowel elimination. Fiber forms the bulk of what passes through the digestive tract. Though fiber is not considered a nutrient, it is an important part of a balanced diet.

Carbohydrates can be divided into two basic types: 1) **complex carbohydrates**, which are found in foods such as bread, cereal, potatoes, rice, pasta, vegetables, and fruits; and 2) **simple carbohydrates**, found in foods such as sugars, sweets, syrups, and jellies. Simple carbohydrates do not have the same nutritional value as complex carbohydrates (**Fig. 22-2**). The only value of simple carbohydrates is as a source of energy for people who eat very little or are malnourished. In other people, simple carbohydrates are stored as fat.

3. Fats. Fat helps the body store energy. Fat contains more energy per unit of measure than other nutrients. Body fat also provides the body with

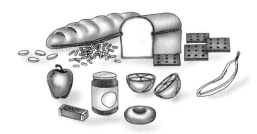

Fig. 22-2. Sources of carbohydrates.

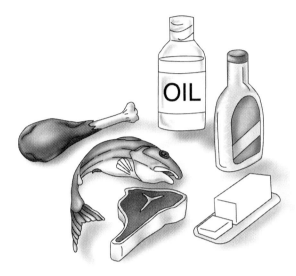

Fig. 22-3. Sources of fat.

insulation and protects body organs. In addition, fats supply the body with essential fatty acids needed for healthy nervous tissue. Fats add flavor to food and are important for the absorption of certain vitamins. Excess fat in the diet is stored as fat in the body.

Examples of fats are butter, margarine, salad dressings, oils, and animal fats found in meats, fowl, and fish (**Fig. 22-3**). Monounsaturated vegetable fats (including olive oil and canola oil) and polyunsaturated vegetable fats (including corn and safflower oils) are healthier kinds of fats. Saturated fats, including animal fats like butter, lard, bacon and other fatty meats, are not as healthy and should be limited in most diets. Saturated fats raise the level of blood cholesterol, which contributes to circulatory disorders like arteriosclerosis.

4. **Vitamins.** Most vitamins cannot be produced by the body. They can only be obtained from food, but they are essential to body functions. Vitamins A, D, E, and K are **fat-soluble** vitamins, meaning they are carried and stored in body fat. Vitamins B and C are **water-soluble** vitamins that are broken

Table 22-2. Source and Function of Essential Minerals

MINERAL	SOURCE	FUNCTION
Iron	egg yolks, green leafy vegetables, breads, cereals, and organ meats	necessary for the red blood cells to carry oxygen; helps in the formation of enzymes
Sodium	almost all foods and table salt	important for maintaining fluid balance (helps the body retain water)
Potassium	fruits and vegetables, cereals, coffee, and meats	essential for nerve and heart function and muscle contraction
Calcium	milk and milk products such as cheese, ice cream, and yogurt; green leafy vegetables such as collards, kale, mustard, dandelion, and turnip greens; and canned fish with soft bones, such as salmon	important for the formation of teeth and bones, the clotting of blood, muscle contraction, and heart and nerve function
Phosphorus	milk, milk products, meat, fish, poultry, nuts, and eggs	needed for the formation of bones and teeth and nerve and heart function; important for the body's utilization of proteins, fats, and carbohydrates

down by water in our bodies. They cannot be stored in the body, but are eliminated in urine and feces. **Table 22-1** summarizes the source and function of vitamins the body needs to stay healthy.

5. Minerals. Minerals, such as zinc, iron, calcium, and magnesium assist with various chemical reactions within the body. They work as co-enzymes in body reactions and are found in many foods. **Table 22-2** summarizes the source and function of minerals the body needs.

6. Water. Because one-half to two-thirds of our body weight is water, we need about 6 to 8 glasses of water a day. Water is the most essential nutrient for life. Without it, a person can only live a few days. Water assists in the digestion and absorption of food, as well as elimination of waste. Through perspiration, water also helps maintain normal body temperature. Maintaining fluid balance in our bodies is absolutely necessary for good health. Fluid balance is discussed more in Chapter 14 and in Learning Objective 3 in this chapter.

The fluids we drink—water, juice, soda, coffee, tea, and milk—provide most of the water our bodies use. Some foods are also sources of water, including celery, lettuce, apples, peaches, meat, chicken, and fish.

❑ 2. List the six food groups on the USDA Food Guide Pyramid and give examples of each

Planning nutritious meals requires a knowledge of the various food groups and the types of nutrients that are concentrated in each of them. Most foods contain several nutrients, but no one food contains all the nutrients that are necessary to maintain a healthy body. Therefore, it is important that we eat a daily diet that is well-balanced, containing several foods selected from each of the following food groups.

The U.S. Department of Agriculture (USDA) has divided the foods that we eat into six groups:

1. grains, including cereals, bread, rice, and pasta

2. fruits

3. vegetables

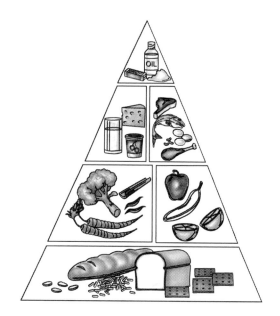

Fig. 22-4. The Food Guide Pyramid was created by the U.S. Department of Agriculture to show the six food groups and how, together, they form a healthy diet.

4. milk and milk products

5. meat, poultry, fish, eggs, dry beans, and nuts

6. fats, oils, and sweets

These six groups have been arranged into the **Food Guide Pyramid** (**Fig. 22-4**). Foods close to the bottom of the pyramid should make up most of our diet. Foods closer to the top should be eaten in smaller quantities.

Grains. Grains found in cereal, bread, rice, and pasta provide the foundation for a healthful diet. These foods, in addition to fruits and vegetables, are an excellent source of carbohydrates. The Food Guide Pyramid recommends eating between six and eleven servings from the grain group each day. Examples of one serving include one slice of bread, one cup of dry cereal, or ½ cup of cooked pasta or rice. When we eat more than our bodies need of any type of carbohydrate, the excess is converted into fat and stored.

Foods containing complex carbohydrates take longer to break down. Therefore, they provide longer-lasting energy than foods containing simple carbohydrates. Whole grain foods, such as whole wheat breads, bran cereals, brown rice, and whole wheat pastas, contain more complex carbohydrates than white breads, rice, pastas, and processed cereals. Whole grain foods also contain more vitamins, protein, and energy. Simple carbohydrates such as sugar, and foods made from processed flour and refined sugar, are poor sources of nutrients and energy.

Vegetables. Vegetables are excellent sources of vitamins and fiber. Choose from green leafy vegetables, including lettuce, spinach, and kale; tomatoes, green beans, peas, corn, cabbage, cauliflower, broccoli, and other vegetables. Vegetable sources of vitamin C include brussels sprouts, green or red peppers, and broccoli. The Food Guide Pyramid recommends eating three to five servings from the vegetable group each day. One serving from this group consists of ½ cup of cooked or chopped vegetables or ¾ cup of vegetable juice.

Fruits. Fruits are good sources of complex carbohydrates, vitamins, and fiber. Fruits are one of the best sources of vitamin C, a nutrient we should eat each day. Good sources of vitamin C include oranges and orange juice, grapefruit and grapefruit juice, strawberries, mango, papaya, and cantaloupe. The Food Guide Pyramid recommends eating two to four servings from the fruit group each day. One serving from this group could include one medium-sized apple, orange, pear, or banana; ¾ cup of juice; ½ cup of canned fruit; or ¼ cup of raisins.

Dairy Products. Milk and milk products, such as cheese and yogurt, are important sources of calcium, a nutrient needed for the development and maintenance of bones and teeth. Milk products also contain other minerals, protein, and vitamins. Other milk products are buttermilk, evaporated milk, and cottage cheese. Because whole milk, cheese, and other products made with whole milk contain a lot of saturated fat, most adults should eat low-fat or nonfat milk and milk products. Adults are advised to have two to three servings from the dairy group each day. A serving of milk equals one cup. Other serving sizes from the dairy group include one cup of yogurt, two cups of cottage cheese, or one-and-a-half ounces of cheese.

Milk can be incorporated into foods, such as pudding, milk shakes, cereal, and cream soups, for peo-

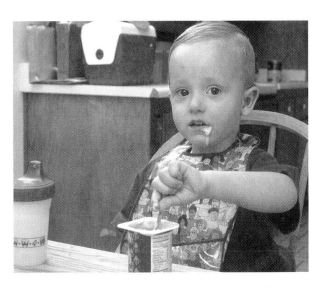

Fig. 22-5. Serving foods made with milk is one way to help clients who do not like to drink milk.

ple who dislike milk (**Fig. 22-5**). Powdered milk can be used in cooking and baking as an economic alternative to regular milk. For clients who need an extra source of protein and nourishment, powdered skim milk can be mixed with milk rather than water for puddings and milk shakes.

Fish, Poultry, Meat, Eggs, Dry Beans, and Nuts. These foods provide protein, minerals, and vitamins. In addition, meat is a good source of iron. Lower fat choices from this group include most fish, chicken or turkey breast, lean cuts of meat, and dry beans. These are the best choices for most adults. The Food Guide Pyramid recommends eating two to three servings from this group each day. One serving from this group equals three ounces of cooked meat, one egg, ½ cup cooked dry beans, or ½ cup of nuts.

Fats, Oils, and Sweets. Fats and oils help the body absorb fat-soluble vitamins. They also provide fla-

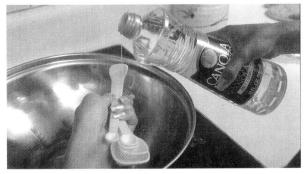

Fig. 22-6. Substitute olive, canola, or corn oil in recipes that call for higher fat oils.

vor and make us feel full. Fats are needed by the body in very small quantities. Most adults eat more fat than their bodies need. Fats contain more than twice as many calories per gram as carbohydrates or proteins. Excess fat is stored by the body as fatty tissue. The best kinds of fats to use in a healthy diet are vegetable oils, including olive oil, canola oil, and corn oil (**Fig. 22-6**).

Sweets, including candy, cookies, cakes, pies, and ice cream, contain large quantities of fat and sugar and should be eaten sparingly. In general, sweets provide no nutritional value. Eating too many sweets will cause weight gain. Some clients, particularly those with diabetes, must avoid sweets altogether.

❑ 3. Identify four ways to assist clients in maintaining fluid balance

As long as they are not on fluid restrictions, all clients should be encouraged to drink six to eight glasses of water a day. As discussed above, water is an essential nutrient for life. Because the sense of thirst often diminishes as people age, all elderly clients should be reminded to drink fluids often. For younger clients, it is important to remember that children can quickly become **dehydrated** or experience **fluid overload**.

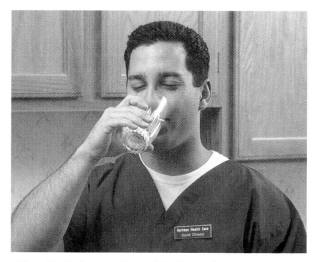

Fig. 22-7. Remember, drinking plenty of water is good for you, too!

Dehydration (dee-high-DRAY-shun) occurs when a person does not have enough fluid in the body. People can become dehydrated not only from not drinking enough, but also if they are experiencing diarrhea or vomiting. Signs and symptoms of dehydration include the following:

▶ poor skin elasticity

▶ flushed, dry skin

▶ coated tongue

▶ decreased urine output

▶ confusion and irritability

▶ elevated body temperature

▶ decrease or absence of tears and/or saliva

Fluid overload occurs when the body is unable to handle the amount of fluid consumed. This condition often affects people with heart or kidney disease. Signs and symptoms of fluid overload include the following:

▶ swelling/edema of extremities (ankles, feet, fingers, hands)

▶ weight gain (daily weight gain of one to two pounds)

▶ decreased urine output

▶ shortness of breath

▶ increased heart rate

▶ skin that appears tight, smooth, and shiny

Fluid balance (having the right amount of fluid in the body) can be measured by monitoring a client's input and output. Chapter 14, Performing Basic Health Care Skills, describes the procedure for measuring intake and output. If you suspect a client is experiencing either dehydration or fluid overload, contact your supervisor immediately.

The following guidelines make it easier to assist clients in maintaining fluid balance:

▶ Keep *fresh* water available. If possible, place it within reach for bed-bound clients.

▶ Encourage the client to keep a log of fluids consumed.

▶ Offer small sips of fluids frequently.

▶ Use adaptive cups to help clients help themselves.

4. Identify nutritional problems of the elderly or ill

Aging and illness can lead to emotional and physical problems that affect the intake of food. For example, people who are lonely or who suffer from physical impairments that affect their ability to chew and swallow may have little interest in food. Special care must be taken in meal planning and preparation to ensure an adequate intake of nutrients.

Clients who have small appetites may consume a better diet if they are fed five or six small meals a day. If you are concerned that a client is not getting enough nutrients in the amount of foods consumed, talk with your supervisor about preparing high-calorie, high-protein foods and beverages. Food should be prepared to look, taste, and smell good, particularly since many people who are elderly and sick may have a poor sense of taste and smell.

Many elderly people who receive certain medications or have limited activity are constipated. Constipation often interferes with appetite. Adding more fiber, fluids, and exercise to the daily regimen can improve this common problem. Many illnesses require restrictions in fluids, proteins, certain minerals, or calories, so always check with your supervisor before changing a client's diet.

In addition, clients who are ill are often fatigued, nauseated, or in pain. Home care aides should make sure these clients get plenty of rest and take prescribed medications for pain or nausea according to instructions. Some medications must be taken with food, others must be taken before meals. These instructions are important both for reminding clients to take medications (through routine), and for avoiding or limiting nausea and upset stomach caused by medications. People who are nauseated may tolerate cold foods better than warm foods, because cold foods have less aroma. Eating small amounts of food throughout the day and eating slowly may also help.

Clients who have had strokes may have difficulty swallowing liquids because of facial weakness. Liquids that have been thickened may be easier to swallow. Thickened liquids include milk shakes, pureed foods, sherbet, gelatin, thin hot cereal, cream soups, and fruit juices that have been frozen to a slushy consistency.

Artificial Feeding

When clients are too ill to receive adequate nutrition by mouth, artificial feeding becomes necessary. Two types of artificial feeding may be administered.

1. Intravenous Feeding. When the digestive system does not function properly, intravenous hyperalimentation (in-tra-VEE-nus high-per-al-ih-men-TAY-shun), or **IVH** may be necessary to sustain life. A solution of nutrients that can be administered directly into the blood stream is infused into the client's veins, which carry the nutrients to the tissues and cells of the body. Intravenous feeding may be temporary or permanent. Home care aides are *not* responsible for IVH. You may be assigned to take the person's temperature or assemble supplies for a sterile dressing change. In addition, you should observe, report, and document any observation of changes in the client or problems with the feeding.

2. Enteral Feeding. Clients who have functioning digestive systems may be fed through a tube that has been passed through the nose and esophagus into the stomach, or through a tube that is placed through the skin directly into the stomach, called a **gastric gavage** (**Fig. 22-8**). This type of feeding

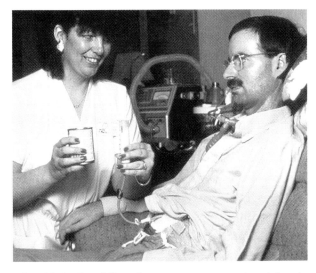

Fig. 22-8. Providing intravenous or enteral feeding requires special training and is performed by a nurse.

may be used when clients cannot swallow. Conditions that may prevent clients from swallowing include coma, stroke, refusal to eat, extreme weakness, or a need for increased calories.

Home care aides are *not* assigned to do enteral feedings. You may, however, be asked to assist the nurse with an enteral feeding. Home care aides *never* insert tubes, do the feeding, or irrigate (clean) the tubes. Home care aides may assemble equipment and supplies and hand them to the nurse. You may position the client for feeding. You may also dispose of used equipment and supplies, or clean and store reusable equipment and supplies. As always, you should observe, report, and document anything unusual about the feeding or anything unusual about the gastric gavage between feedings.

❑ 5. Demonstrate awareness of regional, cultural, and religious food preferences

We all prefer some foods or some types of cooking over others. Our preferences may be formed by the foods we ate as children, by what tastes good to us, or by our beliefs about what we should eat. Sometimes the place or culture we grew up in influences the kinds of foods we like to eat. For example, people from the southwestern US may like spicy foods. "Southern cooking" may include fried foods, like fried chicken or fried okra. Ethnic groups often have certain foods that are common to them and these may be eaten at certain times of the year or all the time. Sometimes religious beliefs influence diet; for example, Jewish people may not eat any pork and may not eat milk products at the same time as meat.

When planning meals and cooking for your clients, it is essential to know about their food preferences. Some of these may be listed in the care plan, but you will also need to find out more before planning meals. You can ask the client or a family member to tell you about food preferences, or you can suggest some sample menus and ask for reactions. Pay attention to what is eaten when you serve meals. If a client never finishes her chicken, it may mean that she prefers other kinds of meats. Cost may also be a factor in choosing foods. Protein-rich foods are generally the most expensive, but also the most

important for the healing process. You will learn to consider all these aspects of meal planning in Chapter 23, Meal Planning, Shopping, Preparation, and Storage.

> ### Part 2
> ### Food Labeling

❑ 6. List and define the five most common health claims on food labels

Food packages often make claims about the health benefits of the food they contain. Remember that food labels are advertising that is designed to convince you to buy a product. Although some regulations exist about what labels can claim, you should evaluate health claims carefully before making a decision to buy (**Box 22-1**).

❑ 7. Explain the information on the FDA-required Nutrition Facts label

The Food and Drug Administration (FDA) requires that all packaged foods contain a standardized nutrition label, called "Nutrition Facts." This label contains information about the nutritional content of food. Because the label is in the same format on all foods, it is easy to compare different products (**Fig. 22-9**).

Regular Frozen Lasagna

Nutrition Facts	
Serving size 1 Package (10.75 oz.)	
Amount Per Serving	
Calories 360	**Calories from Fat 120**
	% Daily Value
Total Fat 13g	20%
Saturated Fat 7g	35%
Cholesterol 35mg	11%
Sodium 960mg	40%
Total Carbohydrate 40g	14%
Dietary Fiber 6g	23%
Sugars 10g	
Protein 21g	
Calcium	35%
Vitamin A	10%
Vitamin C	10%
Iron	6%

Fig. 22-9. The FDA-required Nutrition Facts label contains standard nutritional information that makes it easy to compare different products.

Box 22-1. Key Claims in Food Label Advertising

Low-fat, nonfat, fat-free, reduced fat, or light. If a product is labeled low-fat or nonfat, you can be pretty sure it does not contain much fat. One exception to this is 2% milk, which is often labeled low-fat, but actually gets more than 30% of its calories from fat. You should always read the label anyway to determine the fat content of the food.

Some products are called "reduced fat" or "light," meaning they contain less fat than other versions of the same product. For example, salad dressing labeled "reduced fat" should contain 25% less fat than regular salad dressing, but may still be high in fat. Salad dressing labeled "light" should contain 50% less fat than regular. Read the label to determine fat content.

Some foods labeled low-fat, non-fat, or reduced fat may contain fat substitutes, including vegetable gums or synthetic substitutes. In general, the best food and dollar value is found in products that do not contain these substitutes.

Cookies, cakes, and other treats labeled fat-free or reduced fat usually contain a lot of sugar and calories. Remember that all sweets should be used sparingly, as they provide little or no food value. Also remember that extra calories, especially sugars, are quickly converted to fat by the body.

Low-sodium, sodium-free, or no salt added. For clients who must reduce their sodium or salt intake, foods labeled low-sodium or sodium-free are important. Remember that most foods naturally contain some sodium, but avoid foods that list salt or sodium as added ingredients. In general, canned foods and prepared foods like soups and frozen dinners tend to contain a lot of added salt and should be avoided.

Cholesterol-free. Some foods are labeled cholesterol-free. These may be useful for those clients who must restrict their cholesterol intake. However, the best way to limit cholesterol is to avoid foods containing animal fats, such as butter, cheese, whole milk, eggs,

red meats, and organ meats.

Sugar-free or no sugar added. Clients who must restrict their weight or who are diabetic must be very careful about consuming any product containing sugar. Sugar-free products can be helpful, but you must read the labels carefully. Sugar-free products may contain artificial sweeteners, such as saccharine or aspartame. These have no food value and should be used sparingly. Foods sweetened with fruit juice may still contain a lot of calories. Diabetics may need to avoid fruit-juice sweetened products as well as sugar sweetened ones.

Natural, healthy, or good for you. These claims may have little or no meaning. Buy whole, unprocessed grains, fresh fruits and vegetables, and lean meats, poultry and fish, and you will know you are buying food that is healthy and nutritious. Don't be swayed by the advertising you see on labels; check the facts before you buy.

The Nutrition Facts label gives you the following information.

Serving size and number of servings per container: Check the size of the serving. Remember that a serving may be a different amount than what a client actually eats.

Calories per serving and calories from fat per serving: The number of calories per serving tells you how much food energy a serving contains. It does not tell you how much nutritional value the food has. A candy bar is high in calories, providing quick energy, but has very few nutrients and lots of fat and sugar.

The number of calories from fat tells you a lot about the fat content of a food. In general, no more than one-third or roughly 30% of the total calories should come from fat. Thus, potato chips containing 110 calories per ounce and 80 calories from fat per ounce are not a good food choice. With more than two-thirds of their calories from fat, they are a high fat food.

Amounts and % daily totals: For each of the following items, the label tells you two things. First, how much does a serving contain, and second, what percent of the recommended daily total does a serving contain. For example, crackers that contain three grams of fat per serving contain 5% of the recommended daily total of fat. These recommended daily totals are based on a 2,000 calorie diet. Someone who eats fewer than 2,000 calories per day should have less fat each day; someone who eats more than 2,000 calories per day can have more fat. The FDA-required label gives amounts and % daily totals for the following: total fat and saturated fat, cholesterol, sodium, total carbohydrates, dietary fiber, sugars, and protein.

% Daily totals for vitamins and minerals: Finally, the label lists the percentages of the recommended daily total for certain vitamins and minerals. If the label says one serving contains 50% of the vitamin C needed each day, you know this food is a good source of vitamin C.

Part 3
Special Diets

❑ 8. Describe special or modified diets for common medical conditions

Clients who have illnesses that affect certain organ systems, such as the heart, circulatory system, kidneys, liver, and pancreas, are usually placed on modified diets by their physicians as part of the care plan. Certain nutrients or fluids may be restricted or eliminated. Some medications may also interact with certain foods, which then must be restricted. Clients with nutritional deficiencies may be placed on a special supplementary diet. Diets are also prescribed for weight control and food allergies.

As a home care aide, you will play an important role by ensuring that clients receive the basic nutrients essential to maintaining and improving their health while staying within the dietary modifications prescribed. Several types of modified diets are available for different types of illness, and some clients may be on a combination of restricted diets. For example, clients who have heart disease may be on a sodium-restricted diet in addition to low-cholesterol, low-fat, and restricted potassium diets. Clients with kidney disease may be on low-sodium, low-potassium, and restricted protein diets.

The care plan and your assignments for each client should specify any nutritional problems or special diet the client is on. It should also explain any eating problems that may be encountered and how the client's eating habits can be improved (**Fig. 22-10**). Never modify a client's diet. Therapeutic diets can only be prescribed by physicians and planned by dieticians. Follow the client's diet plan without making judgments, and report your observations to your supervisor.

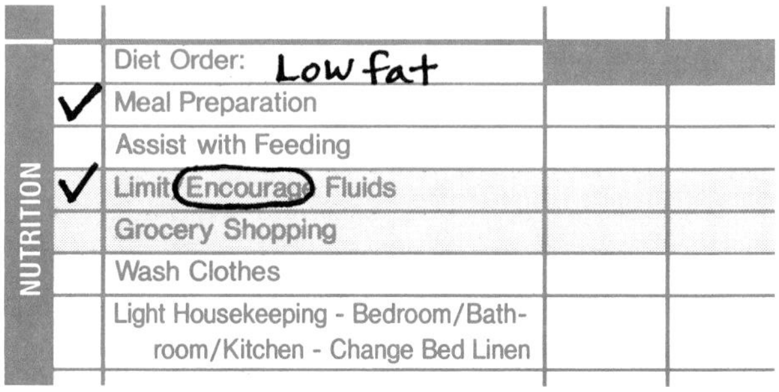

Fig. 22-10. The care plan specifies special diets or dietary restrictions.

Sodium-Restricted Diet (Low-Sodium Diet). Sodium is found in many foods, but people are most familiar with it as one of the two ingredients of salt. Salt is the first food to be restricted in a low-sodium diet because it is high in sodium.

Sodium helps the body retain fluid. Excess sodium causes the body to retain more water in tissues and in the circulatory system than is necessary. This causes the heart to pump harder, a situation that is harmful for clients who have high blood pressure, coronary artery disease, or kidney disease. A modified fluid intake may also be required for people with these conditions, because too much fluid can lead to congestive heart failure.

The human body needs 1,500 to 2,500 milligrams of sodium a day; however, on the average, we consume twice that amount. Excess sodium is excreted in the urine and over the years can erode the kidneys, leading to hypertension and kidney disease.

Foods high in sodium include the following:

▶ cured meats: ham, bacon, lunch meat, sausage, salt pork, and hot dogs

- salty or smoked fish: herring, salted cod, sardines, anchovies, caviar, smoked salmon or lox
- processed cheese
- canned and dried soups
- vegetables preserved in brine: pickles, sauerkraut, olives, relishes
- salted foods: nuts, dips, and spreads
- sauces with high concentrations of salt: Worcestershire, barbecue, chili, and soy sauces; catsup and mustard
- canned foods
- some cereals
- over-the-counter medications and drugs

Read product labels to determine if they contain salt or sodium in any form. Common forms of sodium include monosodium glutamate (GLOO-ta-mayt), often added to meat tenderizers, seasonings, and prepared foods to enhance flavor; and sodium nitrate, a salt used to preserve lunch meats and other cured meats.

You can make low-sodium meals more flavorful by adding lemon, herbs, dry mustard, pepper, paprika, orange rind, onion, and garlic to recipes. The flavor of meats can also be enhanced by the addition of fruits and jellies. Salt substitutes should only be used with the approval of the client's doctor. These seasonings might be high in potassium, a substance that is harmful to people with certain illnesses, such as kidney disease.

Fluid-Restricted Diets. The amount of fluid taken into the body through food and fluids must equal the amount of fluid that leaves the body through perspiration, stool, urine, and expiration. When fluid intake is greater than fluid output, the tissues of the body become swollen with excess fluid. In addition, people with severe heart disease and kidney disease may have difficulty processing large volumes of fluid. To prevent further heart and kidney damage, physicians may restrict a client's fluid intake. For clients on fluid restriction, you will need to take exact measurements of fluid intake, document them, and report excesses to your supervisor.

High Potassium Diets (K+). Some clients who are on diuretics (dye-you-RET-iks), which are medications that reduce fluid volume, or on some blood pressure medications, may be excreting so much fluid that their bodies could be depleted of potassium. Other clients may be placed on a high potassium diet for different reasons.

Foods high in potassium include bananas, grapefruit, oranges, orange juice, prune juice, prunes, dried apricots, figs, raisins, dates, cantaloupes, tomatoes, potatoes with skins, sweet potatoes and yams, winter squash, legumes, avocados, and unsalted nuts.

Low-Protein Diet. In addition to restricted dietary intake of fluids, sodium, and potassium, people who have kidney disease may also be on low-protein diets. Protein is restricted because it breaks down into compounds that may lead to further kidney damage. The extent of the restrictions depends on the stage of the disease and whether the client is on dialysis.

Lists of foods that can be exchanged for one another on a meal plan, or exchange lists, are used extensively in special diets for people with diabetes. But exchange lists have also been developed for clients on diets modified for protein, potassium, and sodium. Follow the instructions for these diets carefully and ask for help whenever you need it.

Low-Fat/Low-Cholesterol Diet. People who have high levels of cholesterol in their blood are at risk for heart attacks and atherosclerosis. People with gallbladder disease, diseases that interfere with fat digestion, and liver disease are also placed on low-fat/low-cholesterol diets.

Low-fat/low-cholesterol diets permit skim milk, low-fat cottage cheese, fish, white meat of turkey and chicken, veal, and vegetable fats (especially monounsaturated fats such as olive, canola, and peanut oils). Clients may be advised to limit their diets in the following ways:

- Eat lean cuts of meat including lamb, beef, and pork, and limit even these to three times a week.
- Limit egg yolks to three or four per week (including eggs used in baking).
- Avoid organ meats, shellfish, fatty meats, cream, butter, lard, meat drippings, coconut and palm oils, and desserts and soups made with whole milk.
- Avoid fried foods and sweets.

People who have gallbladder disease or other digestive problems may be placed on a diet that restricts all fats.

Modified Calorie Diet for Weight Management. Some clients may need to reduce calories to lose weight or prevent additional weight gain. Other clients may need to gain weight and increase calories to meet increased energy requirements caused by malnutrition, surgery, illness, or fever. Clients with certain conditions may need to increase protein intake to promote growth and repair of tissue and regulation of body functions.

Dietary Management of Ulcers. Gastric and **duodenal** (doo-a-DEE-nal) **ulcers** can be irritated by foods that produce gastric distress or increase levels of acid in the stomach. People who have ulcers usually know the foods that cause them discomfort. Physicians will advise them to avoid these foods as well as the following: alcohol; beverages containing caffeine, such as coffee, tea, and soft drinks; and spicy seasonings such as black pepper, cayenne, and chili pepper. Three meals or more a day are usually advised. If alcohol is allowed, it should be drunk with meals.

Dietary Management of Diabetes Mellitus. Calories and carbohydrates are carefully regulated in the dietary management of diabetic clients. Protein and fats are also regulated. The types of foods and the amounts are determined by the client's nutritional and energy requirements. As described in Chapter 20, Common Chronic and Acute Conditions, there are two types of diabetes:

1. Adult-onset or non-insulin-dependent diabetes. This type of diabetes can frequently be controlled by weight control or weight loss in which the level of blood sugar returns to normal. Successful management of adult onset diabetes may prevent the client from becoming insulin-dependent.

2. Insulin-dependent or juvenile diabetes. Management of this form of the illness requires daily doses of insulin, regular patterns of exercise, and regular meals of a prescribed diet that is closely followed.

Eating meals in prescribed quantities at regular times throughout the day is extremely important for people with diabetes. Snacks in the mid-afternoon and at bedtime can prevent blood sugar levels from rising and falling, and they can provide a steady supply of food to balance the effect of insulin. Blood sugar levels are influenced by infection, illness, stress, exercise, diet irregularities, and insulin levels. Diabetes mellitus can be managed by two types of diets:

1. Non-concentrated Sweets Diet. This diet is a regular, well-balanced diet that excludes concentrated sweets, such as sugars, honey, syrup, jellies, jams, preserves, candy, and cranberry sauce. The diet also eliminates cakes, pastries, cookies, puddings, ice cream, gelatin, sweetened fruit juices and beverages, sugar-coated cereals, condensed milk, and candied or glazed fruits and vegetables.

2. Exchange List Diets. Exchange list diets are described in more detail in the discussion of diabetes found in Chapter 20, Common Chronic and Acute Conditions. This type of diet is more restricted than the non-concentrated sweets diet, because it involves more than just the elimination of concentrated sweets. Meals are carefully planned based on exact amounts of food from the six food groups. Exchange lists are then used to determine foods and the exact serving sizes that may be eaten to follow the meal plan. Foods are measured and must be eaten completely at certain times. Eating the necessary carbohydrates, which are found in dairy and bread groups, is very important if the client is too ill to tolerate the other foods. Any variation in eating patterns and routine must be reported to the physician or nurse.

Chapter 23

Meal Planning, Shopping, Preparation, and Storage

Learning Objectives

In this chapter you will learn to:

- ☑ 1. Explain how to prepare a basic food plan....... 317
- ☑ 2. List four ways to find the best food for the best prices... 318
- ☑ 3. List four factors to consider when buying food..... 319
- ☑ 4. List five guidelines for safe food preparation..... 319
- ☑ 5. Identify six methods of food preparation..... 320
- ☑ 6. Identify four methods of low-fat food preparation..... 322
- ☑ 7. List four guidelines for safe food storage 322
- ☑ 8. Describe guidelines for assisting with eating 323
- ☑ 9. Describe eating and swallowing problems a client may have.. 324

You will also learn to perform the following procedure:

- ☑ 1. Assisting a client with eating 323

Part 1
Planning and Shopping

❑ 1. Explain how to prepare a basic food plan

It is very important to plan meals for a week or at least several days before heading to the supermarket to shop. When planning, you need to take into account the client's dietary restrictions, food preferences, number of family members present at meals, and the family's or client's budget.

Sit down with a large sheet of paper and write out the days of the week you are planning for, leaving space under each day for meals and snacks. You may end up serving the meals in a different order, but by planning for each day you will be sure to plan the right number of meals and buy the right amount of food (**Fig. 23-1**).

Fill in breakfasts, lunches, dinners, and snacks for each day. Ask the client or family members for ideas or look in cookbooks. If possible, check store advertisements before you plan meals, so you can take advantage of weekly specials. Usually grocery stores mail

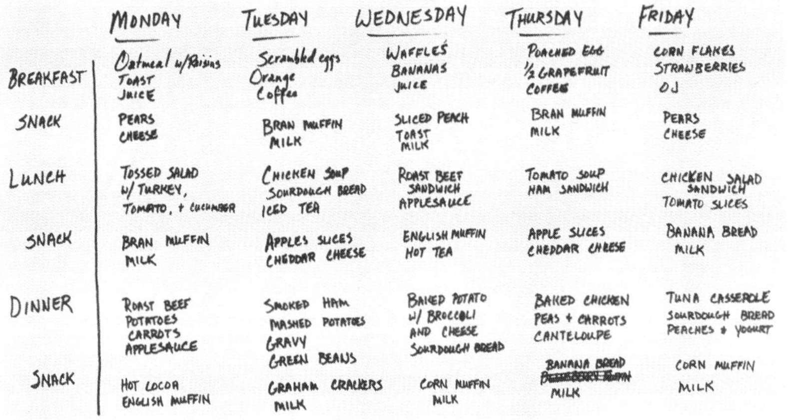

Fig. 23-1. A meal plan will help you know what kinds and quantities of food to buy for a week.

Box 23-1. Nutritious Snacks

All the following make good snacks. Of course you must take into account the client's dietary needs when planning snacks. For example, a client who is diabetic cannot snack on raisins all day.

- low-salt pretzels and tomato juice or vegetable juice
- celery with peanut butter or cream cheese and milk

- graham crackers and milk
- rice cakes with peanut butter and milk
- cereal and milk
- yogurt
- baked tortilla chips with salsa
- carrot or celery sticks with salsa
- crackers and cheese
- gelatin with fruit

- bran muffin and milk
- raisins, dates, figs, prunes, or dried apricots
- trail mix
- "milk shakes" made with yogurt, milk, and fruit blended together
- fresh fruit
- apple with peanut butter
- apple with cheese

Box 23-2. Meals That Make Good Leftovers

- beef stew
- chili
- spaghetti with meat sauce
- casseroles
- red beans and rice
- split pea soup
- lentil soup
- chicken soup
- macaroni and cheese
- lasagna
- meat loaf
- pot roast

Box 23-3. Economical Meals

- pasta dishes
- baked stuffed potatoes
- rice and beans
- tuna casserole
- chicken thighs or legs
- hamburger casserole
- pot roast
- stews
- lentil soup
- split pea soup
- lasagna

a circular with advertised specials once a week. Plan to have leftovers that can be easily reheated on days you will not be in the home to cook. Remember to plan plenty of nutritious snacks; clients may need as many as three snacks a day. Remember to list beverages as well.

When your meal plan is completed, start making your shopping list. On another large sheet of paper, write down categories including produce, meats, canned goods, frozen foods, dairy, and other. Leave space under each category to list the foods you need to buy. Listing items by category will save you time in the grocery store. Go through your plan meal by meal, writing down all of the ingredients you will need to prepare each meal. Remem-

ber to include beverages. Check the refrigerator, cabinets, and pantry for ingredients. Many ingredients you need may already be in the home.

It is a good idea to keep a shopping list going all the time so family members, clients, and you can write down things you run out of during the week.

❑ 2. List four ways to find the best food for the best prices

- Compare foods by reading the unit price tags that are on the shelves in front of the product (**Fig. 23-2**). Store brands are usually cheaper than advertised brands.
- Buy fresh foods that are in season, when they are at peak flavor and inexpensive.

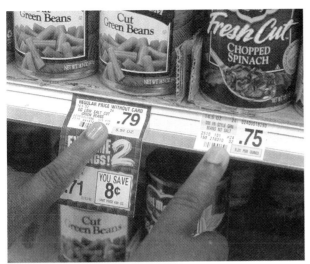

Fig. 23-2. Compare foods by reading the unit price tag.

▶ Buy in quantity. Large amounts or larger sizes are usually more economical. Do not buy more than you can store. Do not buy quantity if it will spoil before you use it.

▶ Buy the store's specials or sale items, but avoid the temptation to buy a special that is still over budget or that you do not need. Stick to your list.

▶ Avoid processed, already mixed, or ready-made foods. They are usually more expensive and less nutritious. When time allows, buy staple (basic) items and start from scratch to make a cake or potato salad, for example.

▶ Buy a cheaper brand when appearance is not important. For example, store brand mushroom bits are fine to use in a casserole and much cheaper than name brand mushroom pieces.

▶ Read labels to be sure you are getting the kind of product and the quantity you want. Read labels for ingredients that may be harmful to your client, for example, excessive salt or sodium.

▶ Estimate the cost per serving before buying. Divide the total cost by the number of servings to determine the cost per serving.

▶ Consider the amount of waste in bones and fat when buying cheaper cuts of meat. Some cuts of less expensive meats yield only half of what leaner cuts yield per pound. Chicken and turkey are usually inexpensive, especially if they are bought whole and cut up. For clients on low-fat/low-cholesterol diets, pick lean meats and take the skin off chicken and turkey parts. The skin holds much of the fat.

❏ 3. List four factors to consider when buying food

When deciding what to buy, keep these four factors in mind:

1. **Nutritional value.** Does this food contain essential nutrients, vitamins, and minerals? Is it unprocessed, without added salt or sugar?

2. **Quality.** Is this food fresh and in good condition? Fruits, vegetables, and meats should look fresh. Canned goods should not be dented or rusted. Milk and dairy products should not have passed their expiration dates.

3. **Price.** Is this the most economical choice? If it costs more, is it worth it?

4. **Preference.** Will my client like this food? Can I make an appealing meal using this food?

Part 2
Preparation and Storage

❏ 4. List five guidelines for safe food preparation

Food-borne illnesses affect up to 100 million people each year. Elderly people are at increased risk partly because they may not see, smell, or taste that food is spoiled; and partly because they may not have the energy to prepare and store food safely. For people who have weakened immune systems because of AIDS or cancer, a food-borne illness can be deadly. Remember the following guidelines for safe food preparation:

1. **Wash hands frequently.** Wash your hands thoroughly before beginning any food preparation. Wash your hands after handling raw meat, poultry, or fish.

2. **Keep everything clean.** Clean and disinfect countertops and other surfaces before, during (as necessary), and after food preparation. Handle raw meat, poultry and fish carefully. Use an antibacterial kitchen cleaner or a dilute bleach solution to clean any countertops on which meat juices were spilled. Wrap paper or packaging containing meat juices in plastic and discard immediately. Once you have used a knife or cutting board to cut fresh meat, *do not* use it for anything

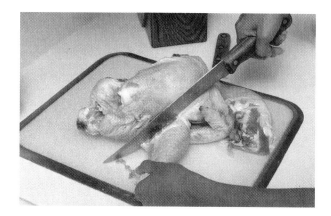

Fig. 23-3. Carefully wash areas used to cut raw meats.

else until it has been washed in the dishwasher or in very hot, soapy water containing bleach. Use plastic cutting boards for raw meat, wooden ones for vegetables and other foods (**Fig. 23-3**). Change dishcloths, sponges and towels frequently. Sponges may be washed in the dishwasher to disinfect them.

3. Thaw in the refrigerator. Defrost frozen foods in the refrigerator, not on the countertop. Do not remove meats or dairy products from the refrigerator until just before use.

4. Wash thoroughly. Wash fruits and vegetables thoroughly in running water to remove pesticides and bacteria.

5. Cook thoroughly. Cook meats, poultry, and fish thoroughly to kill any harmful microorganisms they may contain. Heat leftovers thoroughly. Never leave food out for over two hours. Keep cold foods cold and hot foods hot.

❏ 5. Identify six methods of food preparation

The following basic methods of food preparation will allow you to prepare a variety of healthy meals:

Boiling: Food is cooked in boiling water until tender or done. This is the best method for cooking pasta, noodles, rice, and hard- or soft-boiled eggs (**Fig. 23-4**). Vegetables and meats may also be boiled, but they will lose some of their nutrients and flavor in the water.

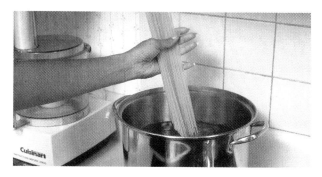

Fig. 23-4. Boiling works well for pasta and other grains.

Steaming: Steaming is a healthy way to prepare vegetables. A small amount of water is boiled in the bottom of a saucepan and food is set over it on a rack (**Fig. 23-5**). The pan is tightly covered to keep the steam in. Vegetables are done when tender. Steaming allows vegetables to retain their vitamins and flavor.

Poaching: Fish or eggs may be cooked by poaching in barely boiling water or other liquid. Eggs are

---

Box 23-4. Cooking Safety

Safety issues are discussed in detail in Chapter 6, Safety and Body Mechanics. Following is a quick review of kitchen safety:

▶ Do not cook with long, loose sleeves that can catch on pot handles or catch fire.

▶ Turn pot handles toward the back of the stove to prevent tipping.

▶ Dry hands before using electrical appliances.

▶ Immediately clean any spills on the floor to prevent slipping.

▶ When lighting a gas stove or oven, light the match before turning on the gas and be sure the match is extinguished and cool before throwing it away.

Never use a match to light a self-lighting gas stove.

▶ Store potholders, dish towels, and other flammable kitchen items away from the stove.

▶ Stay in or near the kitchen when anything is cooking or baking. Never leave stove on and unattended unless temperature is very, very low.

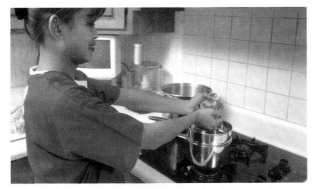

Fig. 23-5. Steaming retains valuable nutrients.

cracked and shells discarded before poaching. Fish may be poached in milk or broth, on top of the stove or in the oven in a baking dish (**Fig. 23-6**).

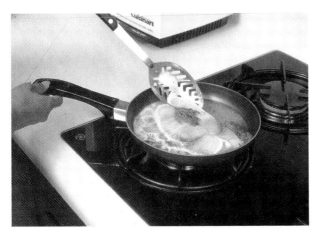

Fig. 23-6. Fish and eggs can both be poached.

Roasting: Used for meats and poultry or some vegetables, roasting is a simple way to cook. Dry heat roasting means food is roasted in an open pan in the oven (**Fig. 23-7**). Meats and poultry are **basted**, or coated with juices or other liquid, during roasting. To roast vegetables such as carrots, potatoes,

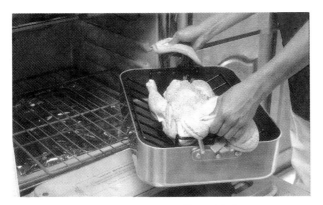

Fig. 23-7. Meats roast well at high temperatures but may need to be basted.

onions, mushrooms, or zucchini, cut into small chunks and coat with vegetable oil. Spread chunks on a flat cookie sheet or roasting pan and cook in a 450° oven until tender.

Moist heat roasting is used for lean cuts of beef such as pot roast. Liquid such as broth, wine, or tomato sauce is poured over and around the meat and the pot is covered. Moist heat roasting may be done in the oven or on the stove top. Use a lower temperature (300–350°) and cook several hours until tender.

Baking: Baking is used for many foods, including breads, poultry, fish, and vegetables. Baking is done in a moderate oven, 350°F to 400°F. Vegetables such as potatoes and winter squash bake very well (**Fig. 23-8**).

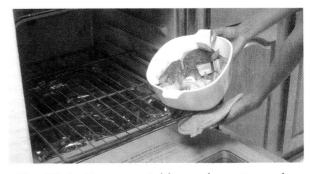

Fig. 23-8. Many vegetables and meats can be baked together.

Broiling: Used primarily for meats, broiling involves cooking food close to the source of heat at a high temperature for a short time (**Fig. 23-9**). Meat must be tender to be broiled successfully; inexpensive and lean cuts are often better cooked using moist heat. The broil setting on the oven can also be used

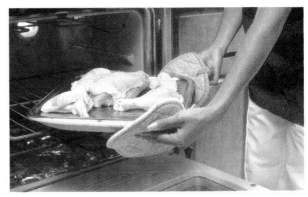

Fig. 23-9. Broiling involves cooking at a very high temperature.

to melt cheese or brown the top of a casserole. Leave the oven door ajar when broiling and never leave the kitchen: things can burn *very* fast when broiling.

Sauteing or stir frying: These are quick cooking methods for vegetables and meats. Use a small amount of oil in a frying pan or wok over high heat. Stir the food constantly to cook it quickly and prevent sticking (**Fig. 23-10**).

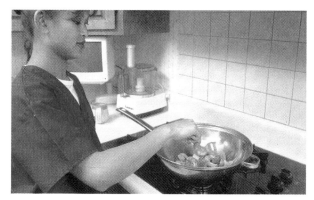

Fig. 23-10. Stir frying is quick and uses very little fat.

Frying: The least healthy way to cook, frying uses a lot of fat. Avoid frying foods for clients (**Fig. 23-11**).

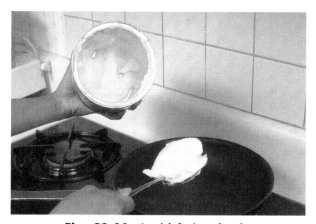

Fig. 23-11. Avoid frying foods.

Fresh, uncooked foods: Many fruits and vegetables have the most nutrients when eaten fresh, as in salads (**Fig. 23-12**). However, fresh fruits and vegetables may be difficult for some clients to chew or digest. Before preparing or serving fresh fruits or vegetables, be sure to wash them well to remove any chemicals or pesticides.

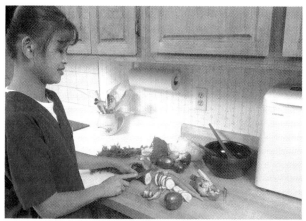

Fig. 23-12. Many fruits and vegetables have the most nutrients when eaten uncooked and fresh.

❏ 6. Identify four methods of low-fat food preparation

1. **Cook lean.** Boiling, steaming, broiling, and roasting are all methods of cooking that require little or no added fat. Broiling also allows fats in meat to drip out before food is consumed, lowering fat content even further.

2. **Drain fat.** When using ground meats for casseroles or other recipes, brown it first, then drain it on paper towels and newspaper to remove excess fat.

3. **Plan lean.** Choosing foods with lower fat content to begin with will make low-fat cooking easier. Planning meals around grains — the base of the food pyramid—will help cut the fat content of meals. Some examples of low-fat meals based on grains include pasta dishes, rice and beans, baked or stuffed potatoes, and soups.

4. **Substitute or cut down.** Sometimes high-fat ingredients can be omitted or replaced to lower the fat content of a recipe. Leave out or cut down the amount of cheese used on sandwiches or to top casseroles. Try substituting plain nonfat yogurt for mayonnaise or sour cream. Nonfat cottage cheese can also be used to make foods creamy without adding fat; try it on a baked potato instead of sour cream.

❏ 7. List four guidelines for safe food storage

1. **Buy cold food last, get it home fast.** After shopping, put away refrigerated foods first.

2. **Keep it safe, refrigerate.** Maintain refrigerator temperature between 36° F and 40° F; maintain freezer temperature at 0° F. Refrigerated items that spoil easily should be kept in the rear of the refrigerator, not the door. Look on the jar or package to determine if a

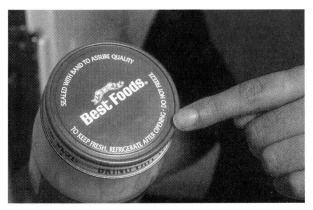

Fig. 23-13. Look for refrigeration guidelines on food labels.

food item requires refrigeration once it has been opened (**Fig. 23-13**). Salad dressings, mayonnaise, and other items with fat in them require refrigeration after they have been opened. Do not refreeze items after they have been thawed.

3. Use small containers that seal tightly. Foods cool more quickly when stored in smaller containers. Never leave foods out for more than two hours. Tightly cover all foods and store with enough room around them for air circulation. To prevent dry foods, such as cornmeal and flour, from becoming infested with insects, store these items in tightly sealed containers. If you find items that are already infested, discard them and use a clean container to store a fresh supply. Check dry storage areas periodically for signs of insects and rodents.

4. When in doubt, throw it out! If you are not sure whether food is spoiled, don't take any chances. Discard it. Check the expiration dates on foods, especially perishables. Check the refrigerator frequently for spoiled foods and discard any you find.

Part 3
Serving and Assisting with Eating

❏ *8. Describe guidelines for assisting with eating*

Clients who must be fed are often embarrassed and depressed about their dependence on another person. Be alert to this and give assistance only as specified in your assignments, when necessary, or when the client requests it. Feeding a client should be undertaken with gentleness and tact.

Procedure 1: Assisting a client with eating

Always make sure the meal is appropriate according to the meal plan before serving it. Check the temperature of the food when you serve it and again when you are ready to feed it.

1. Explain what you will do.

2. Wash your hands.

3. Assemble equipment:
- bib or extra napkin, if appropriate
- eating utensils (adaptive, if appropriate)
- disposable gloves
- appropriate meal

4. Assisting as necessary, see that client is in an upright but comfortable position.

5. If appropriate, cover the client's clothing with a bib or extra napkin.

6. Seat yourself next to the client, on the stronger side if the client has one-sided weakness.

7. Put on gloves.

8. Check temperature of food again.

9. Offer small spoonfuls, pausing between them for client to swallow and breathe. If the client has trouble swallowing, place food on the back of the tongue or the stronger side. Massage the client's throat gently if necessary to help with swallowing.

10. Offer drinks periodically. If you are holding the cup, touch it to the client's lips before you tip it. Give small, frequent sips. The client may prefer to use a straw or an adaptive cup. Training cups are an inexpensive way to make it easier for the client to drink by herself.

11. Use a napkin to wipe the corners of the client's mouth periodically.

Continued on page 324

Continued from page 323

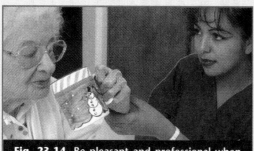

Fig. 23-14. Be pleasant and professional when feeding a client.

12. Try to make the meal pleasant for the client (**Fig. 23-14**). Converse if the client is willing. Feed at the client's pace; do not try to hurry through the meal.

13. When the client is done eating, remove the tray or dishes.

14. Wash your hands.

15. Assist the client in leaving the table or shifting to a comfortable position.

16. Document the client's intake if required, and any observations. How did the client tolerate being upright for the meal? Did the client eat well? What foods did the client eat or not eat?

❑ 9. Describe eating and swallowing problems a client may have

In addition to loss of appetite due to illness, pain, nausea, or medications, clients may experience other conditions that make eating or swallowing difficult. If a client has difficulty swallowing due to stroke or hemiparesis, serve soft foods and thickened liquids. Provide a straw or training cup as needed. Be patient. Assist the client with using a napkin as needed. For the client with mouth sores, serve cold, soft foods, such as milk shakes, yogurt, gelatin, and puddings. Avoid spicy, salty, or acidic foods, as well as crunchy foods. See Chapter 22 for more ideas on helping clients with nausea, loss of appetite, or other eating difficulties.

In some cases, artificial feeding may be required. When a person is completely unable to swallow, a **gastric gavage** (a tube inserted directly into the stomach) may be used for **enteral feeding** (of a liquid nutritional formula). If a person's digestive system will not function properly, intravenous hyperalimentation (in-tra-VEE-nus high-per-al-ih-men-TAY-shun), or **IVH** may be necessary. With IVH, a person receives nutrients directly into the bloodstream. Both of these methods of artificial feeding are described in more detail in Chapter 22. Home care aides are *not* responsible for either type of artificial feeding. As always, however, you should observe, report, and document any changes in the client or problems with the equipment.

Chapter 24

Managing Time, Energy, Money, and Other Resources

> ## Part 1
> ## Managing Time and Energy

❑ 1. Explain three ways to work more efficiently

Taking care of the client and other family members who need assistance and support is your most important responsibility. For this to be accomplished smoothly and effectively, however, certain tasks must be done around the house to maintain an orderly and sanitary environment. To balance these responsibilities, you will need to learn ways to manage your time and energy efficiently. Following are three ways to be sure your work schedule is as efficient as possible.

1. **Distribute Tasks.** Look at the client care plan and your assignments, and note the types of housekeeping services that are assigned. Divide the tasks and schedule them for the week and the month, making sure all your assignments can be completed in the time you have. Some tasks may be best accomplished together. For example, it is most efficient to do all the laundry on one day, so you can do larger loads and fold and iron all at once. Plan one morning or afternoon to do the laundry. For maximum efficiency, plan other tasks to do while loads are in the washer or dryer.

2. **Prioritize Tasks.** Prioritizing your tasks and activities is an important time and energy management skill. Think about the jobs and activities you want to get done throughout the day. Which ones must be done immediately? Which ones must be done at a certain time? Which activities are not absolutely essential and could be put off? Spend time on activities that are most important first.

3. **Simplify Tasks.** Learn to simplify your tasks. Take time to think about how you will go about doing a task and try to eliminate a few steps but still get the same result. For example, when baking a cake, can you mix everything in one bowl? When you clean up, can you stack everything on a tray and take it all to the sink at one time?

Box 24-1. Simple Ways to Conserve Time and Energy

Energize. Use good body mechanics. Take occasional breaks to restore your energy. Alternate longer tasks with shorter tasks, and high-energy tasks with low energy ones. Take care of yourself— eat right, exercise, and get plenty of rest.

Organize. At the beginning of the day, do a mental run-down of the tasks that must be done and rearrange your schedule if necessary. Plan what must be done and do it. Store frequently used items in convenient, accessible places near the work area. Assemble your equipment and materials before you begin a task. Keep clutter in control and work in good light. Think about how to organize activities and equipment to avoid unnecessary work. Make and use shopping lists.

Economize. Save time and energy by doing a little extra ahead of time. Use trays, baskets, or carts to carry several things at once. Prepare often-used food items ahead of time and freeze them. Cook in quantity and freeze meal-size portions. Cook more than one item in the oven at a time.

Minimize. Look for ways to make tasks shorter and easier. Modify your work space if necessary to make your work more comfortable and easier.

Specialize. Use the right tool for each task (for example, a vegetable peeler is more efficient than a knife for peeling carrots). Take pride in what you are doing. Finally, be sure to thank family members who have picked up, cleaned up, or participated in household chores.

Finally, *be realistic*. You may not be able to get everything done even if you plan carefully. Reassess your schedule during the day. Have you finished what you planned or are you behind? Will you be able to finish vacuuming before you have to make lunch, or do you need to quit now to get lunch ready on time? When tasks take longer than you expected, or unexpected tasks need to be done, be realistic about what you can do and don't be afraid to change your plan. It is better to accomplish the highest priority tasks and let others go unfinished than to do everything half way. The key to success is to be flexible.

❑ 2. Describe how to follow an established work plan with the client and family

The client care plan and your assignments will tell you what tasks are required. You can develop your own work plan that will allow you to finish all your assigned tasks as quickly and efficiently as possible. For each day or block of time you will spend in a home, list all the tasks you must complete. Then, prioritize them, marking the most important as "1" and the next most important as "2," and so on. Finally, write out a schedule for the day, filling in the highest priority tasks first. If there are tasks that must be done at a certain time, for example serving a meal or accompanying the client to a doctor appointment, be sure to put those tasks on the schedule at the appropriate time.

Remember to distribute tasks, so that you are not trying to do all the housecleaning on one afternoon and end up with no time to bathe or care for a client. Remember also to simplify tasks whenever possible to allow you to accomplish more.

Following an established work plan will not only allow you to get more done in less time, it will also allow your clients and families to know what to expect of you. You may even want to discuss the plan with a client or family member, either as you're making it up or when it is finished. Some people appreciate knowing what will be happening in their homes at any given time.

❑ 3. Discuss ways to handle inappropriate requests

Because home care aides do so many different kinds of tasks, clients or family members may sometimes be confused about what you are there to do. Occasionally, you may be asked to do something that is not in the care plan or your assignments. Because each client's situation is unique, you will not be assigned to the same tasks for every client. For example, the care plan may specify grocery shopping for Mrs. Salomon, who lives alone and cannot drive. But if another client who lives with family members asks you to run to the store for something, you have to say no if it is not in the care plan or your assignments.

Several things will help you handle requests that you must refuse. First, explain that you are only allowed to do tasks assigned to you in the care plan. Explain that your assignments are delegated by nurses familiar with the client's condition. Emphasize that you would like to help, but you are limited to the tasks outlined in the care plan and your assignments. After explaining this to the client, contact your supervisor and discuss the request. Your supervisor may add the task requested by the client to your assignments. It is possible it was left out of your assignments by mistake in the first place. Be sure to document the client's request and the actions you took to address it.

Establishing a work schedule that you follow in each home will also help you handle inappropriate requests. If a client and family know what to expect of you, they may not be tempted to ask you to do other tasks. Sharing a schedule of everything you must accomplish in a day or visit may help the client understand your job. If inappro-

priate requests continue, refer clients or family members to your supervisor.

> Part 2
> **Managing Money and Other Resources**

❑ 4. List five money-saving homemaking tips

> It is very important that you follow your assignments and the care plan exactly. It is also important to document client requests and the action you took to address it (calling your supervisor and following instructions).

1. **Check store circulars for advertised specials.** Plan your menus around foods that are a good value, for example, raw foods are less expensive than prepared ones. Chapter 23 discusses more ways to plan economical meals.

2. **Use coupons.** If your client receives a newspaper, scan it for coupons from stores or manufacturers (**Fig. 24-1**). Clip and use only those coupons for items you have already planned to buy. Also check that the price of the item less the coupon discount is lower than the price of a store brand. Sometimes store brands are still more economical.

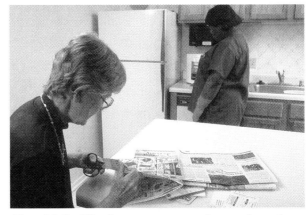

Fig. 24-1. Clipping coupons and scanning store ads can help save your client money on groceries and household items. Some clients may enjoy performing this household management task themselves.

3. Shop from your list. Don't be tempted by items that are not on your list, even if they are on sale.

4. Avoid convenience stores. Shopping at large supermarkets or discount stores usually guarantees you will get the best prices. Be aware of the cost of items you buy regularly so you can compare prices in different stores. Cleaning products and health and beauty aids are often much cheaper at discount stores than in the grocery store.

5. Plan ahead. Knowing what you need and buying before you run out will save you money, because you can buy at the store that has the best prices instead of at a convenience store. Planning will also save you time and energy, because you won't have to make a special trip when you discover you've run out of laundry detergent or scouring powder.

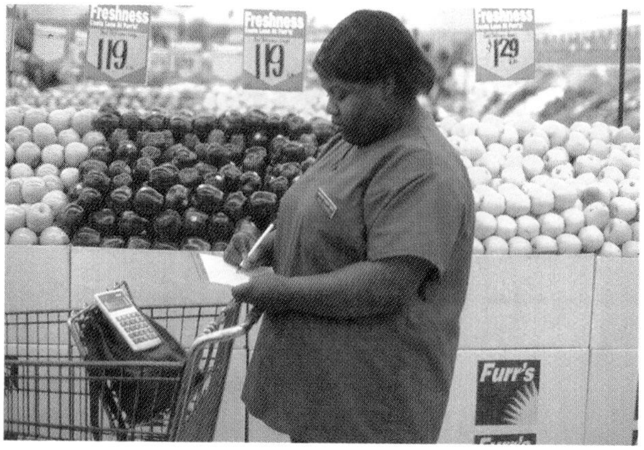

Fig. 24-2. It may be necessary to take a calculator to the grocery store to stay within the client's grocery budget.

❏ 5. Explain the importance of knowing whether you are allowed to handle a client's money

Different states and employers have different regulations and policies regarding health care employees handling clients' money. Find out from your employer whether you will be expected to handle client's money. If you are not allowed to handle money, never agree to do so, even occasionally, as a favor for a client. You could get yourself and your employer in serious trouble.

❏ 6. List guidelines for handling a client's money

If your state and your employer permit you to handle clients' money, there are several guidelines you must follow in doing so:

Never use a client's money for your own needs, even if you plan to pay it back. This is considered stealing. You could end up losing your job and/or being arrested!

Estimate the amount of money you will need before requesting it. If you are making a weekly trip to the grocery store, show the client your list and ask how much he or she is willing to spend on groceries, or how much is budgeted. You may need to take things off your list or estimate the total bill as you go along in the store to stay within the money allotted (**Fig. 24-2**).

Take checks rather than cash, when possible, and have the client or family member fill out the name of the store. A signed check that is not made out is as good as cash. If you lose cash or a signed bank check, you may be responsible for paying back the amount to your client.

Get a receipt for every purchase. This proves how much you spent and gives a record for you and the client.

Return receipts and change to client or family member immediately. Don't wait until the end of the day or week to settle up. Do it right away while everything is fresh in your mind. Forgetting to return change could be viewed by the client or a family member as stealing.

Keep a record of money you've spent. Follow your agency's policies and procedures for documenting money issues. Write down how much you spent and where. Note any change returned to client. The better record you have, the smaller the chance of misunderstanding.

Keep a client's cash separate from yours. If you must use the client's cash, don't put it in your own wallet. Keep it in a separate, safe place. Do the same with change. This will prevent confusion.

Never offer money advice to a client. You should not even refer a client to others regarding their financial matters.

SECTION VII
Where Do I Go From Here?

Chapter 25

Caring for Yourself and Your Career

❏ **1. Explain how to conduct a job search**

To find a job, you must first target potential employers. Then you must contact them to find out about job opportunities. To find

---

Learning Objectives

In this chapter you will learn to:

potential employers, use the newspaper, telephone book, or personal contacts. Try these resources:

▶ Classified or employment sections of the newspaper list jobs currently available. Circle ads for home care aide or homemaker positions and make a list of names and phone numbers to contact (**Fig. 25-1**).

▶ Look in the yellow pages of the phone book under Home Health Services for a list of agencies.

▶ Call the state or local Department of Social Services. Many states hire or place home care aides.

▶ Ask your instructor for potential employers. Some schools maintain a list of employers seeking home care aides.

CNA's & HCA's / Whether you are just starting out in the health care field or you are an experienced professional seeking new challenges, we invite you to join one of the country's leading providers of home health care. Because our HHAs are the backbone of our quality care, we provide a competitive salary, attendance, bonus program and benefits package, as well as opportunities to advance your career. For consideration, apply in person at our downtown facility, 120 Main St., (555)291-3333. Pre-employment drug screening and criminal background check required. EOE Home Health America

Home Health Aides / Part time or full time. 3pm–11pm & 4pm–9pm. CNA or 1 year experience. Send resume to: Las Portales Village, 555 North Cottonwood Pl, City, 87555

Home Care Aides or CNAs with a minimum of 1 year experience as an aide needed immediately for part time Home Care positions throughout city and surrounding areas. Must have proof of current comprehensive/liability auto insurance. Individuals with valid CPR certification preferred. Bilingual a plus. Contact Josh at (555)293-6598 for application info.

Home Health Aid to work as an independent contractor, providing care for elderly patient. Personal care, bathing, meals, LT, housekeeping, certification required. PT hours, incl. over nights, 289-0224

Great opportunities to develop your career CNA RESTORATIVE OPPORTUNITIES EARN UP TO $10/HR FT all shifts. If you're a caring person that's looking for challenging rewarding position that will allow you to expand your career, come to All City Home Care. Must have current cert. in good standing. Call 555-9851 for more information.

Fig. 25-1. Newspaper ads are one way to identify potential employers.

Box 25-1.
Making Contact with Potential Employers

When you call an employer, ask to speak to someone in the personnel department.

"Hello, I am calling about employment opportunities as a home care aide. May I speak to someone in the personnel department please?"

When you get someone in personnel, the first thing to say is who you are and why you are calling.

"Hello, my name is Gina Graham and I am a graduate of Kingston Vocational High School home care aide training program. I am looking for work as a home care aide."

If you are calling an employer who advertised in the paper, you know there is a job opening. After introducing yourself, you can say,

"I saw your ad in the paper. Can you tell me about job opportunities available?"

If you are calling a potential employer that has not advertised a job, be more general.

"Can you tell me about job opportunities you might have?"

If there are jobs available, ask for an appointment to come in and speak to someone. Be sure to write down the time and date of the appointment, and ask where the agency is located and what office to go to.

Once you have a good list of potential employers, you need to contact them about job opportunities. Phoning first is a good way to find out what opportunities are available and what you need to do to apply for a job with each potential employer.

❏ 2. Identify documents that may be required when applying for a job

You may need several documents in order to apply for a job. When making an appointment, ask what information to bring with you. Make sure you have this information with you when you go to an appointment.

Identification. You may need to show a driver's license, social security card, birth certificate, passport, or other official form of identification to prove who you are.

Immigrant or alien documentation. Even if you are a U.S.-born citizen, you will need to show proof of your legal status in this country and proof that you are legally able to work. All employers must have files showing that every single employee is legally allowed to work in this country.

Credentials. You may need your high school diploma or equivalency, school transcripts, and diploma or certificate from your home care aide training course. Have the name and phone number of your instructor with you as well.

Letters of reference. References from former employers or personal acquaintances may be required. References can include former teachers, your minister, or your doctor. Do not use relatives or friends as references. You can save time by asking your references to write general letters for you, addressed "To whom it may concern," explaining how they know you and describing your skills, qualities, and habits. Take copies of these with you for employers to keep.

❏ 3. Demonstrate completing an effective job application

Write down the general information you will need for an application on a sheet of paper and take it with you. This will save time and avoid mistakes as you fill out the application form.

General information to include:

▶ your address and phone number or the number of a neighbor or relative who has agreed to take messages for you

▶ your birth date

▶ your social security number

▶ the name of the school or program where you were trained and the date you completed your training

▶ the names and addresses of your previous employers, and the dates you worked there

▶ the names and phone numbers of your references

▶ the days and hours you are available to work

▶ a brief statement of why you are changing jobs or why you want to work as a home care aide

Fill out the application carefully and neatly (**Fig. 25-2, as seen on page 332**). Read it all the way through once before you write anything. If you are not sure what is being asked, find out before filling in that space.

If it is not already a law in your state, soon most health care agencies will be required to perform criminal background checks on all health care workers. You may be asked to sign a form granting the agency permission to do this. Don't take it personally; it is a law intended to protect patients, clients, and residents.

❏ 4. Demonstrate competence in job interview techniques

To make the best impression at a job interview, be professional (**Fig. 25-3, as seen on page 332**):

▶ dress neatly and appropriately

▶ shower or bathe and use deodorant or anti-perspirant

▶ wear only simple makeup and jewelry or none at all

▶ arrive ten or fifteen minutes early

▶ introduce yourself, smile, and shake hands

▶ answer questions clearly and completely

▶ avoid using slang words or expressions

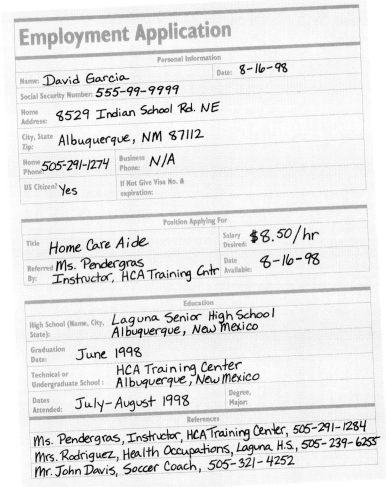

Employment Application

Personal Information

Name: David Garcia   Date: 8-16-98

Social Security Number: 555-99-9999

Home Address: 8529 Indian School Rd. NE

City, State Zip: Albuquerque, NM 87112

Home Phone: 505-291-1274   Business Phone: N/A

US Citizen? Yes   If Not Give Visa No. & expiration:

Position Applying For

Title: Home Care Aide   Salary Desired: $8.50/hr

Referred By: Ms. Pendergras Instructor, HCA Training Cntr   Date Available: 8-16-98

Education

High School (Name, City, State): Laguna Senior High School Albuquerque, New Mexico

Graduation Date: June 1998

Technical or Undergraduate School: HCA Training Center Albuquerque, New Mexico

Dates Attended: July-August 1998   Degree, Major:

References

Ms. Pendergras, Instructor, HCA Training Center, 505-291-1284

Mrs. Rodriguez, Health Occupations, Laguna H.S., 505-239-6255

Mr. John Davis, Soccer Coach, 505-321-4252

Fig. 25-2. A completed job application should look neat and should not have scratch outs.

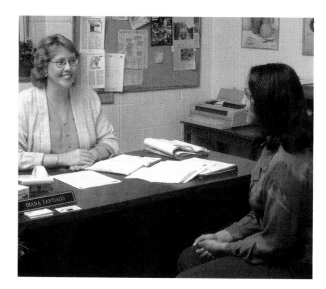

Fig. 25-3. Be professional in job interviews: dress neatly and be confident and polite.

▶ never eat, drink, chew gum, or smoke in an interview

▶ sit up or stand up straight, and look happy to be there

▶ do not bring friends or children to the interview with you

The following are some questions you can expect to be asked:

▶ Why did you become a home care aide? What do you like about working as an aide? What don't you like? (If this is your first job, you may be asked what you expect to like or dislike.)

▶ What are your best qualities? What are your weaknesses?

▶ Why did you leave your last job?

▶ What kinds of clients do you prefer to work with?

Be positive when answering questions. Emphasize what you enjoy or think you will enjoy about being an aide. Do not use a complaining tone when you explain why you left previous jobs. Make it clear that you are willing and able to work with all kinds of clients, even if you may prefer certain kinds of cases.

Usually interviewers will ask if you have any questions. Have some prepared and written down so you don't waste time or forget things you really want to know. Following are some questions you may want to ask:

▶ What hours would I work?

▶ What benefits does the job include? Is health insurance available? Would I get paid sick days or holidays?

▶ How much traveling would I have to do between clients? Do I need a car? Would I be paid for mileage or travel time?

▶ What orientation or in-service training is provided? How much contact would I have with my supervisor?

▶ Later in the interview, you may want to ask about salary or wages if you have not already been told what it would be.

Listen carefully to the answers to your questions and take notes if needed. At the end of the interview, you will probably be told when you can expect to hear from the employer. Don't expect to be offered a job at the interview. When the interview is over, stand up, shake hands again, and say something like, "Thank you for taking the time to meet with me today. I look forward to hearing from you." (**Fig. 25-4**)

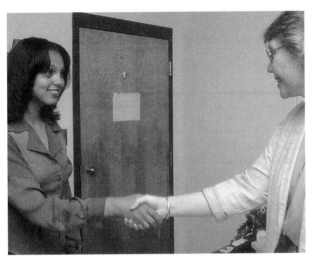

Fig. 25-4. Stand, shake hands, and thank the interviewer when your interview is over.

Send a letter to the employer after the interview to say thank you and to express your continued interest in a job (**Fig. 25-5**). If you have not heard anything from the employer in several days, call and ask whether the job was filled.

❑ 5. Discuss appropriate responses to criticism from employers, supervisors, and others

Handling criticism is difficult for most of us, but being able to accept criticism well and learn from it is the mark of a truly professional person. Here are some ideas for handling criticism and using it to your benefit:

Listen to what is being said. Sometimes we are so upset by criticism that we never really understand what message is being sent.

Differentiate between hostile criticism and constructive criticism. Hostile criticism is angry and negative. Examples are "You did a terrible job!" or "You are lazy and slow." Hostile criticism should not come from your employer or supervisor. You may experience hostile criticism from clients, family members,

August 18, 1998

Marilyn Michaels
4356 12th St.
Rio Huevo, TX 74568

Nancy Proust, Personnel Manager
HomeHelp, Inc.
332 S. Main
Rio Huevo, TX 74568

Dear Ms. Proust:

Thank you for taking the time to interview me last week for a home care aide position with HomeHelp, Inc. It was a pleasure to talk to you and to learn more about your agency. I look forward to hearing from you soon regarding the home care aide openings you are currently advertising for.

Sincerely,

Marilyn Michaels

Fig. 25-5. You should always send a professional thank-you letter to a potential employer after a job interview.

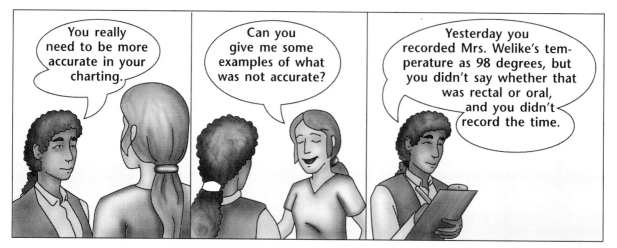

Fig. 25-6. Ask for details when receiving constructive criticism.

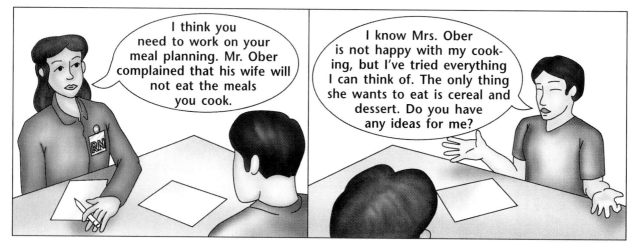

Fig. 25-7. Ask for suggestions for improvement when receiving constructive criticism.

or others. The best response is to say something like "I'm sorry you are so disappointed," and nothing more. Give the person a chance to calm down before trying to discuss what provoked the attack.

Constructive criticism may come from your employer, supervisor, or others. Constructive criticism is intended to help you do better or understand more. Examples are: "You really need to be more accurate in your charting," or "You are late too often; you'll have to make more of an effort to be on time." Listening and acting

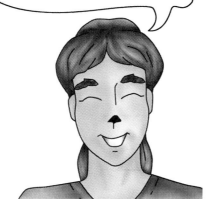

Fig. 25-8. Be willing to apologize if you have made a mistake.

on constructive criticism can help you be more successful in your job, so it is to your benefit to pay attention.

Ask for details. The following dialogue shows how you can learn from constructive criticism by asking for details (**Fig. 25-6**):

Ask for suggestions. Sometimes you aren't sure how to avoid a mistake you have made. Always ask the person criticizing you for suggestions in improving your performance (**Fig. 25-7**).

Apologize and move on. If you have made a mistake, apologize as needed. This may be to your supervisor, your client, or others. Learn what you can from the incident and put it behind you. Don't dwell on it or hold a grudge. You must be able to respond professionally to criticism or you will have a hard time being successful in any job (**Fig. 25-8**).

❑ 6. Identify effective ways to make a complaint to an employer or supervisor

Sometimes you will need to make a complaint or voice a concern about some part of your job. Do not be afraid to do this, but do it carefully.

Think about the problem. Some major problems must be reported right away. For example, if you are threatened or harassed by a client, family member, or coworker, you must report this to your supervisor immediately. Other problems may work themselves out if you give them a little time. If a new client seems to be rude to you, it is possible that he or she feels uncomfortable with new people or doesn't understand your role. You may want to wait several days or weeks to see if things improve before making a complaint. Know which problems should be reported immediately to your supervisor.

Plan what you will say. Think through and even write out what you will say to your supervisor. This will help you present your complaint clearly and completely.

HCA: Ms. Greene, I have a concern about the daughter of my client, Mrs. Paulsen. Last week she asked me to cut her mother's toenails. I explained I was not allowed to do that procedure and she would have to wait for the nurse to come. On Monday she wanted me to take her car out and fill the gas tank while she visited with her mother. I told her that was not in the care plan. Yesterday she dropped a glass and told me to clean up my mess or she would have me fired. I cleaned up the glass, but I think this woman has a problem with me. I wanted to let you know what had happened and ask if you could help me solve this problem.

Don't get emotional. Although some situations may be very upsetting, you will be more effective in communicating and problem-solving if you can keep your emotions out of it. Share your *feelings* about a situation—whether you are mad, hurt, or annoyed—with a friend. Tell your supervisor the *facts*.

Do not hesitate to communicate situations that you feel are important or that may put you or a client at risk. One common problem in home care is aides and other professionals *not* reporting when they feel unsafe at a particular client's home. In this case, *not* complaining can prove dangerous for you and the client. Always report to your supervisor any situation in which you feel you or the client are at risk of harm, even if the situation involves the client's family or friends.

❑ 7. Identify guidelines for making job changes appropriately

If you decide to change jobs, you should act responsibly toward your current employer. Always give your employer at least two weeks' written notice that you will be leaving. Otherwise, assignments may be left uncovered, or other home care aides may have to take on extra work until the agency fills your spot. Keep in mind that you took the job knowing the conditions (such as the hours and the pay), and you must fulfill your end of the agreement. In addition, potential future employers will look at your past work records and may talk with past supervisors. People who change jobs often and seem unable to carry through with a job are less likely to be hired.

❑ 8. List your state's requirements for maintaining certification as an aide

Each state has slightly different requirements for maintaining your certification. You must be familiar with the requirements and follow them exactly or you will not be able to keep working as an aide. Ask your instructor or employer for the requirements in your state. You should know how many hours of in-service education are required per year and how long an absence from working is allowed without retraining or recertification.

Some states do not have a registry for home care aides like the ones they maintain for certified nursing assistants (CNAs). If, for example, you have taken the certification exam for CNAs and are on the state registry, you may need to work a certain number of hours in a long-term care facility to remain on the registry. As a home care aide, ask your employer how best to maintain your certification.

❑ 9. Explain the importance of continuing education

The federal government requires that home care aides have 12 hours of continuing education each year. Some states may require more. "In-service" continuing education courses help you keep your knowledge and skills fresh. Perhaps you haven't worked with a dying client for some time. A class on hospice care can help you prepare for that assignment. Classes may also provide you with more information about certain conditions or challenges that you face in working with clients. Sometimes treatments or regulations change. You need to be up-to-date on the latest that is expected of you.

If you feel you could benefit from further instruction in some particular area, speak to your supervisor. Perhaps he or she can arrange for an in-service continuing education class to be offered on that topic. Many agencies offer in-service education. It is your responsibility as a home care aide to adhere to the education requirements.

❑ 10. List the responsibilities a home care aide has for receiving continuing education

Your employer may be responsible for offering continuing education courses, but you are responsible for successfully attending and completing them. Specifically, you must:

▶ Sign up for the course or find out where it is offered (**Fig. 25-9**).

▶ Attend all class sessions.

▶ Pay attention and complete all the class requirements.

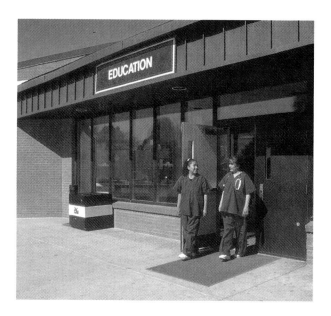

Fig. 25-9. You may want to go outside the in-service programs offered by your employer to get some continuing education courses you want to take.

▶ Make the most of your time in in-service programs. PARTICIPATE!

▶ Keep records of your successful attendance so you can prove you took the class.

Part 2
Managing Time, Stress, and Money

❑ 11. Define stress and stressors, and list examples

Stress is the state of being frightened, excited, confused, in danger, or irritated. Although we usually associate stress with negative situations in our lives, positive situations can cause stress too. For example, getting married or having a new baby are usually positive situations, but both can bring enormous stress from the changes they bring to our lives.

You may be thrilled when you get a new job as a home care aide, but starting work may also cause you stress. You may be afraid of making mistakes, excited about earning money or helping people, or confused about how to perform your new duties. Learning how to recognize stress and what causes it, and mastering a few simple techniques for relaxing and managing stress can be helpful for all of us.

A **stressor** is something that *causes* stress. Anything can be a stressor if it causes you stress. Some examples include:

◗ divorce
◗ marriage
◗ a new baby
◗ children growing up
◗ children leaving home
◗ losing a job
◗ a new job
◗ problems at work
◗ new responsibilities at work
◗ supervisors
◗ co-workers
◗ clients
◗ illness
◗ finances

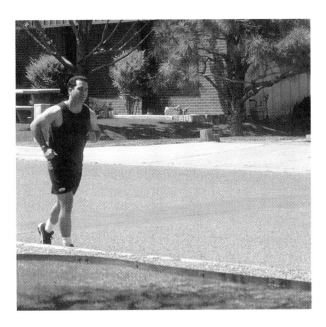

Fig. 25-10. A regular exercise routine can help your body handle stress.

❏ 12. Explain how diet and exercise affect stress

Stress is not only an emotional response, but a physical response. When we experience stress, certain changes occur in our bodies. The endocrine system may produce more of the hormone adrenaline (a-DREH-na-lin), which can increase nervous system response, heart rate, respiratory rate, and blood pressure. This is why, in stressful situations, you may feel your heart is beating fast, you are breathing hard, and you feel warm or perspire.

Each of us has a different tolerance level for stress. In other words, what one person would find overwhelmingly stressful might not bother another person. Your level of tolerance for stress depends on your personality and life experiences, but also on your general physical health.

Research has shown that people who exercise regularly, eat a nutritious diet, and lead a healthy lifestyle are better able to handle stress. Exercise, diet, and lifestyle affect physical health, and a healthy body is more able to cope with the physical effects of

stress (**Fig. 25-10**). In addition, exercise promotes relaxation, providing relief from the emotional effects of stress.

To manage the stress in your life, start by establishing healthy habits of diet, exercise, and lifestyle. Eat nutritious foods, exercise regularly, get enough sleep, drink only in moderation, and do not smoke.

❏ 13. Demonstrate two effective relaxation techniques

What do you do to relax? Many of us turn to food, alcohol, or smoking to take a break. Although these may feel good in the short run, usually their effects are negative. These are not healthy habits to depend on. In addition, drinking on the job is not allowed. More and more, smoking is not allowed in the workplace either. Exercise can be a great way to relax and is certainly healthy. But what can you do when you have only a few minutes to take a break at work?

Sometimes when you need a break, using a relaxation exercise can help you feel refreshed and relaxed in only a short time. The following are two simple relaxation exercises, the body scan and the waterfall. Try them out and see if either one helps you feel more relaxed.

The body scan. Close your eyes. Pay attention to your breathing and posture. Be sure you are comfortable. Starting at the balls of your feet, concentrate on your feet. Discover any tension hidden in the feet and try to relax and release the tension. Continue very slowly, taking a breath between each body part. Move up from the feet, focusing on and relaxing the legs, knees, thighs, hips, stomach, back, shoulders, neck, jaw, eyes, forehead, and scalp. Take a few very deep breaths and open your eyes.

The waterfall. Breathe deeply and imagine you are under a waterfall. The force of the water is washing away your tension. Imagine the tension is being washed away, one body part at a time, from the head through the soles of the feet. Visualize the tension being washed far away by the rushing water.

Either of these relaxation techniques takes only about two minutes. If one is helpful for you, you might want to try it the next time you need a break, whether you are at work or at home.

❑ 14. Identify seven sources of help in managing personal and job-related stress

Stress can seem overwhelming when we try to handle it ourselves. Often just talking about the stress you are experiencing can help you manage it better. Sometimes another person can offer suggestions for managing stress. Sometimes you will think of new ways to handle stress just by talking it through with another person.

Where can you turn for help managing stress? Try the following:

▶ your supervisor or another member of the care team for work-related stress

▶ your family

▶ your friends

▶ your church or synagogue

▶ your physician

▶ a local mental health agency

▶ any phone hotline that deals with related problems (check your local yellow pages)

It is not appropriate to turn to your clients or their family members to help you manage personal or job-related stress.

❑ 15. Describe how to develop a personal stress management plan

One of the best ways of managing stress in your life is to develop a plan for managing stress. The plan can include things you will do every day and things to do in stressful situations. When you think about a plan, you first need to answer the following questions:

▶ What are the sources of stress in my life?

▶ When do I most often experience stress?

▶ What effects of stress do I see in my life?

▶ What can I change to decrease the stress I feel?

▶ What do I have to learn to cope with because I cannot change it?

When you have answered these questions, you will have a clearer picture of the challenges you face. Then you can try to come up with strategies for managing stress. Following are some examples:

Situation #1. Anita is a home care aide and a single mother. After work, she picks up her two children at day care and heads home. She is tired, the children are hungry, and supper isn't ready. Sometimes she gets so stressed out she wants to yell at her children to get their own supper. What can she do?

Response. Planning and preparing ahead of time can make the after work/before supper time go more smoothly. If Anita can plan and prepare suppers ahead of time for every night she works, she will feel less stress. Keeping made-ahead meals in the refrigerator or freezer is a good way to eliminate a stressor (**Fig. 25-11**).

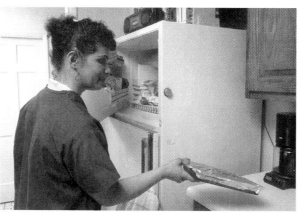

Fig. 25-11. Keeping made-ahead meals in the refrigerator or freezer is a good way to eliminate a stressor.

Situation #2. Juan is a home care aide with a new job at an agency. Because he is new, his schedule gets shifted frequently so he cannot predict from week to week when he will have to work. He likes to go out with his friends in the evenings and on weekends, but when he has to work weekends or early mornings he is exhausted before he even starts work. This makes the day much more stressful for him.

Response. Not having a routine can be very stressful. If you cannot predict when you will have to work, it is hard to plan the rest of your life. But going out and staying out too late before you have to work will make things more stressful. Juan needs to establish a routine for the times he can control. He needs to get to bed at roughly the same time every night and get eight hours of sleep. Drinking and smoking should be avoided or limited. And Juan should try to get into a regular exercise routine. Maybe he could convince his friends to work out or play sports with him, so he could do his socializing while getting his exercise (Fig. 25-12).

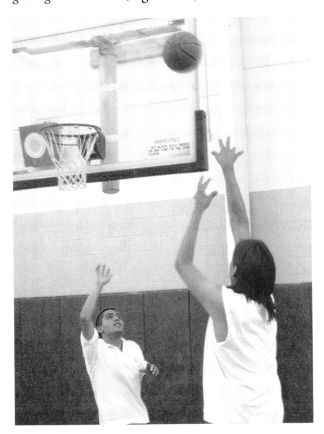

Fig. 25-12. Combining exercise with socializing is a good way to relieve stress.

Situation #3. Martha is a home care aide and a mother and grandmother. Her husband Chuck lost his job so she must support them both. Last year Martha decided she had a stress problem and started going to Nurse Aide support group. She feels much better since she started, and would like to get more control in other areas of her life to reduce her stress level.

Response. Martha wrote a personal stress management plan for herself:

Every day:
Eat breakfast, take an apple and a granola bar or other healthy snacks with me to work. Take breaks to stretch, sit down, and relax for several minutes two or three times.

Monday, Wednesday, Friday:
Go for a walk after supper. Invite Chuck to go with me.

Tuesday, Saturday:
Go to support group (Fig. 25-13).

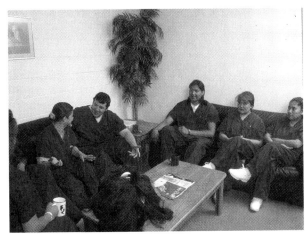

Fig. 25-13. Support groups can help you deal with stress of different types.

Sunday:
Go to church. Visit grandchildren. Plan menus for the week, clip coupons from the paper and go grocery shopping.

Every week:
Do one thing I want to do, like see a movie, take a bubble bath, read a magazine.

Martha's plan is a great start in managing stress. It helps her fit in all the things she wants to do each week. It includes healthy habits like eating breakfast and nutritious snacks, walking regularly, and taking breaks. She may not stick to her plan exactly every week, but it gives her something to try for.

❏ 16. List five guidelines for managing time

Many of the ideas for managing time on the job can be used to manage your personal time as well. The following are five basic strategies for managing time:

1. **Plan ahead.** Planning is the single best way to help you manage your time better. Sometimes you may feel you don't even have the time to plan, but take five minutes to sit down and list everything you have to do. Often just making the list will help you feel better and get you focused on accomplishing what you need to do.

2. **Prioritize.** Identify the most important things to get done and do these first.

3. **Make a schedule.** Write out the hours of the day and fill in when you will do what. This will help you be realistic. If you only have twenty minutes between getting off work and picking up your children, you will not be able to get the grocery shopping done. Schedule that activity for later, when you have at least an hour.

4. **Combine activities.** Can you read the paper while you're on the bus? Can you prepare tomorrow's supper while the laundry is in the dryer? Or help your son with his homework while you do the dishes? Work more efficiently when you can (**Fig. 25-14**).

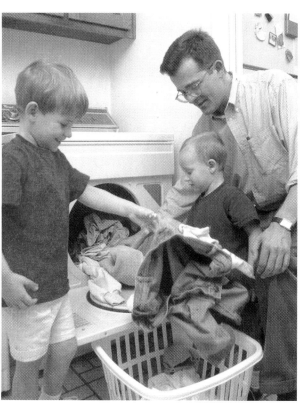

Fig. 25-14. Managing time effectively may include combining activities, such as doing housework while catching up with your children.

5. **Get help.** It is not reasonable for you to do everything. If children are old enough to help, give them chores that they can be responsible for. If other family members are available, make a plan for who will cook or clean up each night. If you have no one to help you, give yourself a break. You cannot do everything, so some things just may not get done.

❏ 17. Demonstrate an understanding of the basics of money management

Money can be a real source of stress. Not being able to buy the things we need or want, getting into debt, or facing emergencies without a cash reserve can be very difficult. Understanding a little bit about money management can help you avoid money problems before they arise.

Make a budget. Making a personal or household budget is not complicated and is the starting point for solving money problems. To make a budget, you need to know total income and total expenses, including rent or mortgage, transportation, utilities, insurance, debts, food, clothing, medical and dental, entertainment, and miscellaneous. Expenses may be calculated as weekly, monthly, or annual.

Reduce or avoid debts. When you owe money, whether to a bank, a mortgage company, or a credit card company, you pay interest. Interest is the money you pay for the right to use someone else's money. When you can avoid borrowing money, you can avoid paying interest. Whenever you can, save up the money to buy something instead of borrowing the money. For instance, saving the money to buy a new television rather than borrowing the money means the television will end up costing less because of the money you save in interest.

Most people must borrow money for major purchases, like a house or a car. In these situations paying interest is unavoidable. But whenever you can avoid borrowing money, it is smart to do so. If you have debts already, pay them off as soon as possible to avoid the expense of interest. Furthermore, when you apply for a loan to buy a house or a car, you will have to show that you can handle debt responsibly. If you have too much debt on credit cards or other loans, you may not be able to get a loan for a house or a car.

When you apply for a mortgage or car loan, the bank or lender will check your credit report. A credit report is a document that lists all of the loans or debts you have ever had and shows how you paid them off. If you were ever late paying bills, this will appear on your credit report. You are legally entitled to see your credit report and have it corrected if it is wrong.

Credit cards can make it especially hard to manage money well. It is easy to get and use a credit card, so many of us buy things we do not need or could wait and save for. The interest charged on credit card debt is often the highest interest charged on any loan. If you have trouble controlling what you buy with credit cards, consider getting rid of them altogether.

Save as much as you can. No matter how small your income or how great your expenses, always try to put something away in a savings account every time you get a check. Ten percent is a good savings goal, but if you can only save one percent of your check, do it. Open a savings account at your bank and when you take your check to cash or deposit, deposit your savings in the savings account right then.

There are many advantages to saving. You can avoid debt if you save rather than borrow. In fact, if you save up the money to buy that new television, not only will you avoid paying interest, but the bank will pay you interest on the money you save while it is in the bank. The more you save, the more interest you get.

Another important reason to save is that having savings allows you to face emergency situations. If your car breaks down, or you have unexpected medical bills, or your work hours are cut, having savings means you have a safety net to fall back on. Get into the habit of saving right from the start. It can mean the difference between financial independence and financial disaster.

Control miscellaneous expenses. Sometimes we get to the end of the week or month and wonder, "Where did all my money go?" If this happens to you, you may be spending too much on miscellaneous items, like snacks, coffee, lottery tickets, or cigarettes during the day, unnecessary items at the grocery store, or eating out when your budget cannot support it. Cash cards make it easy for us to get cash, which makes it easier to spend more cash.

Try writing down what you spend money on each day. A cup of coffee and a donut, a lottery ticket, a candy bar, and two sodas can add up to more than $4.00. That may not seem like a lot, but if you spend that every day for five days, that's $20.00 a week. Can your budget support that? Consider eliminating these kinds of expenses by bringing coffee and other snacks from home and skipping the lottery tickets.

Plan your cash for the week and stick to it. Figure out how much cash you need in a week, counting bus fare, tolls, children's lunch money, any other regular expenses, and including some emergency cash. Withdraw this amount at the beginning of the week and make it last. Use your cash card for emergencies only.

Be proud of your efforts to manage money. We live in a society where very few people manage their money well. Most of us have too much debt, buy more than we need, and don't save enough money. It is hard to be responsible and control expenses when you see people around you spending freely, using credit cards, and living beyond their means.

But if you can manage your money well, you will help make sure that you and your family will be well taken care of and will never have to face emergencies without a safety net. You can also help yourself become wealthier by saving. You can live a more comfortable life, and get satisfaction from knowing that your belongings are paid for.

❑ 18. Demonstrate an understanding that money matters are emotional

Money problems are often listed as the number one cause of family and marital arguments. Money carries great meaning for most of us. Not only do we need money to live, but money has come to represent value for many of us. That is, we think that the more money we have, the better people we are. We may try to show off by driving fancy cars or wearing expensive clothes or jewelry. We may try to make ourselves feel better by buying something, often something we don't really need or cannot afford. The images we see on television, in the movies, or in magazines make us feel we ought to have certain possessions. Many of us feel we deserve certain things, even when we really cannot afford them. All these emotions come into play whenever we think about or talk about money matters (**Fig. 25-15**).

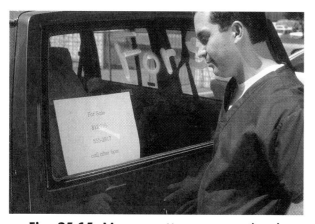

Fig. 25-15. Money matters are emotional.

Money also equals security for many of us. When we cannot pay our bills, or when debts get too high, we feel a lot of anxiety about how we will make ends meet. The best way to avoid this anxiety is to budget, plan, and manage money matters wisely. But in order to manage our money well,

most of us need to spend less and save more, which means we must give up the pleasure, satisfaction, or self-esteem we get from spending money. If you can look at your financial situation realistically, and decide what you will and will not spend your money on, you can get even greater satisfaction from being responsible and independent (**Fig. 25-16**).

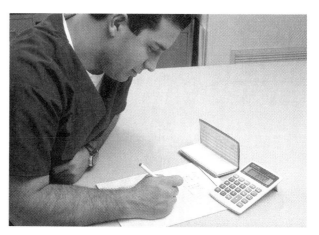

Fig. 25-16. Being responsible about money can be very satisfying.

Separating emotions from realities about money will help you make good decisions and stick to them. You may very reasonably feel that you deserve to eat out. You work hard, you are tired, and you don't want to have to cook every night. But the reality may be that your budget only allows you to eat out once a month. Or, you may have decided you would skip eating out altogether until you saved the money for your vacation or another expense. Recognize the feelings of being tired and wanting and even deserving to eat out, but try to focus on the reality of needing to stick to your budget and save.

❑ 19. List ways to remind yourself that the work of a home care aide is important, valuable, and meaningful

This is the only learning objective in this text that does not include all of the information you need to master it. It requires you to review what you have learned, use your imagination, and be creative. The answers will also change as you gain more work experience.

Look back over all you have learned in this program. Your work as a home care aide is vitally important. Every day may be different and challenging. In a hundred ways every week you will offer help that only a caring person like you can provide.

Don't forget to value the work you have chosen to do. It is important. Sometimes your work can mean the difference between living at home and living in an institution. It can mean living with independence and dignity versus living without. The difference you make is sometimes life versus death.

Look in the face of each of your clients, and know that you are doing important work. Look in a mirror when you get home, and be proud of how you make your living.

An important life skill is being able to reflect on how you spend your time. Learn ways to fully appreciate that what you do has great meaning. Few jobs have the challenges and rewards of home health care. Congratulate yourself for choosing a path that includes helping others along the way.

INDEX

This index lists all of the key terms and topics found in this book. Page numbers in **bold** text refer to the page containing a definition or pronunciation of the word. Looking up unfamiliar words in this manner will give the reader not only a definition and pronunciation, but also the context for usage.

BRAT diet
defined, **105**
children and, 257

breast milk, 248

breastfeeding
assisting with, 248

broiling, 321

bronchi, **99**

bronchioles, **99**

bronchitis
acute, 100
chronic, 100
respiratory system disorder,
100

bronchus, **99**

Buddhism, **39**

budgeting
see money management

bulimia
adolescence, **120**

burns
see also accidents
prevention, 58

C

caffeine, 31

calculi
see also kidney stones
urinary system disorder,
102

calories
nutrition facts label, 313

cancer
defined, **262**
care guidelines, 264
communicating with
client, 263
community resources, 265
HCA role, 264
observing and reporting,
265
risk factors, 262
treatments, 263
warning signs, 263
canes
types, 144

capillaries, **88**, **97**

carbohydrates
basic nutrient, 306
client with diabetes, 267
complex, 306
simple, 306

cardiovascular system
see also circulatory system
common disorders, 97

observing and reporting,
99
signs and symptoms, 99
structure and function, 96

care plan
defined, **11**
care team and, 8, 10, 13
family involvement, 24
formulating, 13
HCA role, 13, 37
purpose of, 11
sample form, 12

care team, 10

carotid artery, **68**

cartilage, **89**

case conferences, 37

case manager, 10

cast
fiberglass, 213
plaster of paris, 213

cataracts, **95**, **234**

catastrophic reaction
in Alzheimer's disease, 286

catheter
cleaning, 197
condom, 195
drainage, 197
indwelling, 195
urinary, 195

catheter care
guidelines, 195-196

catheterization, 7

CDC (Centers for Disease
Control and Prevention),
47

cells, **87**

center of gravity, 54, **55**

Centers for Disease Control
and Prevention (CDC)
see CDC

central nervous system
(CNS)
see nervous system

cerebellum, **92**, 93

cerebral cortex, **92**, 93

cerebral palsy
defined, **230**
see also disability(ies)
birth defect, 115
nervous system disorder,
94
related care, 230

cerebral vascular accident
(CVA)
defined, **269**

see also stroke
cardiovascular system disorder, **98**

cerebrospinal fluid, **92**

cerebrum, **92**, 93

certification
maintaining, 335

certify, 15

cerumen, **95**, 125

cervix, **110**

Cesarean section
defined, **246**
herpes outbreak and, 111

chain of command, **15**, **16**

chain reaction, 86

chancres, **111**

change
observing and reporting,
86, 113

changes in health care, 3

changing a baby
guidelines, 253

chemicals
cancer and, 262

chemotherapy
see also cancer: treatments,
263

chest thrusts, 72

chicken pox
childhood disorder, **118**

child abuse
defined, **118**
see also abuse
reporting, 259
signs and symptoms, **259**

child neglect, **259**

child proofing, **116**

childhood
common disorders, 117
development, 116

childhood illnesses
signs and symptoms, 257

childhood infection, 118

children
care guidelines, 256
diarrhea, 257
fever, 257
signs of abuse and neglect,
259
special needs of, 256
understanding, 256
vomiting, 257
working with, 258-259

chlamydia
sexually transmitted disease,
110
signs and symptoms, 111

Christianity, **39**

chronic, **86**

chronic bronchitis, **100**

chronic kidney failure
urinary system disorder,
103

chyme, **104**

circulatory disorders
care guidelines, 273
dementia and, 279
signs and symptoms, 273

circulatory system
see also cardiovascular system
care guidelines for aging
client, 126
normal changes of aging,
126

circumcision, **256**

claustrophobia, **240**

cleaning
see housekeeping

cleaning body fluids/waste,
44

cleaning products
proper use, 292

cleaning schedule
see also housekeeping, 297

cleaning solutions
preparing, 297

cleaning spills, 44

clichés, **29**, **85**

client
abuse, 24
comfort measures, 153
decision making, 23
documenting, 34
financial information, 23
payment, 6
privacy, 23
responsibilities, 23
rights, 23, 24

Client Bill of Rights, **23**

client preferences
housekeeping, 290

client requests
inappropriate, 327

client rights, supporting, 25

clinical depression
see depression

clinical notes
see documentation

clothes care
see also housekeeping, 298-300

cognition, **279**

cognitive development, **117**

cognitive impairment, **279**

cold applications
benefits of, 198
  cold compresses, 202
  ice packs, 202

cold compresses
see cold applications

colitis
gastrointestinal system disorder, **105, 106**

colon, **104**

colorectal cancer
gastrointestinal system disorder, **106**

colostomy
defined, 202
  treatment of ulcerative colitis, **106**

combative behavior
guidelines for reporting, **39**

combing/brushing hair
see hair care

combustible, **222**

comfort
dying and, 136
  observing and reporting, 156

comfort measures, 153

communication
defined, **26**
  barriers, 29
  body language, 28
  client, 37
  client with cancer, 263
  client with stroke, 271
  cultural behavior, 28
  cultural diversity, 38
  demented client, 282
  facts and opinions, 31
  families, 37
  guidelines, 30
  interpersonal relationships, 31
  nonverbal, 27
  of HCA, 8
  oral reports, 33
  religious differences, 38
  telephone, 37
  verbal, 27
  within the agency, 32

communication problems
stroke and, 270

community resources
aging, 132
  cancer, 265
  illness, 84

community support
see also hospice, 139

compassionate, **20**

complaint
to an employer, 335

complex carbohydrates, **306**

condom catheter, **195**

condoms, 110

confidentiality
see also client: rights, 25

Confucianism, **39**

confusion
stroke and, 270

congestive heart failure (CHF)
defined, **275**
  cardiovascular system disorder, **98**
  care guidelines, 275
  side effects of medication, 276
  signs and symptoms, 275

conscientious, **20**

conserving energy, 326

conserving time, 326

constipation
aging and, 128
  gastrointestinal system disorder, **104, 105**

constrict, **88**

contact precautions
see also infection control, isolation precautions, 48

contagious
see infectious

continuing education, 336

contractures, **90**

cooking safety, 320

coping
see also adjustments, 84

coping mechanisms
types, **239**

cornea, **95**

coronary arteries, **97**

coronary artery disease

(CAD)
defined, **274**
  cardiovascular system disorder, **98**

coronary thrombosis
see also myocardial infarction, **274**

cost control
health care, 2

CPR (cardiopulmonary resuscitation)
see emergency care

crime
see also safety
  avoiding, 65

criminal background
checks, 6

criticism
responding to, 333

crutches
guidelines for proper use, 146

C-section
see Cesarean section

culture
death and, 135
  food preferences, 312

CVA (cerebrovascular accident)
see also stroke, 32

cyanotic, **32, 70, 275**

cystic fibrosis
birth defect, 115

cystitis
urinary system disorder, **102**

D

dairy products
food group, 309

dangle, **143**

dangling position
procedure, 142

deafness
see also hearing impairment, 96

death
see also dying
  approaching signs, 135-136
  attitudes towards, 135
  culture, 135
  religious beliefs, 135

debilitating, **86**

debts
reducing/avoiding, 340

decubitus ulcers
see also pressure sores, **88**

deep breathing exercises
assisting with, 216

defrosting, 294

degenerative, **87, 279**

dehydrated, **192**
  aging and, 128

dehydration
signs and symptoms, **310**

delegation
from team members, 11

delusions
defined, **242**
  in Alzheimer's disease, 286

dementia, **93, 279**

denial
grieving and, 134
  stages of dying, 133

denture care, 173

dentures
inserting, 174

dependable, **20**

depression
defined, **241**
  in adolescence, 120
  in Alzheimer's disease, 286
  in older adult, 129
  major depression, **241**
  manic depression, **241**
  postpartum, 247
  signs and symptoms, 241
  stages of dying, 134

dermis, **75, 88**

development
see human development

developmental
disability(ies), 229

diabetes, **7, 107**

diabetes mellitus
defined, **265**
  care guidelines, 267
  care plan, 108
  complications, 266
  endocrine system disorder, **108**
  foot care, 267, 268
  meal plans, 268-269
  observing and reporting, 266
  related health problems, 108
  signs and symptoms, 108, 265

employer responsibilities
infection control, 53
  to HCA, 20, 21

employers
contacting potential, 330

employment
changing jobs, 335
  interview questions, 332
  interview techniques, 331-332
  job application, 331-333
  maintaining certification, 335
  making complaints, 335
  required documents, 331
  responding to criticism, 333-335

employment applications, 331

empty nest, 120

endocardium, **97**

endocrine system
care guidelines for aging client, 128
  common disorders, 107
  normal changes of aging, 128
  observing and reporting, 108
  pronounced, **265**
  signs and symptoms, 108
  structure and function, 106

endometrium, **109**

enteral feeding, 311, **324**

environmental contamination, 43

enzymes
nutrition and, 305

epidermis, 75, **88**

epididymis, **109**

epilepsy
nervous system disorder, **94**

epinephrine
see adrenaline

episiotomy, **246**

epistaxis, 77

equilibrium
dangling position, **143**

erectile tissue, **109**

esophagus, **103**, **104**

estrogen
see also endocrine system, 107

cancer and, 263

ethical behavior, 22

ethics, **22**

eustachian tube, **95**

evacuation, 73, **79**

exacerbations, **232**

exchange lists
diabetes and, 268, 269, 315

exercise
stress and, 337

expiration, **99**, **186**

exposure report
infection control and, 53

extension, 207

external catheter
see condom catheter

external ear, **95**

external rotation, 207, 210

eye
see also nervous system: sense organs
  common disorders, 95
  observing and reporting, 96
  signs and symptoms, 96
  structure and function, 94

eye shield, 45

F

face mask
see mask

face shield
emergency care and, 71

facilities, **1**

fallacy, **238**

falling client, 56, 143

fallopian tube, **109**

falls
see also accidents, falling client
  prevention, 58

family assistance
client with cancer, 265

family contact
of HCA, 8

family roles
health care, 83

family support, 13

family(ies)
adjustments to illness/disability, 84
  community resources, 84
  emotional needs, 84
  establishing a work plan, 326
  functions, 84
  housekeeping, 291

farsightedness, **234**

fats
basic nutrient, 306
  food group, 309

fat-soluble, **307**

feces, **104**

feeding
client with stroke, 271
  infants, 248-251

fee-for-service, 2

female reproductive system
see reproductive system

fertilized, 109

fiber, **306**

fire
see also safety: fire, 63

fire extinguishers
see safety: fire

flexibility
of HCA, 9

flexion, 207

flossing
procedure, 172

flotation pads, 212

fluid
conversion tables, 193

fluid balance
defined, **192**
  see also urinary system, **101**
  assisting with, **310**
  importance of, 192-195

fluid overload
signs and symptoms, **310**

fluid retention
see nephritis

food
planning and shopping, 317
  pricing, 318
  purchasing, 319
  storage, 294

food additives
cancer and, 262

Food and Drug Administration (FDA), 312

food groups, 308-309

food guide pyramid, **308**

food handling
AIDS and, 277

food labeling, 312

food labels
health claims, 312, 313

food plan
preparing, 317

food preferences
culture and religion, 312

food preparation
AIDS client, 277
  guidelines, 319
  low fat methods, 322
  methods, 320

food storage
guidelines, 322

foot and nail care, 165-166

foot care
client with diabetes, 267, 268

footboards, 156

formula
infants, 250

forward flexion, 207

Fowler's position, **150**

fracture, **91**, **212**

fracture pan, **175**

fruits
food group, 309

frying, 322

fulcrum, **55**

fundus, **110**

G

gallbladder, **104**

garment care
see clothes care

gastric gavage, **311**, **324**

gastric reflux
gastrointestinal system disorder, **105**

gastric ulcer, 105, **316**

gastrointestinal system (GI)
see also digestive system
  common disorders, 104
  observing and reporting, 106

tub bath
see also bathing
  infants, 253

tuberculosis (TB)
defined, **51**
  infection control guidelines, 52
  respiratory system disorder,
  101
  signs and symptoms, 51
  transmission, 51
  types, 51

tumor
defined, **262**
  benign, 262
  malignant, 262

turning
see positioning

turning sheet
see draw sheet

tympanic membrane
see also vital signs, **95**

tympanic temperature
adults, 184
  infants, 255

tympanic thermometer, **182**

U

U.S. health care system, 1,
3

ulcer, 105

ulceration, **105**

ulcerative colitis
gastrointestinal system disorder, **106**

ulnar flexion, 207

undressing
guidelines, 168

uninvolved side, **270**

universal precautions, 47

unoccupied bed
see bedmaking: unoccupied
bed

unprejudiced, **20**

upper respiratory infection
(URI)
respiratory system disorder,
100

uremia
see chronic kidney failure

ureter, **102**

urethra, **102**

urinal
see also toileting, **175**, 178

urinal use, 178

urinary catheter, 127, **195**

urinary system
care guidelines for aging
client, 127
  common disorders, 102
  normal changes of aging,
  127
  observing and reporting,
  103
  signs and symptoms, 103
  structure and function,
  101

urinary tract infection
(UTI), **102**

urination, 178

urine
collecting, 191-194

uterus, 107, 109

V

vaccination, **112**

vaccination schedule, 118

vagina, 102, 109

vaginitis
reproductive system disorder, **110**

validating, **287**

validation therapy
in Alzheimer's disease, 287

vas deferens, **109**

vegetables
food group, 309

veins, **97**

veneral diseases
see sexually transmitted diseases

ventricles, **97**

venules, **99**

verbal abuse
see also abuse, **24**

verbal communication, **27**

vertebrae, **89**

vertigo, **96**

villi, **104**

violent behavior
in Alzheimer's disease, 286

vision impairment
related care, 234-235

visit form, 16, 36

visit records
see also documentation, 36

visually impaired
communication with, 234

vital signs
defined, 14
  basic health care skill,
  180-190
  blood pressure, 186-188
  importance of, 181
  infants, 255
  measuring, 181
  normal ranges, 181
  pulse, 185-186
  respirations, 186
  temperature, 181
  weight/height, 189-190

vitamins
basic nutrient, 307

source and function, 306

voluntary muscles
see muscles

volunteers
hospice, 139

vomiting
see also emesis
  AIDS and, 278

W

walker, 144

wandering
in Alzheimer's disease, **285**

warm applications
see also heat applications,
196

warm compresses
see heat applications

warm soaks
see heat applications

washing
see bathing, handwashing,
laundry

washing hands
see handwashing

water
basic nutrient, 308

water-soluble, **307**

weak/involved side, **270**

weight
recording, 189

weight loss
AIDS and, 277

wheelchair
transfers, 147

white blood cells
see also cardiovascular system, **96**

whooping cough
see vaccination schedule

withdrawal
mental illness and, 239

work plan
establishing, 326
  following, 326

working environment
of HCA, 9

wrist pulse
see radial pulse

Y

yarmulke, **39**

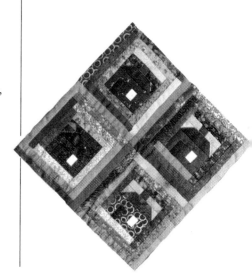